The Psychology of Yoga

The Psychology of Yoga

Integrating Eastern and Western Approaches
for Understanding the Mind

GEORG FEUERSTEIN

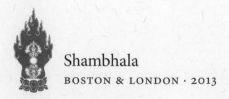

Shambhala

BOSTON & LONDON · 2013

Shambhala Publications, Inc.
Horticultural Hall
300 Massachusetts Avenue
Boston, Massachusetts 02115
www.shambhala.com

9 8 7 6 5 4 3 2 1

First Edition
Printed in the United States of America

⊛ This edition is printed on acid-free paper that meets
the American National Standards Institute z39.48 Standard.
♻ This book is printed on 30% postconsumer recycled paper.
For more information please visit www.shambhala.com.

Distributed in the United States by Penguin Random House LLC
and in Canada by Random House of Canada Ltd

Designed by Michael Russem

Library of Congress Cataloging-in-Publication Data

Feuerstein, Georg.
The psychology of yoga: integrating Eastern and Western approaches
for understanding the mind/Georg Feuerstein.—First Edition.
Pages   cm
Includes bibliographical references and index.
ISBN 978-1-61180-042-5 (pbk.: alk. paper)
1. Yoga—Psychology. I. Title.
BL1238.54.F48 2014
181'.45—dc23
2013010150

In memoriam Lee (Liberatore) Sannella, visionary, author, and dear friend. And to Brenda, my beautiful wife and spiritual partner, for sharing with me the difficult path of inner growth and illumination with great love and compassion.

Contents

PART FOUR Analysis and Relevance

Preface

The psychology of Yoga in its Hindu, Buddhist, and Jaina forms (see Appendix 1) is a much-neglected area of research but one that is potentially rewarding to write about and harvest for the benefit of both dedicated students of Yoga and specialists in psychology wishing to become acquainted with Yoga's psychological concepts. Both the breadth of my subject and the depth to which I am exploring it are challenging, and I would probably not have dared to attempt this study if I had gauged its difficulty before embarking on it with my usual enthusiasm and boldness.

To state my position clearly up front, I understand psychology in a non-behavioristic manner as the study of the mind in the broadest sense of the term. In other words, I am advocating a nonmaterialist viewpoint. It is impossible to bracket philosophy when considering psychology. In the West, the philosophical presuppositions of psychology are usually implied rather than stated for everyone to witness. The framework in question is, of course, a one-dimensional materialism, which a priori deems the mind to be an epiphenomenon of the brain and nervous system and therefore routinely dismisses all claims to the contrary.

That René Descartes's dualistic model, which underlies the reigning scientific paradigm with its supposedly inviolable dogma of objectivism, is not universally applicable has become clear to all but the most inflexible adherents of the ideology of scientism. Yet even those who do not subscribe to the Cartesian paradigm have so far not unanimously agreed on a strong contender for a new one. Thus, there is a theoretical gray area, which is another way of talking about the crisis in present-day science. I believe that presenting the psychological teachings of the Eastern wisdom traditions as clearly and honestly as possible can prove helpful in this transitional phase in the unfolding of science. I am open to an explanation of the mind-matter relationship that does not follow the ruling paradigm of Cartesian dualism. I have not, however, found the existing alternatives—many of them influenced by or based on quantum-theoretical speculations—entirely convincing. But they all gesture toward a new paradigm that will fully emerge sooner or later.

The West's interest in the psychology of Yoga dates back to the Roaring Twenties and to the fateful fascist thirties. From that time on, treatments of the psychological dimension of Yoga have been published sporadically in both Western countries and India, with a focus either on Indology (the study of Indian culture) or on psychology (see Appendix 2). Of more recent writings, I wish to single out Karl Baier's incisive 1998 exploration in German of the reception of Yoga in the field of depth psychology, which comprises chapter 8 of his fine monograph *Yoga auf dem Weg nach Westen* (Yoga on the Way to the West). I have also greatly profited from his colossal two-volume study on meditation (2009), also in German, which examines the historical pathways leading from the medieval Christian contemplative tradition to the sixteenth-century meditation system of Saint Ignatius of Loyola to seventeenth-century quietism to eighteenth-century mesmerism to nineteenth-century occultism, theosophy, and New Thought (also called Mind Cure and Mental Science), and from there to twentieth-century depth psychology, autogenic training, the New Age movement, Buddhism, and Yoga. Baier's splendid survey ends with the countercultural developments of the 1980s. Unfortunately, he only touches on Tibetan Buddhism, which succeeded the introduction of Buddhism and Yoga into the West and became singularly prominent on the North American continent in the 1970s.

Parallel to Baier's searching monograph but focusing on the English-speaking world is Elizabeth de Michelis's *A History of Modern Yoga* (2004). She traced the historical roots of modern Yoga to the Bengali renaissance movement and the publication of Swami Vivekananda's relatively free but popular translation of the *Yoga-Sūtra* in 1896 along neo-Hindu/Vedāntic lines. Few know that his commentary was originally spoken, because he regarded writing a "botheration" (Vivekananda 1972, 293).[1]

All the books mentioned here have offered valuable parameters for my own investigation into the psychology of Yoga. The present study is the most comprehensive foray to date into the subject matter. It is based on my many years of delving into the Hindu and Buddhist forms of Yoga—both theoretically and practically—and, to a much lesser degree, Jaina Yoga from a historical, literary, and philosophical viewpoint. My layman's grasp of modern psychology, which I have acquired over a lifetime but mainly while preparing my book *Structures of Consciousness* (1987), is largely limited to the field of depth psychology, humanistic psychology, and transpersonal psychology. I draw primarily on these disciplines here, because they seem singularly relevant to my discussion.

It remains to me to thank Dr. Roger Walsh and Ken Wilber, who generously offered their helpful feedback on the manuscript. I also wish to kindly thank Karl Baier, Douglas Brooks, Edwin Bryant, Christopher Key Chapple, Dr. James Fadiman, Amit Goswami, Reginald Ray, Kenneth Ring, Henry Skolimowski, Stuart Sovatskzy, Michael Washburn, and Allan Watts. I also thank Shambhala Publications and their editorial staff, notably Dave O'Neal and Julia Gaviria, for their vision and support of my writings.

A special thank-you goes to my beloved wife and spiritual partner, Brenda, who has walked this path with me, offering more love, compassion, and support I ever thought possible.

Abbreviations

B.C.E. = before the common era
c. = circa; approximately
C.E. = common era
pron. = pronounced
Tib. = Tibetan
Skt. = Sanskrit

All references to the *Mahābharata* are to the critical edition of the Sanskrit text by S. K. Belvalkar (1950). All references to the *Hatha-Yoga-Pradīpikā* are to the ten-chapter edition by M. L. Gharote and Parimal Devnath (2001), which is available online.

Introduction

> The time has come to realize that the Eastern
> spiritual traditions are part of our tradition.
>
> —HENRYK SKOLIMOWSKI (1994, 378)

HISTORICAL GLIMPSE

Modern psychology, the systematic study of the mind, traces its origins back
to ancient Greek and Christian philosophy, and so it may be useful to review
the progress since then. Among the Greek thinkers, it is the empiricist Aristotle who has won the reputation of being one of the cornerstones of the
sprawling edifice that we call psychology. Among the early Christian thinkers, it is first and foremost Saint Augustine who is looked upon as the second
cornerstone. He was just as speculative as Aristotle before him, though he
admired the metaphysician Plato and, like him, thoroughly distrusted sensory experiences. We cannot but be deeply touched by Saint Augustine's confession about what he deemed an abject failure of will during his profligate
youth. We also can be impressed by his insight that doubt is a sure sign of our
ability to think, which, in turn, shows that we exist—vaguely anticipating
Descartes's philosophical axiom.

With Greek philosophical inquiry and the reflections of the early church
fathers fading out of focus, psychological concerns assumed a backseat
during much of the European Middle Ages. Then, thanks to Muslim scholars, Christian thinkers rediscovered the Greek heritage. First they became
enamored of the idealist Plato, but in the thirteenth century the balance
dipped in favor of the realist Aristotle, especially because of the Domini-
can monk Saint Thomas Aquinas. His twenty-volume *Summa Theologica*
became the gospel truth, as it were, for the next several centuries. In psychological matters, Saint Thomas took his cue from the conjectures of Aristotle
but merrily mixed them with Christian doctrines, notably the belief in an
afterlife and the unbridgeable gap between body and mind that still riddles
modern psychology and popular thought.

1

Saint Thomas's overwhelming authority stifled not only the further development of theology but also that of psychology. The Renaissance promised to change all this. Then, in the fifteenth century, nonclerical scholars began to appear, pursuing their thoughts without the doctrinal straightjacket of the church. In the sixteenth century—the era of Andreas Vesalius (anatomy), Nicolaus Copernicus (astronomy), Galileo Galilei (physics and astronomy), Georgius Agricola (mineralogy), Johannes Kepler (astronomy), Ferdinand Magellan (geography), and Juan Luis Vives (education and psychology)—a strong new wind was blowing, which ushered in the scientific revolution. Many naive beliefs and assumptions were jettisoned, and empirical fact came to stand for truth.

Building on this novel trend, the seventeenth century witnessed an efflorescence of intellectual activity. The great figure was Sir Isaac Newton, who proved that matter—wherever it may be—follows the same natural laws of motion and gravitation. His scientific model, which is found explained in his *Principia* (*Philosophiae Principia Mathematica*, 1687), reigned supreme until the formulation of relativity theory and quantum theory at the dawn of the twentieth century, and it is still deemed valid in physics when it comes to phenomena above the scale of subatomic processes. The church authorities understandably reacted to such scientific mavericks and their followers with condemnation, the threat of excommunication, and the infamous Inquisition. But the new attitude proved uncontainable and a century later culminated in the Enlightenment movement, which relied on reason (rationalism) to answer the important questions of life and openly challenged established religious authority.

Historically, the eighteenth century was a restless era riddled with wars and revolutions and punctuated with numerous discoveries and inventions that brought about the Industrial Revolution. The cultural elite, which carried the Enlightenment movement forward, celebrated knowledge, independent thinking, criticism, and a cosmopolitan spirit. This orientation reached its peak in, and was symbolized by, the German philosopher Immanuel Kant. Significantly, in his *Kritik der Reinen Vernunft* (*Critique of Pure Reason*, 1781), he explained metaphysics as knowledge of the limits of reason rather than as knowledge of the Absolute—a major step forward in philosophical thinking.

The Industrial Revolution, which was spearheaded by Great Britain, continued vigorously in the nineteenth century. Technological discoveries and inventions—especially steel, electricity, and the internal combustion engine, along with the inevitable deadly weapons—altered the world in significant ways. Scientists and scholars, embracing the scientific method, professionalized their trade. What Isaac Newton had been to the seventeenth century, Charles Darwin was to the nineteenth. Both giants of science taught a form of naturalism that does not require the causative principle of a deity. As the philosopher Friedrich Nietzsche declared dramatically in *Die Fröhliche Wissenschaft* (*The Gay Science*, 1882), God was dead. In less scandalous terms, the concept of the paternal creator-deity that had dominated the Western world ever since the spread of Christianity under Constantine I in the fourth century C.E. was busy being pulverized by science.

At the sociopolitical level, old empires crumbled, and new ones (mainly Great Britain and Germany) emerged. At the same time, it was becoming clear that the eighteenth-century optimism of human perfectibility was little more than an illusion, but the idea of progress flourished undiminished. Not everyone was capable of following the dictates of the critical mind. In fact, most people felt disoriented and disheartened and reverted to authority—scientific, medical, educational, moral, and even religious.

This was the ideal breeding ground for the new science of psychology. The nineteenth century saw a radical break with the preceding tradition of largely *speculative* psychology and the beginning application of the so-called scientific method (modeled after the physical sciences) to the study of elusive mental phenomena. Early research into the workings of the mind focused on concrete (measurable) physiological processes, such as sensory functions and reflex reactions.

The German physician and physiologist Wilhelm Wundt is usually looked upon as the founder of modern psychology, though perhaps this discipline had more than one creator. Wundt did, however, establish the first psychology laboratory in Leipzig in 1879, and this after Kant, the supreme rationalist, had confidently declared less than ninety years before that psychology could never be an experimental science. Before Wundt, his compatriots Hermann Helmholtz (a surgeon and physiologist) and the fascinating Gustav Theodor Fechner (who started out in medicine only to move on to physics and later metaphysics) also had quantitatively explored the physiology of the mind. But Wundt, who had studied under Helmholtz, turned experimental psychology into a veritable science. His work seemed promising enough to entice William James, already a renowned professor of psychology at Harvard University, to leave the United States and visit various German universities for half a year.

James, ever the nonconformist, assimilated as much as he could on that fact-finding sabbatical but continued to go very much his own way. Although he promoted experimental psychology, he never really saw himself as a psychologist but primarily as a philosopher. Yet his monumental two-volume magnum opus titled *Principles of Psychology* (1890) and his widely read *Varieties of Religious Experience* (1902) continue to stand as remarkable milestones in psychological studies.

Then, in the late nineteenth to early twentieth centuries, a shift occurred within the new science of psychology that opened up higher mental processes (thinking and the will) to psychological investigation. The German philosopher Wilhelm Dilthey brought *Erlebnis* (lived experience) and *Verstehen* (understanding) into focus, which then inspired the explorations of the Gestalt psychologists. The notion of *Gestalt* (a German word meaning "configuration"), suggesting the idea of wholeness, was introduced because understanding always happens in context. Speculatively, it probably became attractive because of the growing need to overcome the fragmentation of scientific data and also the fragmentation of the modern psyche.

Ignoring these developments, the quantifying physicalist trend simultaneously acquired a new life under the name of behaviorism. Rejecting introspection and self-observation, the behaviorists focused only on what was objectively measurable in terms of stimulus and response. This approach, which was launched in the United States with the nonvolunteered help of thousands of animals (dogs, rats, pigeons, and so forth), is still popular.

The holistic, mentalist trend to which we have already referred led to, among other things, the work of Sigmund Freud, the founder of psychoanalysis, which aspired to bring wholeness to broken psyches. After years of working in relative obscurity, Freud published his widely read book on psychoanalytic dream interpretation in 1900. His approach as a whole, however, suffers from the same physicalist bias that also afflicted his immediate forerunners; the Freudian model has often been criticized for its "hydraulic" nature. Yet Freud, who had originally been fascinated with physiology and the nervous system in particular, went deeper into the mind and showed that, through skillful assistance, the mind could heal itself. Such assistance, he held, should mainly consist of unearthing repressed materials that manifested in neuroses and psychoses.

Freud's intellectual labors, in turn, led to the establishment of various approaches in what came to be known as depth psychology. From among his close students, Carl Gustav Jung and Alfred Adler particularly stand out. The former especially has been widely influential in the twentieth century, and I will have occasion to draw on his work on more than one occasion in this book. Mention must also be made of the sagacious Italian Roberto Assagioli, who studied under the eminent psychiatrist Eugen Bleuler at the Burghölzli psychiatric hospital in Switzerland. Bleuler adopted some of Freud's ideas and, in the early period of psychoanalysis, lent his professional prestige to the promotion of psychoanalysis. Although Assagioli never met Freud in person, he corresponded with him; he also knew Carl Jung personally and thought that Jung's approach came closest to his own. Assagioli's psychosynthesis went far beyond psychoanalysis and anticipated later transpersonal psychology, yet it has been largely ignored by mainstream depth psychology.[1]

In the 1950s, humanistic psychology emerged in the English-speaking world and was promoted chiefly by Abraham Maslow, an intellectual giant and irrepressible innovator. He was instrumental in, among other things, getting Assagioli's first book in English published.[2] In the late 1960s, Maslow's efforts led to the formation of transpersonal psychology, which was ushered in by Maslow himself, as well as Roberto Assagioli and Anthony J. Sutich. Early principal developers include Charles Tart, Roger Walsh, Stanislav Grof, Ken Wilber, and James Fadiman. These two developmental branches of psychology—the humanistic and the transpersonal—serve as the principal theoretical framework for the approach taken in this book.

I am also drawing on Henryk Skolimowski's participatory philosophy and Ervin Laszlo's systems approach, as well as Jean Gebser's cultural-historical model of structures of consciousness. I feel fortunate to have had the opportunity of several years' lively correspondence with Gebser before his passing in 1973 and also to have been in touch with Skolimowski, whom I heard speak animatedly at the California Institute of Integral Studies in San Francisco.

WEST MEETS EAST

It is not easy to grasp what the encounter between the two cultural hemispheres means to India; in many ways that country is still recovering from the trauma of the British Raj and can be thought of as still being in the process of redefining its own identity. I have therefore opted to choose "West Meets East" as the subtitle for this second section. By comparison, it is easier to determine how the Western world has reacted to India, even though this process is also as yet incomplete.

As I mentioned earlier, psychology can look back on a long history in close association with philosophy. In the West, speculative, metaphysical psychology dates back to the ancient Greeks. In the East, it was integral to the closely related systems (*darshana*) of Yoga and Sāmkhya that, I maintain, have their roots in the long-lasting pre-Buddhist era prior to 500 B.C.E.

The Sanskrit language, in which most Yoga texts are written, does not have a word for *psychology*, because psychology was never viewed as a separate field of inquiry from traditional knowledge; the same holds true of philosophy.[3] But this does not mean that the Indian traditions were ignorant of psychological and philosophical thought or that their conclusions are irrelevant to our postmodern world. In his book *Modern Man in Search of a Soul*, written in German in 1933, Carl Jung astutely observed,

> Psychoanalysis itself and the lines of thought to which it gives rise—surely a distinctly Western development—are only a beginner's attempt compared to what is an immemorial art in the East.
>
> (Jung 1933, 216; from the English ed.)

We can appreciate this comment all the more when we know of Jung's keen interest in the occult tradition of Kundalinī-Yoga, an obscure but sophisticated branch of the tradition of Hindu Tantra.[4] Surely, it must mean something when one of the West's shrewdest observers of the psychological scene and also one of the most incisive critics of the uncritical adoption of India's Yoga makes such an admission. It therefore behooves us to follow Jung's wise advice to study India's heritage carefully. "The wisdom and mysticism of the East," he assures us, "have, therefore, very much to say to us."[5]

The concept of Yoga psychology, like that of Yoga philosophy or Hinduism, is admittedly a Western notion that was invented because we like to understand non-Western traditions in terms of our familiar Western categories—a somewhat presumptuous tactic. From the perspective of traditional Yoga, there is only Yoga, which includes many psychological and philosophical as well as practice-related concepts. In the present context then, Yoga psychology is Yoga viewed through a Western psychological lens but, I think, with reasonable fidelity to the Indian traditional heritage.

Yoga has long intrigued curious Westerners, beginning with the ancient Greeks, who witnessed yogic "demonstrations," such as the spectacular self-immolation of a certain Kalanos, who was traveling in Alexander the Great's entourage when that emperor returned from his military campaigns in India. Apparently, without showing the least sign of fear or pain, Kalanos stepped onto a pyre he himself had built and lit, and he was soon engulfed by flames. The Greek philosophers of the day, who aspired to perfect happiness (*eudaimonía*) and upheld the ethical ideal of unshakability (*ataraxía*) were wondering just how Kalanos could remain so calm when terror should grip him and unbearable pain should riddle his body.

For centuries, the extraordinary feats of Indian ascetics captured the imagination of the Mediterranean sages, philosophers, and church fathers. Unquestionably, the Indian wisdom traditions exerted a lively influence on Western spirituality and esotericism, though the exact lines of influence are difficult, if not impossible, to trace for sure. Some scholars think that "Oriental" ideas infiltrated the West early on and helped shape early Christianity primarily through gnosticism.

Throughout the Middle Ages, India was looked on as the land of untold wealth, exotic peoples, and fantastic phenomena. On the material level, it was particularly valued for its spices, which were trafficked along the famous Silk Route. In the fifteenth century, this led the Portuguese trader Vasco da Gama to look for a sea route to India. He made landfall in Kappad near Calicut in southwest India in 1498, after sailing around the African coastline and then boldly plunging into the unknown Indian Ocean, a stretch of about forty-five hundred miles (in a straight line). His success stimulated the growth of the Portuguese seaborne empire, which lasted from 1415 to the first quarter of the nineteenth century.

In the sixteenth century, the first Christian missionaries arrived on the Indian peninsula, also by sea, making an all-out effort to convert the heathens but persistently failing to do so. Instead, some of the missionaries learned native Indian languages and started importing Indian ideas to the West under the ever-watchful eyes of the church. Then, under Queen Victoria, imperialist British arrived in India and, in 1858, established the ill-famed British Raj (British colonial rule), which lasted until 1947 when India achieved political independence. The rest, as they say, is history. In 1851, an Indian physician (perhaps Babu Nobin Chander Paul) under the name of N. C. Paul published *A Treatise on the Yoga Philosophy*, which achieved considerable influence in the Theosophical Society.

There is a little-known episode in which Queen Victoria granted no fewer than eighteen audiences to the long-lived Shivapuri Baba (alias Swami Govindananda Bharati, 1826–1963). His visits to Queen Victoria and other heads of state around the world may have been meaningful to him and perhaps to the individuals involved, but they did not make an obvious impact on the public. This changed only with the Parliament of Religions in 1893, which he claimed to have attended unofficially.

Indian nationalism, which was born in the final decades of the British Raj, spawned its own brand of missionaries, notably Swami Vivekananda, who disseminated yogic ideas and practices in the late nineteenth century in America and Europe. His unexpected participation at the Parliament of Religions in Chicago happened at the right time. Many people were hungry for metaphysics and the practical pursuit of inner knowledge, which they hoped could lift them out of the ordinariness and ennui of daily living in an increasingly stressful modern society. A lecture bureau offered to represent Swami Vivekananda. Innocently, he accepted and found himself addressing people in many cities across the states, earning him the nickname Cyclonic Hindu. His public talks drew hundreds and even thousands. Watching the swami's meteoric rise to popularity, fanatical Christian missionaries took exception and began to slander him, which only urged this fiery apostle on.

As is well-known, Swami Vivekananda's dazzling success in the United States and other Western countries opened the floodgate to other Hindu missionaries eager to propagate Yoga and Vedānta (metaphysical nondualism) outside their homeland. They brought with them a host of philosophical and psychological notions, as well as a battery of meditation practices and physical routines that they readily mixed with Western ideas, including nineteenth-century materialistic science, popular Christian beliefs, and New Thought (the precursor of the New Age movement). Swami Vivekananda's fellow renouncers of the Ramakrishna movement, who had lost the saintly Ramakrishna in 1886 and whom the swami himself had helped gather into a monastic order, were obvious candidates. With the support of fervent Western disciples, Vedānta "societies" were founded in major metropolitan areas, especially Chicago, Boston, St. Louis, and New York. Vedānta has at its heart the branch of Yoga that is known as the nondualist path of liberating wisdom (Jnāna-Yoga). Among this ensemble of Hindu spokespersons were influential men like Swami Abhedananda (who was a direct disciple of Sri Ramakrishna, ran the Vedānta society in New York, and wrote several books, including *How to Be a Yogi*); Swami Nikhilananda (the most illustrious of the swamis, who took over in New York after Swami Abhedananda's death and wrote many important presentations of Vedānta, including a brilliant biography of Swami Vivekananda); Swami Prabhavananda (who ran the societies in Portland and Los Angeles and who worked with Christopher Isherwood on widely read translations of Hindu classics); and Swami Satprakashananda (founder of the Vedānta Society of St. Louis, who wrote several key books, including his brilliant *Methods of Knowledge According to Advaita Vedanta*). Today, the Western-born Swami Yogeshananda offers inspiring and touching vignettes of the lives of some of the principal figures of the Ramakrishna movement in *Six Lighted Windows* (1997).[6]

But members of the Ramakrishna movement, representing Vedānta (that is, Jnāna-Yoga), were not the only Indian teachers heading westward. There was the Jaina Yoga teacher Virchand Gandhi (no relation to the Mahatma), who was also a delegate at the Parliament of Religions; the Vaishnava teacher Baba Bharati, who established a Krishna temple in Los Angeles and returned to India in 1907; and Swami Rama Tirtha, who was a former professor of mathematics and a great spiritual master, visiting the United States in 1903 and 1904. Yogendra Mastanami arrived in America in 1919 and stayed in New York for three years before returning to Mumbai.

One of the first nonacademic publications on Yoga by a Westerner was Carl Kellner's twenty-one-page booklet in German *Eine Skizze über den psychologischen Teil der alten indischen Yogalehre* (A Sketch about the Physiological Part of the Old Indian Yoga Teaching), which was printed in Munich in 1896. Its text is distorted by numerous printing and other mistakes. Kellner (1850–1905), known in Vienna as a strongman, was a fascinating person. As far as we can tell, he was a self-taught electrochemist, who made a fortune by inventing a paper-making method. He also taught Hatha-Yoga and was involved with theosophy, freemasonry, alchemy, and (according to some researchers) the Ordo Templi Orientis, which had the infamous Aleister Crowley for its eventual head. Kellner introduced various Hindu Yoga masters to Viennese society and makes particular mention in his booklet of Bheema Sena Pratapa of Lahore, whom he seems to have met during his travels in India. He had for his teacher the Panjabi Sri Mahatma Agamya Paramahansa, who visited Austria several times during 1900 and 1905. Agamya was allegedly a supreme court judge in India before renouncing the world and teaching "Paramanu Yoga" (Atom Yoga). He initiated Kellner into the secret Tantric art of artificially prolonging life, but when Kellner's disciple allegedly disclosed the relevant techniques to his family members, Agamya ritually cursed Kellner. A year later, in 1905, Kellner met with a horrible accident in his chemical lab. It killed two other technicians and seriously wounded Kellner, who died the same year. Those close to Kellner had no doubt that Agamya's curse was responsible for the fatal accident. Most parapsychologists would have no difficulty pondering the possibility of this explanation.

In 1903, Swami Ramacharaka published his first book, titled *Hindu Science of Breath*; each year thereafter, he released a new book filled with a mixture of Yoga and New Thought (the forerunner of New Ageism). Swami Ramacharaka, whose many books are still selling well, was not a swami at all; the name is a pseudonym of William Walker Atkinson (1862–1932), who was an erstwhile lawyer.

A seminal Western Yoga teacher who was also intimately involved with Tantra was the notorious Pierre Bernard ("Oom the Omnipotent"),[7] who with his wife Blanche de Vries (a former dancer) founded the equally notorious and rather luxurious Nyack Country Club in 1919. De Fries intensively taught Hatha-Yoga and, historically, is perhaps more entitled to the laudatory title "First Lady of Yoga" than the later Latvian-born Indra Devi, who taught in Los Angeles in the 1960s and 1970s. While de Vries busied herself with teaching and serving as Bernard's compliant girl Friday, Bernard saw himself in the weighty role of the *guru*. Together they attracted large numbers of well-to-do women and men (in that order), who for many years willingly financed the extravagant club and its programs. Bernard had been educated for about eighteen years by the little-known Tantric adept named Sylvais Hamati, said to be a Syrian-Indian who spoke English fluently and also seems to have been well educated but avoided the limelight. Bernard had the uncanny ability to enter into a deathlike state at will. He had demonstrated this skill, which he called "Kali-Mudra," before an audience of physicians back in 1898. Shortly after this spectacular demonstration, Hamati and Bernard opened a private clinic for the treatment of "nervous disorders." The clinic initially served as the public face of the Tantrik Order, which was founded in 1905.

A few of Bernard's Western disciples, who had reached the highest (or seventh) level, were permitted to engage in the ritual of the Five M's of the Kaula tradition involving sexual congress. In a general climate of distrust about *gurus* in the United States, abundant rumors of immorality flew, and complaints by two former female students led to Bernard's arrest in 1910. After serving just over three months, he was released from jail on his own recognizance. Five months later, the charges were dropped. For many years, the country club was the fulcrum of Yoga in the United States, and de Vries trained numerous Yoga teachers who, in turn, catered to many early Hollywood stars.

In 1911, a Swami A. P. Mukerji published *Yoga Lessons for Developing Spiritual Consciousness*. Eleven years later, he founded the Yogi Publication Society, which acted as the publisher for his other works. His book *The Doctrine and Practice of Yoga* (1922) is written in a somewhat peremptory style, epitomized in his opening statement that "[n]ot one useless or superfluous sentence is written" (Mukerji 1922, 1). Sri Ananda Acharya, a former philosophy professor and Yoga master as well as a poet, settled in Norway in 1912 and lived and taught there until his death on V-E Day in 1945. Another early Yoga teacher from the East was Yogi Hari Rama, who toured throughout the United States in the 1920s, apparently demonstrating the yogic art of levitation. This was also the period in which Sir John Woodroffe published the first Sanskrit editions and translations of Tantric scriptures, which inadvertently boosted the popular fascination with, and flummoxed reaction to, the antinomian teachings of Tantra.

In 1920, Paramahamsa Yogananda arrived in the states and was incredibly successful due to his appealing personality and his willingness to adapt his teachings of Yogoda to Western audiences. His organization—Self-Realization Fellowship—claimed in 1937 to have already initiated 150,000 people. His spiritual autobiography was not published until 1946 but, probably because of its Christianity-friendly attitude, significantly boosted interest in Yoga in the West. The influx of Indian wisdom into North America received a temporary but significant setback when, in 1924, the United States passed the Immigration Act, which essentially forbade all nonwhites entry into the country. This act, which was based on quotas, was the culmination of many years of anti-Indian sentiment by the general public. The law was formally repealed in 1965.

In 1930, a certain Rishi Singh Gherwal (1889–?) published a book on the *kundalinī*, one on the *Yoga-Vāsishtha*, and several more on other topics. A kind of Yoga strikingly different from Paramahamsa Yogananda's Kriya-Yoga—namely Hatha-Yoga—had been taught ever since Swami Abhedananda's days in New York. Hatha-Yoga was reintroduced in 1936 by the hugely popular Yoga teacher Selvarajan Yesudian (1916–1990), the son of an Indian physician, whose book *Yoga and Health* is said to have sold something like one million copies in many languages. Yesudian, who understood Yoga as a spiritual teaching, coauthored all his books with his Hungarian student, Elisabeth Haich. Escaping from Communist Hungary and on the way to North America, they were persuaded by students to settle in Switzerland, which they did.

In 1937, the infamous Aleister Crowley, head of the Ordo Templis Orientis (since 1912), wrote eight essays on Yoga that were published two years later under the title *Eight Lectures on Yoga*. Crowley (alias Mahatma Guru Sri Paramahansa Shivaji) attempted to integrate, not without a great deal of biting humor and irony, Yoga with his own particular strain of Western occultism and magic.[8] Crowley correctly wrote that "[t]here is more nonsense talked and written about Yoga than about anything else in the world," and he spoke of the "Yoga mongers" and "charlatans." The lectures he delivered to small groups were perceptive but also indiscriminately witty, which created confusion among his listeners. He indulged in a great deal of obscurantism by dragging astrological symbolism and the inevitable kabbalah into the discussion, treating Yoga's moral disciplines as "magical practices." He made misleading statements such as "[t]here is no true discrimination between good and evil"; Mantra-Yoga (the yogic path of the recitation of special sounds) is "really a branch of *prāṇāyāma*"; and *pratyāhāra* (sensory inhibition) "may be roughly described as introspection." Apart from adding to the public's confusion about Yoga, Crowley's main contribution to Western Yoga and occultism was his unfortunate yogic sexual magic, with which he was preoccupied and that loosely linked him with Pierre Bernard's neo-Tantric cult.

Since the days of Swami Abhedananda, Pierre Bernard, Yogi Ramacharaka, and Yesudian, Yoga in the West has been progressively promoted as Modern Postural Yoga (MPY). Today tens of millions of people around the globe—mostly women—use it to promote fitness, health, and beauty, with only a small contingent practicing Yoga as a lifestyle or spiritual discipline. In the 1950s, MPY received a major boost, primarily through the emergence of Iyengar Yoga, which established itself as the leading "style" around the world. Elizabeth de Michelis, who coined the useful term Modern Postural Yoga, concludes her study as follows:

> The ultimate teleology of "God-" and "Self-realization" may or may not be adopted by followers, but it will nevertheless remain as a possible background option. Even if practitioners' commitments and beliefs are differently structured, it is likely that MPY will be able to offer some solace, physical, psychological or spiritual, in a world where solace and reassurance are sometimes elusive. As such, MPY has obviously found a place in our society. (de Michelis 2004, 260)

I agree. At the same time, we ought to make an effort to understand, and promote as best we can, Yoga as a spiritual tradition, since fitness, health, and beauty surely cannot give us lasting happiness and deep-level freedom.

Mark Singleton, in his controversial book *Yoga Body* (2010, 18), opts to dismiss de Michelis's typology. He disagrees that modern Yoga has an identifiable unity. While it is true that it comprises many strands, which make any hope of unity illusory, I would argue that the majority of these strands suffer from the same uninspiring commercialism that is ably critiqued in John Philp's 2009 book, *Yoga, Inc.: A Journey through the Big Business of Yoga.*[9] It is both appropriate and necessary to simplify by making use of a Weberian ideal type and contrast the various forms of "McYoga" with "traditional Yoga." Singleton makes ample use of such simplifications, as when he employs the concept of Hinduism, "Transnational Anglophone Yoga," or "Mainstream Western Physical Culture." Many of Singleton's historical observations are pertinent and duly corrective, but on this point, he goes beyond mere academic exercise. Anyone who is familiar with the contemporary Yoga scene knows what is meant by Modern Postural Yoga. If it waddles and quacks, surely it is a duck. But my stance implies more of a spiritual commitment and caring than the academic ethos allows.

In this book, I speak of traditional Yoga in terms of Hindu, Jaina, and Buddhist Yoga. While this inevitably makes this book more challenging to read, for the convenience of my readers, I have organized the materials in such a manner that each tradition is given voice in clearly differentiated sections. It behooves me to say a brief word about the immigration of these three spiritual and cultural traditions to the West as well. Jaina Yoga has never had many occidental representatives, which is regrettable, since Jainism has some fine Yoga teachings. Buddhist Yoga has been with us since the late nineteenth century, largely through the efforts of the Theosophical Society. At the Parliament of Religions in Chicago in 1893, two delegates attracted the most attention: Swami Vivekananda (Hinduism) and Anagarika Dharmapala, alias David Hewavitarne (Theravāda Buddhism). Both attempted to win disciples in the post-Parliament days and succeeded. Dharmapala converted one solitary American to Buddhism, a Jewish-born man by the name of C. T. Strauss, who subsequently vigorously promoted the Buddha's teachings in New York. Swami Vivekananda won many disciples over to Hinduism.

Dharmapala was dynamic—perhaps too dynamic and confrontational for some. The German-born Paul Carus, who had attended the Parliament of Religions and was serving at the time as the editor of Open Court Publishing, invited the more measured Rinzai Zen master Soyen Shaku to his home in LaSalle, Illinois. Carus authored, among other books, *Buddhism and Its Christian Critics* (1897) and *The Gospel of the Buddha* (1894). He was hoping that Soyen Shaku would agree to become involved in a new line of Eastern books. But Soyen Shaku, who was the abbot of the Engakuji Zen monastery in Japan and spoke no English, recommended his disciple D. T. Suzuki, who had successfully translated for him at the Parliament.

D. T. Suzuki conformed to his teacher's request, moved into Carus's rambling house, and started his work with the *Tao Te Ching*. Even though he was writing about Zen and its Chinese precursor Ch'an in the early decades of the twentieth century, these forms of Buddhism did not captivate the American public in a bigger way until the 1950s. In his instructive book *Thirty Years of Buddhist Studies,* published in 1967, the renowned (if controversial) Buddhist scholar Edward Conze made this comment about Suzuki's contribution:

> Stirred by his message, a vast literature on "Zen" arose in England, France, Italy, Germany, and the U.S.A., ranging from positively stuffy to ultra respectable "square" Zennists to the wild whoopees of Mr. Kerouak and his Beatniks. All that there is in these books about Zen comes from Suzuki, and he is held responsible for the misunderstandings they contain. If Suzuki is to be blamed for anything, it is an insufficient awareness of the aridity of the desert into which he transplanted his lovely azalea tree.
>
> (Conze 1967, 28–29)[10]

Tibetan Vajrayāna, another form of Buddhism, has been abundantly represented in the West since shortly after the perilous 1959 exodus of many Tibetans from their mountainous homeland, including the Dalai Lama and many other high lamas, including His Holiness the Karmapa XIV, His Holiness Sakya Trizin, His Holiness Dudjom Rinpoche, Ato Rinpoche, Namkhai Norbu Rinpoche, Kalu Rinpoche, Tai Situ Rinpoche, Trungpa Rinpoche, and Lama Thubten Yeshe. Tibetan Buddhism has thrived on the North American continent particularly since the 1970s and today can claim a few hundred thousand followers in the United States and Canada. It is, however, exceedingly difficult to provide reliable demographics, because not all Tibetan Buddhists are affiliated with a center.

Here I wish to provide a wider context for the preceding discussion. Because the diplomats of the British Raj were naturally interested in ruling as efficiently as possible, they were eager to know native Indian law as well as possible. So the East India Company (a trading company later taken over by the Crown) commissioned scholars to study Sanskrit and translate texts. They also translated texts that belonged to literature and philosophy. Thus it came to be that in 1785, the *Bhagavad-Gītā* (Lord's Song), perhaps the single most significant Hindu Yoga scripture, was translated into English. Other texts followed, and the scholarly discipline of Indology was born and, through the Romantic movement, reached large audiences in the nineteenth century. The German-British scholar Max Müller (1823–1900), who was highly influential and rather idealistic, was one of the last ambassadors of the Romantic movement. Swami Vivekananda paid him a visit at his Oxford home and saw in him a reincarnation of the famous Vedic scholar Sāyana, who had lived in the fourteenth century and whose Sanskrit commentary Müller had edited. In an enthusiastic article on Müller, written in 1896 for the Indian magazine *Brahmavādin,* the swami called him a "Vedantist of Vedantists" who had "caught the real soul of the melody of the Vedanta." Little wonder that this savant was later nicknamed (and in a way honored) as *moksha-mūla* ("root of liberation") by his numerous Indian admirers.

As explained earlier, in the early decades of the twentieth century, Hindu swamis and yogis already used the same sea route that had brought Westerners to the shores of India in order to export Yoga teachings to an eager audience across the ocean. These included masters of Hatha-Yoga, the "forceful" (*hatha*) path to spiritual freedom and immortality.

Little did Western adherents of this branch of Yoga, which emerged in India c. 1000 C.E., suspect that it had been reshaped in the early twentieth century under a nationalistic agenda and was thus singularly equipped for international dissemination, particularly at a time when nationalism was ripe in other parts of the world. Hatha-Yoga focused on physical fitness and was greatly influenced by Indian approaches to bodybuilding and gymnastics, which clearly suited Western expectations and needs. This piece of history about Hatha-Yoga, which is now practiced in a despiritualized form by upward of forty million people around the globe, has come to light only recently through books like Elizabeth de Michelis's *A History of Modern Yoga* (2004), Joseph S. Alter's *Yoga in Modern India* (2004), and Mark Singleton's *Yoga Body* (2010).

Jung, who had warned about "imitating" Yoga, failed to recognize that the Yoga exported to the Western hemisphere was in many ways already thoroughly westernized. Therefore, his caveat has not been especially applicable to most Yoga practitioners. The overwhelming majority of them have little interest in adopting Yoga's ideas and practices other than postures for promoting fitness, beauty, and health. There seems to be a growing trend, however, that puts Yoga's philosophical and psychological heritage before Western students. Therefore, it appears to be appropriate to reconsider briefly what this means in Jung's terms.

Yoga, which in the past was an initiatory tradition, has gone worldwide and become a popular movement. This implies that practitioners apply popular expectations and standards to Yoga rather than the aspiration to actualize the "meta-values" of traditional Yoga. This is an unfortunate historical reality. One can only hope that as the environmental, social, economic, and political world crisis sharpens, there will be a growing interest in what Yoga really has to offer. Of course there are those who, often under the influence of New Age ideology, are prone to misinterpret Yoga and engage only in its outermost practices. I am reminded here of an astute observation by Pabongka Rinpoche, who died in 1941 at the age of sixty-three. This great Buddhist teacher of the twentieth century remarked,

Don't let your mouth start watering every time you hear somebody spout some meaningless chatter about some new and very oh-so-very "profound" Dharma [teaching] they've discovered.

Rather take yourself through the great texts and special advices of the wise and accomplished masters of our own tradition, all in the proper order of learning, contemplation, and meditation. (Tsongkhapa 1995, 104)

He also said,

Now there are false teachings that some persons simply make up on their own, out of an ignorant desire for gain. There are paths that are absolutely backwards, and there are paths that will lead you astray.

(Tsongkhapa 1995, 92)

These are uncompromising, tough words that need to be heard and heeded. The teachings of Yoga, which include many secret instructions, must not be treated lightly and casually. Too many yogic concepts are misunderstood, and yogic techniques are applied frivolously and far below par. Those who misconstrue the Eastern teachings are the ones whom Jung rightly decried as "imitators." But then, it must be said, there are others who endeavor to practice Yoga as a spiritual discipline and do so in the context of our own complex culture.

The following passage makes it clear that Jung would have summarily and erroneously dismissed their approach as well:

> What is the use of imitating yoga if your dark side remains as good a medieval Christian as ever? If you can afford to seat yourself on a gazelle skin under a Bo-tree or in the cell of a *gompa* for the rest of your life without being troubled by politics or the collapse of your securities, I will look favourably upon your case. But yoga in Mayfair or Fifth Avenue, or in any other place which is on the telephone, is a spiritual fake. (Jung 1978, 128)

This is true enough if a Western Yoga practitioner were to do no more than pursue Yoga's psychotechnology without adequate self-knowledge or even the desire for it and without making an effort to change his or her emotional and moral life. Just to sit in meditation for one or more hours a day does not a yogi make. This is as disingenuous as a daily posture routine unaccompanied by any desire for spiritual transformation. However, if a Westerner can pursue a yogic discipline as part of an overall orientation of self-transformation, surely it does not matter whether this occurs in the context of a modern household with all the usual trappings—telephone, computer, television, and what not. When these items turn out to be intrusive to the spiritual work, the practitioner will most certainly limit their impact on his or her life. Even traditional India gave people the option to be either world-renouncing ascetics or world-engaging householder-yogis. This was the big issue with which the *Bhagavad-Gītā* wrestled. It would seem that the harshness of Jung's stance was due to a personal Eurocentric bias and inadequate acquaintance with the Indian sources. We cannot, however, quibble with its essential message:

> Western imitation is a tragic misunderstanding of the psychology of the East, every bit as sterile as the modern escapades to New Mexico, the blissful South Sea islands, and central Africa, where "the primitive life" is played at in deadly earnest while Western man secretly evades his menacing duties.... It is not for us to imitate what is foreign to our organism

or to play the missionary; our task is to build up our Western civilization, which sickens with a thousand ills. This has to be done on the spot, and by the European just as he is, with all his Western ordinariness, his marriage problems, his neuroses, his social and political delusions, and his whole philosophical disorientation. (Jung 1978, 10)

Jung wrote this in 1929 as part of his commentary on *The Secret of the Golden Flower* by Richard Wilhelm. He confirmed these observations in an article published in *Prabuddha Bharata,* an Indian magazine, in 1936:

[The Westerner] will infallibly make a wrong use of yoga because his psychic disposition is quite different from that of the Oriental. I say to whomever I can: "Study yoga—you will learn an infinite amount from it—but do not try to apply it, for we Europeans are not so constituted that we apply these methods correctly, just like that. An Indian guru can explain everything and you can imitate everything. But do you know *who* is applying this yoga? In other words, do you know who you are and how you are constituted?" (Jung 1978, 82)

While we may not agree with Jung that Europeans (his "Westerners") are uniquely constituted, we can agree that our historical experience has left us mentally, emotionally, and spiritually adrift, so that before we can engage Yoga properly, we must do a certain amount of preliminary psychological work. Otherwise we are apt to carry our confusion over into our yogic discipline. Also, if we are thoroughly Western in our disposition, we are likely to be steeped in Western (mostly Christian) values and symbols, and this, as he correctly saw, might prove an obstacle to a no-holds-barred practice of Yoga. I believe, though, that it is possible for a Westerner to practice Yoga without succumbing to mere "imitation," just as it is possible (but by no means easy) for a Westerner to live a Christian spiritual life intensively, authentically, and successfully.

What would Jung have said about those Westerners who, since the 1970s, have delved headfirst into the rich spiritual culture of Tibetan Buddhism? Certainly his criticism applies to them, and Westerners' involvement with Buddhism has not been without its problems. After many years of Buddhist practice, Westerners see merit in a course of psychotherapy.[11]

With these crucial considerations clearly expressed, we are equipped to turn to the substance of this book.

PART ONE Foundations

CHAPTER 1

Yoga Psychology and Modern Psychology
Orientation and Goals

> Yoga is the most eloquent expression of the Indian mind.
>
> —CARL G. JUNG (1978, 160)

DIFFERENTIATIONS

Since this book will be read primarily by lay readers, it may be useful to begin by providing a brief overview of the spectrum of major present-day psychological orientations. As a thriving branch of modern humanistic science, psychology consists of various subdisciplines, notably the following, in alphabetical order:

- *Abnormal psychology* is concerned with malfunctions (psychopathology) of the mind, such as neurosis and psychosis, and it is also referred to as *psychiatry*.
- *Cognitive psychology* investigates the functioning of the normal mind, especially intelligence and memory.
- *Cross-cultural psychology* looks for significant psychological insights on the basis of comparative research done among people of diverse languages and sociocultural environments.
- *Depth psychology* explores the hidden features of the mind and covers such approaches as *psychoanalysis* (based primarily on the work of Sigmund Freud and his students) and *psychotherapy* (based primarily on the work of Carl Jung and his students).
- *Developmental psychology* is concerned with psychological processes as they unfold in the course of an individual's life from cradle to grave.
- *Educational psychology* focuses on the mental processes involved in teaching and learning.
- *Environmental psychology* is concerned with the psychological implica-

tions of environmental design (mostly by questionnaire and observational studies).

· *Industrial and organizational psychology* applies psychological principles to working life (such as personnel selection and workplace or equipment design).

· *Integral psychology,* as developed by Ken Wilber, is an attempt to synthesize the various psychological approaches by creating a template that meaningfully covers all of them. In his book *Integral Psychology* (2000a), Wilber based his "master template"—which he agrees is merely a heuristic device—on an examination of more than one hundred psychologists from both hemispheres of the globe and from antiquity to modern times. His orientation represents a further development of the ideas first presented in his book *The Spectrum of Consciousness* (1977), which he wrote at the age of twenty-three.

· *Neuropsychology,* a relatively new discipline, investigates the neurological aspects of the mind. It has two camps: one has a materialistic bias, and one favors spiritual interpretations. The latter is favored by Mario Beauregard and Denyse O'Leary in their book *The Spiritual Brain* (2007).

· *Parapsychology* focuses on extraordinary human abilities, such as telepathy, telekinesis, and clairvoyance.

· *Physiological psychology* studies the biological foundations of human thought and behavior, primarily by means of laboratory research of perception and brain functions.

· *Positive psychology* is an approach that is midway between a model and a scientific discipline. It investigates and emphasizes the value of positivity in the affective field. Barbara L. Fredrickson (2009), the genius behind this approach, is the author of the key text.

· *Psychopharmacology* is interested in the influence of drugs on the functioning of the brain and nervous system.

· *Psychosomatic medicine* is especially interested in the connection between cognitive processes (such as thoughts and attitudes) and the state of an individual's physical health.

· *Social psychology* explores how individuals are shaped by society and how cultural norms and values are translated into individual thought and behavior.

· *Transpersonal psychology* is concerned with those cognitive processes that occur beyond the range of both normal and abnormal functioning, notably experiences of ego transcendence and illumination.

Yoga psychology has, of course, none of this differentiation into specific subdivisions, although Yoga itself has many branches, each of which can be said to represent—analogously—a particular focus of interest or psychological competence: Rāja-Yoga (Patanjali's Classical Yoga of higher mental disciplines); Jnāna-Yoga (the "intellectual" approach of discernment); Hatha-Yoga (primarily physical discipline, including postures and breath control); Karma-Yoga (self-transcending action in everyday life); Bhakti-Yoga (the devotional-emotive path); Mantra-Yoga (the path of transformative sound); and Tantra-Yoga (an integrative approach). Traditionally, these diverse branches are viewed as bands of a common spectrum addressing the different capacities of students of Yoga. In practice, each branch has its own historical trajectory and considers itself a path to spiritual enlightenment in its own right. It is, however, correct that disciples of various capacities are drawn to a given path, which helps them develop self-transcendence in a unique way that corresponds to their particular personality. Thus, those who have a natural capacity for introspection may be drawn to the meditative approach of Rāja-Yoga; those who have a particular propensity toward bodily exercise may be attracted to Hatha-Yoga; those with an intellectual bent may find Jnāna-Yoga especially appealing, and so on.

So much for Hindu Yoga. The story of Jaina Yoga's immigration to the West is far simpler. Jainism came to be known to Western scholars in the late nineteenth century but never attracted much public interest. The first four chapters of Hemacandra's magnificent *Yoga-Shāstra* were first translated into German by Ernst Windish in 1884 based on a single manuscript. The rendering is inadequate, because it did not take into consideration Hemacandra's autocommentary, the *Svopajña-Vṛtti*. Another attempt to edit and translate Hemacandra's work was made for the *Bibliotheca Indica* series in 1907 but was abandoned halfway through in 1921. Other efforts were made subsequently, the last in 2002 by Olle Quarnström in a handsome edition by Harvard University. Since that time, other works on Jaina ethics, philosophy, and Yoga have been translated and printed in small numbers.

The situation with Buddhist Yoga is more complex. Pāli, the language of the scriptures of Southern Buddhism, first came to be of grammatical interest to the Wesleyan missionary Benjamin Clough, who published his study in 1824. Eugène Burnouf, a linguistic genius, published his *L'Introduction à l'histoire du Buddhism indien* in 1844. His premature death in 1852, at the age of fifty-one, disrupted his plan to append two further volumes to this formidable scholarly work. His translation into French of the *Lotus*

Sutra, a Mahāyāna text of the first century C.E., fortunately was published in 1852. Almost single-handedly, Burnouf managed to establish Buddhism as a field of study, and his investigations gave rise to a slew of other academic efforts and popular writings. He inspired, among others, the German philosopher Arthur Schopenhauer, who published his best-known work *Die Welt als Wille und Vorstellung* (*The World as Will and Representation*) in 1818, which, despite all sorts of misunderstandings, spread the fame of Buddhism in Europe. In 1854, the German composer Richard Wagner was given a copy of Schopenhauer's work, and it had an electrifying effect on him that was symbolic of a larger receptivity toward Buddhism at the time.

As early as 1878, the celebrated English poet Edwin Arnold lionized and also Victorianized the life of the Buddha in *The Light of Asia,* which has sold a million copies. Scholarly interest in Buddhism soared in the last two decades of the nineteenth century, partly because it was associated with the Theosophical Society, which was founded in 1876. Because of the society's connection with occultism, which was widespread, interest in Buddhism grew rapidly early on in the West. In 1880, Helena Petrovna Blavatsky, the cofounder of the Theosophical Society, took Buddhist vows in Sri Lanka. One year later, the Pāli Text Society was founded in London and aspired to print and translate the entire Pāli canon. In 1888, Vincent van Gogh painted himself with the slanted eyes of a clean-shaven Japanese Buddhist monk in *Self-Portrait Dedicated to Paul Gauguin.* He ended his own life the following year, obviously having been unable to replace his derelict Christian faith with bona fide Buddhist spiritual practice.

Although the notable Zen master Soyen Shaku, abbot of the Engakuji Monastery in Kamakura, was present at the World Parliament of Religions in Chicago in 1893, he was eclipsed by the young Hindu master Swami Vivekananda. The great Zen scholar D. T. Suzuki, who had served as Soyen Shaku's translator at the Parliament, created various foundational books on Zen for several years afterward. In 1911, Blavatsky accompanied by her sixteen-year-old future *buddha,* Krishnamurti, lectured to a rapt audience of four thousand at the Sorbonne. Buddhism was definitely proving attractive to all those who felt they had outgrown Christianity. Also in 1911, Oxford University released W. Y. Evans-Wentz's book *Fairy-Faith in Celtic Countries.* It was Evans-Wentz who, in collaboration with Kazi Dawa-Samdup, worked on the *Bardo Thödol,* which is best known in the Western hemisphere as *The Book of the Dead.* Their joint translation (Evans-Wentz knew precious little Tibetan and was more responsible for editing) was published in 1927 and, with a psychological commentary by Carl Jung, made a substantial impact on the English-speaking world.

Yet neither Blavatsky's occult Buddhism nor Suzuki's Rinzai Zen nor Evans-Wentz's Vajrayāna Buddhism proved more than stepping-stones toward widespread Buddhist practice among the American public. This was to happen several decades later.

Analogous to Wilber's integral psychology, which seeks to integrate the diverse psychological subdisciplines, Sri Aurobindo's Integral Yoga—which he formulated between 1915 and 1920—is a modern attempt to integrate and thereby transcend the limitations of the diverse branches of traditional Hindu Yoga (see Chaudhuri 1975 and Chaudhuri and Spiegelberg 1960). As Aurobindo wrote,

> Yoga, as Swami Vivekananda has said, may be regarded as a means of compressing one's evolution into a single life or a few years or even a few months of bodily existence. A given system [or branch] of Yoga, then, can be no more than a selection or a compression into narrower but more energetic forms of intensity....It is this view of Yoga that can alone form the basis for a sound and rational synthesis of Yogic methods. For then Yoga ceases to appear [as] something mystic and abnormal. (Aurobindo 1976, 2)

He also said,

> The true and full object and utility of Yoga can only be accomplished when the conscious Yoga in man becomes, like the subconscious Yoga in Nature, outwardly conterminous with life itself and we can once more, looking out both on the path and the achievement, say in a more perfect and luminous sense: "All life is Yoga." (Aurobindo 1976, 4)

Aurobindo correctly recognized the "specialising and separative tendency" in traditional Yoga and the need for synthesis. At the same time, he recognized that traditional Yoga itself has a synthetic trend that is certainly within the compass of its own culture. Aurobindo sought to accomplish a more sweeping synthesis on the basis of the modern idea of natural evolution: Yoga achieves for the individual what nature, much more slowly, endeavors to accomplish for everyone.

In *Integral Psychology,* Ken Wilber states that he sees in Integral Yoga "a concerted effort to unite and integrate the ascending (evolutionary) and descending (involutionary) currents in human beings, thus uniting other-worldly and this-worldly, transcendent and immanent, spirit and matter." From the hindsight of the last six or more decades, it is fair to say, as Wilber put it, that Aurobindo did not "fully assimilate the differentiations of modernity." I also agree with Wilber that Aurobindo "was India's greatest modern philosopher-sage" (Wilber 2000a, 83–84).

In the present book, I consider Aurobindo's integrative endeavor as a valid branch, or subdiscipline, of Yoga that deserves special attention because of its evolutionary thrust. Aurobindo's Yoga also shows that the development of Yoga is not yet concluded. Some people point to Modern Postural Yoga as another instance. I would indeed like to think that, perhaps against all odds, contemporary Yoga can mature in time to include the age-old ideal of spiritual freedom as a choice for at least some people.

To make a related point, the late Mircea Eliade (1973, 361) viewed Yoga as a "living fossil." The problem with this characterization is that a fossil—even a living one—is evolutionarily static, whereas Yoga is arguably undergoing at least a certain degree of dynamic change in modern times in some niches of both the East and the West, such as among the followers of Sri Aurobindo, Swami Satyananda, Pandit Gopinath Kaviraj (all three representative of Hindu Yoga), and the late Chögyam Trungpa (representative of Buddhist Yoga). Perhaps the teacher who most blatantly diverged from the traditional pattern was Aurobindo. While Eastern teachers of Buddhism tend to be conservative, some of their Western disciples seek to apply the Buddha Dharma in the context of modern society and the world's environmental crisis.

A MATTER OF ORIENTATION

I will next turn to the basic character of modern psychology versus Yoga psychology. It is *versus,* because the contrast between both orientations to psychological realities is considerable—some would say as much as the contrast between black and white. But there is at least one important similarity, which is pragmatism. This word comes from the Greek word *pragma,* meaning "action/practice." In other words, both modern psychology and Yoga psychology are interested in applying their respective understanding; they are not merely abstract theoretical enterprises.

There are also many differences. The most striking difference concerns the respective orientations of modern psychology and Yoga psychology. Whereas the former, for the most part, seeks to make its knowledge relevant to the proper functioning of the ordinary individual, the latter is designed to transform the ordinary personality so significantly that it is utterly transcended in the condition of enlightenment. Only transpersonal psychology and integral psychology are constituted to relate to this seemingly outlandish view. The goal, then, of traditional Yoga is to create a being who, in some way, is superhuman: identical with the transcendental Reality and endowed with all its capacities (in the form of paranormal abilities).

At best, modern psychology talks about liberating the individual from undesirable character traits or neuroses. In Yoga psychology, in which spirituality is writ large, the liberative process does not concern merely an aspect of the human personality but the human being as a whole. This is not a religious agenda; it is understood in a spiritual sense. The self-transformation aimed at in Yoga is radical rather than merely partial: it seeks to expose the core of the human being behind all conditional facets of the personality. In the language of Hindu and Jaina Yoga, this means freeing the transcendental Self from the body-mind or recognizing that it has always been free.

In Buddhist parlance, the intended transformation simply signifies the transcendence of the personality, without any substantive implications of a stable essence. From the time of Gautama the Buddha, who lived nearly twenty-five hundred years ago, Buddhism has favored a nonessentialist philosophy and psychology that are reminiscent of the process system of the British philosopher-mathematician Alfred North Whitehead. By contrast, both Hindu and Jaina Yoga subscribe to an ontology (science of being) that corresponds to the Wilberian "Great Nest of Being"—internesting levels (*tattvas,* or "principles") of phenomenal reality.

An obvious major difference between modern psychology and Yoga psychology is their respective methodologies. While both proceed empirically (that is, by means of experience), Yoga psychology takes as its principal tool rigorous introspection rather than external experimentation, possibly by means of gadgets, such as test tubes, the electroencephalogram, or the electrocardiogram. Important to note, it pursues introspection more completely than those subdivisions of modern psychology that rely on an introspective method, because Yoga approaches self-understanding primarily—though not exclusively—by means of intensive meditation leading up to the ecstatic state (*samādhi*) in which subject and object become merged.

The practitioner of Yoga—*yogin* (if male) or *yoginī* (if female)—is his or her own laboratory. This self-understanding is one reason why Yoga and alchemy became assimilated at a certain time (after 1000 C.E.) (see White

1996, 76). The body-mind is analogous to the alchemist's cauldron in which the alchemical elixir is generated that grants the Yoga adept immortality. The alchemical notion of immortality is equivalent to the yogic concept of enlightenment, or liberation, and the two became providentially merged in the tradition of Tantra.

Furthermore, modern psychology has the goal of *objectively* advancing our understanding of the mind with its various automaticities but also with its unique capacities for insight, intuition, empathy, interest, decision making, love, compassion, and so on. Yoga has no interest in objective knowledge for its own sake. It does not aim to contribute to any culture's pool of knowledge or data bank. Yoga's heritage has, from the start, been intended for those few who "are called and chosen," that is, who are ready and able to embark on the spiritual adventure of inner transformation. All yogic knowledge is designed to serve this purpose.

A further major difference between modern psychology and Yoga psychology relates to the latter's initiatory structure, which has no equivalent in the former. The typical psychologist undergoes academic training with periodic tests of professional competence; this leads to an academic degree culminating in a PhD or MD, normally between the ages of twenty-eight and thirty. The spiritual "career" of a *yogin* can start at any age and has no formal academic title associated with it. The Yoga student is considered "graduated" when the teacher (*guru*) considers him or her so, which usually coincides with the teacher gently or abruptly and unceremoniously pushing the student out of the protective nest of the hermitage (*āshrama*) and asking him or her to start teaching. Before then, any number of years of pupilage (*shishyatā*) may have passed. In Hindu Yoga, if the period of pupilage is completed more ceremoniously, then it is likely to take the form of the kind of final admonition as we find it in the *Taittirīya-Upanishad* (1.11.1): "Speak the truth; practice virtue (dharma); let there be no neglect of study (*svādhyāya*)."

In the era of the Vedas up to the early Upanishads, the young student lived in the teacher's household—a practice known as *antevāsin* (literally, "dwelling near")—for however many years. Following the stipulation of the ethico-legal literature, it was thought that life ideally (though seldom in practice) unfolded in periods of twenty-one years, with *brahmacarya*, or a period of chastity, claiming the first twenty-one years. During this time, the teacher imparted whatever knowledge and wisdom he felt the student was capable of receiving. In exchange, the student made himself as useful as possible, gathering firewood, tending the teacher's herd of cattle, and doing whatever other menial service was asked of him—undoubtedly a character-building time. During this phase, a student would particularly have learned the value of self-transcendence, self-restraint, kindness, and what in modern terms is called "voluntary simplicity."

In the early days, spiritual training and religious upbringing were intermixed. The main task of a pupil was to learn by heart as many of the Vedic texts as he could. Only members of the higher social estates (*varna*)—brahmin, warrior, and merchant—qualified for pupilage. Members of the servile estate (*shūdra*) were excluded, although it appears that this law of exclusion was applied with a certain leniency in antiquity. With the emergence of the caste system later on, there was less flexibility. A student who came out of the customary pupilage in religious training with the intention of devoting his life to spiritual matters next had to find a master of Yoga.

Demanding prerequisites were stipulated for the spiritual novice or neophyte, and they all had the same purpose: to notify prospective aspirants that they should not approach a *guru* ("weighty one") casually but only if they were serious about self-transformation through an inevitably demanding course of yogic disciplines. Traditionally, once a person embarks on the sacred ordeal of discipleship, he or she is charged with loyal devotion to the *guru* and the path revealed to that teacher. In turn, he or she receives in due course full initiation (*dīkshā*) into the secrets that the master has to impart.

Most important, yogic initiation consists not merely in divulging doctrinally important intellectual knowledge (such as the Vedāntic "Thou art that" axiom). But through the teacher's grace (*prasāda*), the aspirant is endowed with actual *experiential* participation in the spiritual Reality around which all the teachings revolve. This would be like a professor of psychiatry evoking in students a schizophrenic state by means of hallucinogenic drugs or a professor of quantum physics plunging students into the perplexing actuality of the paradoxical quantum state instead of just jotting mathematical formulas on the chalkboard and then obliging students to grasp their meaning through the rational mind and by big intuitive leaps.

The teacher's grace also bears the designation of "transmission" (*sancāra*), which is a parapsychological intervention by which the adept teacher retools the mind of the disciple, so that it becomes more firmly focused on and capable of spiritual transformation. In the tradition of Tantra and Kashmiri Shaivism, for instance, this transmission is often called "descent of Power" (*shakti-pāta*), which is the equivalent of the awakening of the esoteric serpent power (*kundalinī-bodhana*). The *kundalinī* is understood as a form of the Goddess, or divine Power (*shakti*), within the body of each person. I will say more about this phenomenon in chapter 11.

Here is a first-person, traditional description of an ecstatic realization from the nondual perspective resulting from initiation. It is found in the *Ashtāvakra-Samhitā* (2.1–2.4, 2.11, 2.17, 2.20, 2.23), a post-fourteenth-century Vedānta text:

Oh! I am untainted, calm gnosis (*bodha*) beyond the Cosmos! All this time I was duped by illusion!

Just as I alone illuminate this body, so also [do I illuminate] the universe. Hence this entire universe is mine, or indeed nothing [is mine].

Oh! Having abandoned now the universe along with the body, I behold the supreme Self by means of some skill [given to me by my guru].

As waves, foam, and bubbles are not different from water, so the universe emerging out of the Self is not different from the Self.

Oh! I! Salutation to Myself for whom there is no destruction [and who] survives even upon the destruction of the universe [at the end of time, which comprises everything] from Brahma down to [the least] lump of grass.

Oh! I am mere gnosis (*bodha*)! Out of ignorance, I imagined [the presence of all kinds of limiting] assumptions (*upādhi*). Ever contemplating thus, My state [of being] is in the transconceptual (*nirvikalpa*) [Reality].

Body, heaven and hell, bondage and freedom, as well as fear—what should I whose nature is Consciousness/Awareness (*cit*) do [with all] this, [which is] mere imagination (*kalpanā*)?

Oh! In Me the limitless ocean, diverse waves of worlds (*bhuvana*) are instantly generated [even as] mind's wind [or energy] is rising.

A better-known and more dramatic description of an ecstatic realization is given in chapter 11 of the *Bhagavad-Gītā*. It was induced by the God-man Krishna in his disciple Prince Arjuna who, unprepared for such an overwhelming experience, asked his *guru* to mercifully cause the ecstasy to subside again, which he did. Although the *kundalinī* phenomenon is not mentioned in either passage, the descriptions are in keeping with the kind of realization triggered by the aforementioned initiatory procedure of *shakti-pāta.*

This brings me to my final point of difference between modern scientific psychology and Yoga, which is the nonseparation of fact from value. Science purports to be value-free. It assumes that it deals only in facts. Nothing could be further from the truth. "All science and technology," states Alan Drengson (1995, 187), "is conducted according to specific values and within a range of assumptions constituting a worldview, which is not itself science but philosophy." When we look at the world, we look not just with our eyes but with our mind, and our mind is not merely a matter of thoughts; we have emotional impulses, feelings, motives, biases, and so on. We can never look at facts without our whole personality, which charges facts with meaning and value. As Johann Goethe put it, "Every fact is theory." Abraham Maslow explained it this way:

> Facts don't just lie there, like oatmeal in a bowl; they do all sorts of things ... Facts have authority and demand character. They may require of us; they may say "No" or "Yes." They lead us on, suggest to us, imply the next thing to do and guide us in one direction rather than another. (Maslow 1971, 118)

Maslow spoke of the "vectorial nature" of facts (117). Each fact is an "ought," which is not the same as the Freudian superego's "should."

Certainly, Yoga is far from value neutral. It is embedded in moral considerations. It proceeds along an ethical pathway. Thus, the Vedānta tradition, which represents Jnāna-Yoga (or the path of wisdom), expects an aspirant to demonstrate a capacity for discernment (*viveka*), a degree of dispassion (*virāga*), a desire for liberation (*mumukshutva*), as well as the following six qualities:

- Tranquillity (*shama*)
- Self-restraint (*dama*)
- Inner renunciation (*uparati*)
- Patience (*titikshā*)
- Concentration (*samādhi*)
- Faith (*shraddhā*)

It may seem strange that an aspirant should be expected to possess these qualities, which we associate with the virtues of a mature *yogin*. But a preceptor of Yoga wants to see them—at least in seed form—in prospective students, so that the *guru* has some assurance that students will make some progress in their yogic training. If this is not the case, they will merely incur suffering in the course of their studies.

Authorities differ about the precise meaning of each of the aforementioned six qualities. Some of them seem self-explanatory, and I will address only the last one: faith. This is often understood as belief in the Vedic heritage, but faith, which the *Yoga-Bhāshya* (1.20) states protects the *yogin* like a caring mother, is perhaps more of a positive, buoyant attitude toward one's spiritual potential and the liberative capacity of Yoga.

Many Hindu Yoga texts mention prerequisites similar to those in the Vedānta works. Thus, the major scriptures of Hatha-Yoga usually distinguish between mild, middling, and acute practitioners. The latter are typically associated with behavioral capacities, or virtues, such as simplicity, moderation in eating, and perseverance, which are qualities ascribed to accomplished adepts.

Jainism and Buddhism make similar demands on monastic novices but are more lenient toward laypeople. The Jaina monk or nun is expected to live absolutely by the five moral norms of the "great vow" (*mahā-vrata*), which are the same as its yogic equivalent (see *Yoga-Sūtra*, 2.30–31), although individual components are understood somewhat differently: nonharming, truthfulness, nonstealing, chastity, and greedlessness. They also have to adopt the five kinds of "care" (*samiti*), or practices of mindfulness, relative to walking, speaking, begging, receiving and declining (a seat, and so on), and excretion (of feces, urine, phlegm, and so on).

Buddhism is particularly interesting here, because its moral practices have become more extensive in the course of its evolution from the Buddha's teaching to those of Mahāyāna and Vajrayāna (Tibetan) Buddhism. The moral norms of early Buddhism are enshrined in the Buddha's eightfold path, which is described in chapter 14.

Even though there were other, more specific rules for moral behavior, such as abstention from intoxicants, eating after midday, avoidance of adornments, and the like, the Buddha himself seems to have laid the greatest emphasis on kindness or friendliness (*maitrī*). Certain offenses, such as killing and sexual intercourse, are irremediable. Other numerous offenses, such as lascivious language and causing a schism in the community, require either forfeiture of any disallowed item and confession or confession only. Minor infractions simply call for behavioral change.

Mahāyāna added to the early Buddhist ethics many additional vows to be kept by an aspiring bodhisattva. A bodhisattva is someone who engages the Buddhist path in order to liberate all other beings. This is often misunderstood as deferring one's own enlightenment, but it is actually only upon one's own that one can fully accomplish the task of a bodhisattva. Before then, whatever spiritual assistance one can give to others is somewhat limited. The path of the bodhisattva comprises ten stages of moral and spiritual unfolding that are described differently in the literature. This is also described in chapter 14.

CHAPTER 2

The Reality of Suffering

Existentialism in Practice

> [That which is] to be overcome is future suffering.
>
> —PATANJALI, *Yoga-Sūtra* 2.16

One of the cornerstones of Yoga psychology is the recognition of the overwhelming reality of suffering in life—that is, the life of the unenlightened individual. This is acknowledged by all forms and branches of Yoga. It is closely allied to the philosophical notion of the phenomenal world (*samsāra*) as an unending round of complexities driven by the law of moral causation (karma), which is a second cornerstone and is closely related to the idea of rebirth (*punarjanman*). Suffering and karmic necessity (along with rebirth) are associated with the idea of the ego-personality of the unenlightened being. I discuss these three cardinal concepts together here.

SUFFERING

In the eyes of some observers, Yoga's concern with the predictable presence of suffering in the world aligns it with the philosophical approach of existentialism. This diversified and somewhat protean style focuses on the individual and is the opposite of system building; it can even include irrationalism. It is best explained by the themes to which it typically pays attention: alienation, anxiety, being, choice, conscience, death, despair, finitude, freedom, guilt, meaning, purpose, responsibility, and so on. These topics are treated in Yoga, and hence the label *existentialism* is appropriate enough. I have added "in practice" to the chapter's title for the simple reason that Yoga does not present itself as a philosophy and cannot be understood merely as such, even though it includes plenty of philosophical matter.

Suffering is called *duhkha* in Sanskrit. This word, which is found in the pre-Buddhist *Kaushītaki-Brāhmana-Upanishad* (for example, 2.10, 3.5–6), means literally "having a bad axle hole (*kha*)." A cart that does not have its axle well aligned within the wheels' axle holes, or hubs, is bound to wobble and give an uncomfortable ride. It is, therefore, desirable to ensure that axle and wheel are properly aligned, causing the mood of ease and happiness (called *sukha,* the antonym of *duhkha*). The widely used Sanskrit prefix *su* suggests "good/easeful/pleasant." The preceding quotation makes the point that when the body is connected with consciousness, it experiences joy or suffering.

In his 1930 book *Das Unbehagen in der Kultur* (*Civilization and Its Discontents*), Sigmund Freud laconically states:

> Life, as we find it, is too hard for us; it brings us too many pains, disappointments and impossible tasks. In order to bear it we cannot dispense with palliative measures: powerful deflections, which cause us to make light of intoxicating substances, which make us insensitive to it. Something of the kind is indispensable. (Freud 1961, 22)

Freud uses hyperbolic language to impress on us that life is indeed difficult, and like most of conventional society, he excuses our flight into intoxication. At the same time, he argues that we search for happiness but typically confound happiness with pleasure. Hence there is his notion of the "pleasure principle" that dominates the mind.

According to Freud, the universe is designed to frustrate our quest for happiness and to yield unhappiness more readily than happiness. While he admits that Yoga generates the "happiness of quietness," it does so by "killing off the instincts" (Freud 1961, 26). This opportune opinion about Yoga can be excused when we take into account the relative sparsity of good portrayals of Yoga in 1930, when Freud wrote this book. Today, however, we must note that Yoga does not proceed simply by neutralizing our innate reflexes. Besides, for Freud, the instincts were resolvable into the two basic instincts of *eros* and *thanatos,* which is problematical. Certainly the latter has come under consistent attack and is considered to belong to one of the shakier aspects of his theory. The various instinct theories themselves have declined in prominence, because they failed to provide an explanation for instinctual behavior.

The neurotic, claims Freud, is alienated from reality and incapable of enjoyment—this means 99 percent of us. Freud himself wrote, "Thus a healthy person, too, is virtually neurotic."

"Suffering," states the psychotherapist Robert Gerzon dryly in his popular book *Finding Serenity in the Age of Anxiety*, "is not highly respected today." He continues, "Much of our culture considers suffering the province of losers, something to be avoided, a punishment for making mistakes in life" (Gerzon 1997, 202). This negative attitude toward suffering is as prevalent as the fact that people commonly indulge in it. Gerzon regards suffering as a blessing, which "brings us deeper into our spiritual life." He reminds readers that "to suffer" comes from the Latin *sufferre* (or *subferre*), which translates as "to carry below," that is, to carry below the surface of life.

Suffering commonly stands for the dis-ease that arises from physical or emotional pain. We tend to undergo suffering whenever we encounter an unpleasant, disagreeable, difficult, disturbing, limiting, frustrating, or stressful experience. In his *Yoga-Sūtra* (2.15), Patanjali associates suffering with (1) the universal experience of change (*parināma*) in regard to the phenomenal world; (2) anguish (*tāpa*) in the face of loss; (3) the unconscious in the form of the subliminal activators (*samskāra*) that foster unenlightenment; and (4) the conflict (*virodha*) inherent in the very building blocks—*gunas*—of the phenomenal world, which are the principal factors behind all change. Thus, Patanjali's understanding of suffering and its experiential underpinning is rather philosophical and very broad. It captures, however, the basic sentiment of Yoga.

In the present context, then, I give the term *suffering* a special slant: that of a cognitive response to pain. In ordinary parlance, the phrase "pain and suffering" stands for "physical pain and emotional pain." But in the present sense, suffering involves the ego sense to whatever degree. In *The Meaning and End of Suffering for Freud and the Buddhist Tradition*, Gordon E. Pruett (1987, 11) remarks, "[T]he nature of suffering is not physiological but what we shall call, at least for the moment, psychological." Jon Kabat-Zinn, in his widely read book *Full Catastrophe Living*, seems to be saying the same thing:

Aversion to pain is really a misplaced aversion to suffering. Ordinarily we do not make a distinction between pain and suffering, but there are very important differences between them. Pain is a natural part of the experience of life. Suffering is one of many possible responses to pain.... It involves our thoughts and emotions and how they frame the meaning of our experiences.... Even a small pain can produce great suffering in us if we fear that it means we have a tumor or some other frightening condition. (Kabat-Zinn 1990, 285)

Suffering is an experience we humans share with some other higher animals. I say *some,* because one creature (say, a microbe) may just experience pain, while another (a dog, for instance) may experience both physical and emotional pain and perhaps even cognitive dis-ease. For example, a dog may start to shake from terror when expected to approach open water or some other situation that he or she perceives as potentially dangerous. Even within a species, there can be considerable variation from one individual to another. To the degree that a being has inwardness (a psyche), there is also suffering, or cognitive distress.

When it comes to humans, we inevitably encounter the question "Why me?" which epitomizes a cognitive response to a significant painful experience, whether physical or emotional, regardless of whether or not this question is consciously articulated. We want our suffering to be meaningful. This is a basic axiom of Victor Frankl's logotherapy, which he says is trifocal: "It focuses on three fundamental facts of human existence: there is a will to meaning; there is a meaning in suffering; and there is a freedom of will" (Frankl 1965, 126). In his book *The Unconscious God,* which was first published in German in 1948, Frankl makes this further remark (130–31): "Even in diehard positivists the wisdom of the heart may supersede the knowledge of the brain and allow for recognizing the unconditional meaningfulness of life through the potential meaning of suffering."

From a yogic perspective, *everything* is suffering, because the adept confronts existence with full awareness. What does this mean? Here is the Buddha's simple explanation, as given in the *Mahāsatipatthāna-Sūtra* (22.18) of the *Dīgha-Nikāya:*

> Birth is suffering, ageing is suffering, death is suffering, sorrow, lamentation, pain, sadness and distress are suffering. Being attached to the unloved is suffering, not getting what one wants is suffering. (Walsh 1987)

Unless we experience supernal joy, whatever experiences we may have are directly or indirectly connected with suffering. Even in moments of extreme pleasure, we may still mournfully compare our experience with someone whose pleasure is even greater, which then spoils our experience. The *Bhagavad-Gītā* (5.19), which is one of the early scriptures of Yoga, is clear: worldly experience/pleasure (*bhoga*), which is inevitably connected with an object (whether internal or external), is invariably a source of suffering (*duhkha*). This text also gives the antidote—namely, a mind that is not troubled by passion, fear, and anger. Basically the same message is furnished in stanzas 5.23 and 5.24. The latter contrasts "inner joy" with the fleeting pleasures we can find, especially outside ourselves. The inescapable fact that our life is finite, that any experience (however sublime) will end, makes a mockery out of joyous experiences.

For Patanjali, as for Gautama the Buddha, life is suffering, but he specifically states in his *Yoga-Sūtra* (2.15), "Everything is indeed suffering for the discerner" (*duhkham eva sarvam vivekinah*). The discerner is the person who is capable of distinguishing the Real from the unreal, the Self from the nonself, which occurs at various levels of acuity and competence. In his Sanskrit commentary on aphorism 2.16, Vyāsa likens the *vivekin* (the discerner) to an eyeball, which is hypersensitive; it has a painful reaction to even a speck of dust. In other words, the person who has trained him- or herself to keep a bead on the transcendental Self recognizes egoic stuff—self-centered emotions, impulses, motivations, and thoughts—as soon as it arises. By holding apart the Self (*purusha, ātman*) and the nonself (*anātman*), the Hindu Yoga adept moves forward into the freedom of Selfhood rather than the bondage of egoism. Thus, while ordinary, prejudicial discrimination is binding or limiting, yogic discernment is liberating.

The Sāmkhya tradition, with which Pātanjala-Yoga (or Classical Yoga) is closely allied, acknowledges three kinds of suffering: *ādhyātmika, ādhidaivika,* and *ādhibhautika,* that is, suffering derived from oneself, from subtle influences (such as deities or the stars), and from the material elements. In his book *Classical Sāmkhya,* Gerald James Larson (1969, 167) explains these three terms as "personal," "supernatural," and "external." What they suggest is that suffering can originate from within, from above, and from outside. This notion matches Patanjali's idea of the omnipresence of suffering in the conditional realms.

Jainism, which is slightly older than the earliest teachings of Buddhism but finalized its early scriptures in the Buddhist era, shares Buddhism's philosophy of suffering. It treats suffering as a fact of life but, unlike Buddhism and Hinduism, does not highlight *duhkha* doctrinally. Thus, in Hemacandra's twelfth-century scholastic summa titled *Yoga-Shāstra* (4.3), we have this straightforward statement:

Suffering, [which exists owing to] ignorance of the Self, is removed through Self-knowledge (*ātma-jnāna*). Without Self-knowledge, it is impossible to sever suffering even through [the most stringent] asceticism (*tapas*).

Suffering is a pivotal doctrinal issue in Buddhism, and in the *lam rim* (stages of the path) presentations of the way it is used as a platform for detailing the diverse transformative disciplines. In fact, one of the subtlest and most comprehensive appraisals of suffering can be found in Buddhism (which is a form of Yoga). This is indicated in the so-called four noble truths: (1) there is suffering; (2) there is a cause to suffering (nothing comes about ex nihilo); (3) there is potentially an end to suffering; and (4) there is a way to end suffering (by means of the Buddha's eightfold path).

Generally, eight types of suffering are distinguished as follows:

- The suffering of birth
- The suffering of old age
- The suffering of illness
- The suffering of death
- The suffering of encountering pleasant experiences
- The suffering of separation from pleasant experiences
- The suffering of not attaining one's desires
- The suffering inherent in the five aggregates, or "heaps" (*skandhas*)

The last type deserves further explanation. Scholastic or Abhidharma Buddhism categorizes existence into five basic, interdependent psychophysical phenomena: form/body (*rūpa*); sensation (*vedanā*); perception (*samjnā*); subliminal karmic impulses (*samskāra*); and consciousness (*vijnāna*). As the great Tibetan adept and scholar Je Tsongkhapa explains in his *Lam-Rim Chen-Mo* (Great Treatise on the Stages of the Path), these five aggregates are inextricably connected with suffering and hence ought not to be grasped (or fixated on):

- They are vessels of future suffering.
- They are vessels of suffering based on what exists at present.
- They are vessels of suffering pain.
- They are vessels of suffering change.
- They are vessels of suffering conditionality (limitation).

Only complete disenchantment with the conditional world—that is, deeply felt renunciation—can lead to enlightenment and thus to the end of suffering. Hinduism affirms this view as well. In the *Bhagavad-Gītā* (6.23), Krishna defines Yoga as one's "separation from the connection with suffering." Patanjali's *Yoga-Sūtra* (2.16) includes this statement as a single aphorism: "[That which is] to be overcome is suffering yet-to-come."

There can be no more optimistic attitude than the preceding scriptural affirmations. Therefore it makes little sense to characterize Yoga and Hinduism in general as representing a pessimistic outlook, as Albert Schweitzer did in various books.[1] He stereotyped Indian philosophy as life-negating and therefore unsuitable for Westerners. This tenuous opinion was, unfortunately, echoed in many philosophical, religious, scientific, and literary writings throughout the twentieth century. We should at long last put it to rest.

The universality of suffering is a fundamental insight that is shared by all spiritual traditions of India. The same holds true of the teaching about moral causation, which we discuss next.

THE "LAW" OF KARMA

Karma is the mysterious factor that links one lifetime to the next. This Sanskrit word stems from the verbal root *kri,* "to do"; thus, *karma* means literally "action." Most Indologists agree that the teaching of karma, which exists in one form or another in many parts of the world, made its first appearance in Indian literature in the ancient *Brihadāranyaka-Upanishad,* the earliest text of its genre. This Sanskrit scripture is usually placed in the period immediately preceding Buddhism—600 to 500 B.C.E.; some scholars, however, favor an earlier date.

The secret teaching about karma was disclosed by the prominent Upanishadic sage Yājnavalkya to a fellow brahmin named Jāratkārava Ārtabhāga (*Brihadāranyaka-Upanishad* 3.2.13). The two were discussing the postmortem destiny of people. When Ārtabhāga, who knew the basic Vedic teachings as well as Yājnavalkya did, asked specifically about what happens after death, the sage answered, "Ārtabhāga, dear, take my hand. We two alone shall know of this. This is not for us [to speak of] among people." After the two had left the village, Yājnavalkya felt free to disclose the teaching about karma. Basically, he told Ārtabhāga that "one becomes virtuous (*punya*) by virtuous deeds and evil (*pāpa*) by evil [deeds]." The Sanskrit words *punya* and *pāpa* can also be rendered in more contemporary terms as "good" and "bad" or "meritorious" and "demeritorious," respectively.

It appears that Yājnavalkya, who spoke authoritatively about the nature and realization of the Self (*ātman*), spoke with the same authority about karma. If he actually was an enlightened, or liberated, being as tradition presents him, he would have known of the karmic mechanism from personal experience. He would, in other words, have seen into the heart of things. This would make him perhaps the first Self-realizer, which is hard to imagine. Alternatively, we can see him as a realized adept standing in a long line of transmission whose initiates were bound by secrecy. He would have received the secret teaching of karma along with other teachings about Self-transcending discipline, which he could then have realized for himself. Reading the earliest Upanishads, one cannot avoid the impression that they were preceded by many generations of sages who were privy to all kinds of esoteric knowledge.[2] The Upanishadic passage in question states that the moral quality of one's actions determines the quality of one's being in the postmortem state. In his monograph *The Vedic Origins of Karma* (1989), Hermann W. Tull relates the doctrine of karma—implying moral causation—to the sacrificial culture of the era preceding the Upanishads, specifically to the relationship between ritual actions and their consequences for the sacrificing priest. Mistakes made in the ritual were thought to have unfortunate consequences for the performing priest, his family, and the larger society on whose behalf the ritual was conducted.

The karma doctrine applied this belief or actual observation to a much more comprehensive context: Our actions matter not only to ritual success or failure but to the nature of our being in the after-death state (that is, our experience of that state). Combined with the idea of rebirth, which Yājnavalkya also apparently first articulated, karma has implications for all of a person's future lifetimes. The idea implicit in this is that there is a karmic continuum between this life, the postmortem state, and the next life.

Karma is not inevitable destiny. As Christopher Chapple says in the preface of *Karma and Creativity*:

Because texts mentioning karma often state that actions of the past and present will carry over and influence actions of the future, some interpreters have seen only damning possibilities in this operation. However, the mechanics of karma can also be regarded as incentive to better oneself, to strive to create action in a purposeful fashion. (Chapple 1986, xi)

This is a very important point: karma as opportunity to improve one's short-term and long-term lot. This possibility, which makes nonsense of interpretations that look on the Indian wisdom traditions as pessimistic or fatalistic, provides the rationale for all Yoga: by controlling the mind, we improve its quality, and this in turn allows us to intervene in the otherwise automatic karmic process. Chapple also helpfully explains that suffering need not inevitably grind us down but can "prompt one to desire transcendence, to strive for enlightenment (*nirvāna*)" (2). In this way, karma and creativity (or human effort, *paurusheya*) stand in dynamic relationship to each other, which also explains the title of Chapple's book. He rightly states that "this doctrine of action is thoroughly benevolent and philanthropic" (91).

The *Yoga-Sūtra* (4.7), echoing the Buddha,[3] distinguishes four kinds of karma: white, black, mixed, and neither white nor black (applying to a *yogin*). At the simplest level, karma can be meritorious (*punya*) or demeritorious (*apunya*) depending on the volitional activity causing it. In other words, even meritorious activity has karmic consequences, although the egoic involvement is less—perhaps far less—than that in demeritorious activity. As meritorious karma accumulates, we have the possibility of transcending karma altogether through a limpid mind that flows into enlightenment. In aphorism (*sūtra*) 3.22, a distinction is made between karma that is acute (or approaching) and karma that is deferred. In Pātanjala-Yoga, we have a lengthy discussion about karma in Vyāsa's commentary on aphorism 2.13. He reviews a debate, current at his time, about whether a single karmic cause is responsible for one or more lives. He seeks to apply logic to this and other similar arguments. Vyāsa concludes that karma is "mysterious and not easily intelligible."

The important part of Classical Yoga's understanding of karma, which unquestionably derived its inspiration from Buddhism, is that the psychological carrier of karma is the mass of unconscious activators (*samskāra*) in the depth of the mind. Any volitional activity causes a corresponding activator. The karmic aggregation, or "deposit" (*āshaya*), hails from time immemorial, which is why only a fully enlightened being can comprehend the unbelievable complexity of this karmic web.

The teaching of karma is developed at considerable length in Jainism and Buddhism. I will examine the former tradition first. Here we find that the Jaina scriptures have a rather complex doctrine that is closely associated with Jainism's archaic ontology and cosmology, which we need to discuss in passing first. The Jaina philosophers distinguish three main categories of being: (1) sentient, immaterial beings; (2) insentient, material substances; and (3) things that belong to neither the first nor the second category. The first category comprises numberless entities (*jīva*), often called "souls," who consist in pure Consciousness/Awareness. The second category, called *ajīva*, is composed of matter (*pudgala*) that is made up of atoms (*paramāṇu*) that have qualities perceivable by the senses. The last category consists of space, movement, rest, and time.

The most important aspect of existence is the multitude of sentient beings, or souls, who occupy a body of a certain size and have three primary characteristics: consciousness (*caitanya*), joy (*sukha*), and vitality or energy (*vīrya*). These are unlimited in the enlightened state. Embodiment, however, exercises a limiting influence on these characteristics. You could say that embodiment is a karmic condition. The soul, which is inherently formless, is coextensive with a given body that obscures its transcendental properties. We can easily appreciate that, in comparison with a human being, a microorganism has a low degree of consciousness (or sensitivity) that allows it just enough sensitivity to maneuver in its environment but not to explore the solar system by means of telescopes or spaceships. We can probably also agree that a bottlenose dolphin has a consciousness that surpasses that of a grasshopper or a rat.

How the living being is experienced (by oneself and others) depends on the impact of karma, which the Jainas understand as a subtle form of matter rather than some intangible psychological factor. Karma, as subtle matter, floats in space like dust and is ingested by the living beings, or souls. This occurs as a result of their volitional activity, which represents a specific vibrational quality. Everyone vibrates according to the quality of energy manifested in him or her—a thought that will thrill New Agers. This causes the "influx" (*āsrava*) of karmic "matter." That is to say, we attract that with which we resonate. This universal karmic dust can stick to a living being only when it is "moist" with the "taints," or passions (*kashāya*) of attraction (*rāga*) and repulsion (*dvesha*). Attraction comprises anger (*krodha*) and pride (*māna*), while repulsion is made up of deceit (*māyā*) and greed (*lobha*). Karma cannot find a foothold in someone who is "dry," that is, free from passion (*vītarāga*[4]), which is only the case with a liberated being.

The dual passions keep the karmic process in motion. When karma has fructified, it drops off again, which is known as *nirjarā* ("exhaustion"), thus becoming available once again for further use by the same or some other living being. This is an ongoing process, which is beginningless and endless. Since living beings, or souls, are immaterial and only their body belongs to the material realm, there can be no actual physical contact between them and subtle karmic matter. This relationship is analogous to the correlation (*samyoga*) between the transcendental Self (*purusha*) and the cosmic existence as a whole (*prakriti*) that is assumed in Patanjali's Yoga.

Jaina philosophy makes a careful distinction between the following:

- Four "destructive" karmas that give rise to false view and wrong behavior due to the involvement of the passions and subsidiary passions (like sexual pleasure, fear, disgust, and so on)
- Karmas that obstruct knowledge
- Karmas that restrict perception
- Karmas that limit energy
- Four "nondestructive" karmas that affect feeling (whether pleasant or unpleasant), individuation as a particular being, life span, and genetic environment (*gotra,* or "clan")

Jaina scholastics elaborated on this to the point where they had up to 148 kinds of karma. All of these types must be removed in the course of the fourteen-step path to enlightenment, so that enlightenment—often spoken of as "omniscience"—can occur. Jainism does, however, teach that some souls are constitutionally unfit and will never attain it, which is why the karmic process can be considered endless.

Cosmologically, the universe (*loka*) is conceived as a vast, three-dimensional structure comprising various levels of existence (such as seven hell realms, the human world, and sixteen heavenly realms, as well as the abode of the perfected adepts at the top). This is surrounded by negative space (*aloka*) in which nothing exists.

If we find Jainism's materialistic version of karma unappealing (and it is, indeed, an archaic feature), we can always interpret it along psychological lines. This problem does not exist in Buddhism, which has a fairly sophisticated understanding of the karmic process, to which we turn next.

The Buddhist doctrine of karma can be properly understood only in relation to the teaching of dependent origination (*pratītya-samutpāda*): All things are interdependent and have no unique essence (*ātman*). For instance, by "wagon wheel," we mean a rim with spokes fixed to a hub through which an axle passes in order to locomote a vehicle. By extension, the wheel would not exist without a wheelwright, and he would not exist without his helpful family; they would not exist without the farmer, baker, tailor, shoemaker, and so on. Buddhists would analyze the concepts of "rim," "spoke," and "hub" in a similar manner. In the final analysis, everything is connected to everything else—a message that has become more meaningful in modern times thanks to the new discipline of ecology. Are things, then, mere names? Is Buddhism a form of nominalism? There is no simple answer to this question, because in the course of its long history, Buddhism evolved many divergent schools and explanations.

Perhaps the most sophisticated answer was given in the fourteenth century by Je Tsongkhapa, who sought to do justice to the Middle Path perspective of the Buddha without succumbing to the Madhyamika school's tendency to show the absurdity of all teachings (in terms of either essentialist or nihilist positions) without espousing a thesis of its own on one hand or to the kind of idealism that marks the Buddhist schools of Vijñānavāda and Cittamātra, which resemble Hindu Vedānta, on the other hand. He argued that dependent origination and the emptiness (or absence) of intrinsic existence in Mahāyāna coexist; that is to say, there are two ways of apprehending the same thing. Thus, while the Madhyamika position of, say, Nāgārjuna rightly applies the teaching of dependent origination, it must not be overinterpreted by denying the reality of phenomena.[5]

In contrast to his Hindu contemporaries, the Buddha refused to speculate about a transcendental Reality and unknowable facts in general. He was a pragmatist who was interested chiefly in the most expedient way of ending suffering. Like the Jainas, the Buddhist monk-scholars devoted considerable attention to the concept of karma. We need not concern ourselves with their speculations here, except to say that the Abhidharma (Pāli: Abhidamma) teachings make the following distinction: of the twenty-nine types of consciousness recognized in Buddhist scholasticism, every one produces karma. Just as an object in daylight has a shadow, so every volitional activity is inevitably karmic. Only a buddha (a fully enlightened being who has the function of bringing the liberative teaching into the world) or an arhat (an enlightened being who does not have a major teaching function) produces no karma when engaging in action, because there is no "I" that could give rise to volition. The emphasis on *volition* as the karmic culprit is the key.

At the same time, not all occurrences in the present life necessarily have a karmic cause, as the Buddha himself admitted in his dialogue with the wanderer Moliya-Sīvaka.[6] It is one thing to interpret (or, rather, overinterpret) a painful or unpleasant happening in one's own life as the result of karma and another to do the same in regard to other beings. In the former instance, the explanation, even if wholly wrong, can serve to generate an attitude of bravery in the face of pain or unpleasantness such as mistreatment; in the latter instance, there is the possibility of the explanation merely excusing an attitude of moral indifference or superiority.

According to Buddhist scholasticism, karma can be (1) heavy or "weighty," such as murder; (2) "death proximate," due to an intention or aspiration at one's last hour; (3) habitual, the most common type; and (4) residual, meaning karma that is not covered by the other three types. Karma inevitably leads to a corresponding moral consequence, which is known as *vipāka* (ripening) or *phala* (fruition). In early Buddhism, the relationship between karma and its fruition was understood in a literal sense. Later on, the monk-scholars accepted a more symbolic/psychological link. This allows for the fact that we do not inevitably deserve what we get; shockingly, we can get less or more. By understanding the karmic process primarily as a mental one, we can avoid odious literalism. This understanding also affirms that the personality is not a fixed thing but adaptable, so a spiritually mature person may not experience the same consequences that an ordinary person might incur from the same karma.[7]

In his conclusions to *The Varieties of Religious Experience,* the archpragmatist William James stated that he agrees in principle with the doctrine of karma. In the next paragraph, he admits,

> I state the matter [about karma] thus bluntly, because the current of thought in academic circles runs against me, and I feel like a man who must set his back against an open door quickly if he does not wish to see it closed and locked. In spite of its being so shocking to the reigning intellectual tastes, I believe that a candid consideration of piecemeal supernaturalism and a complete discussion of all its metaphysical bearings will show it to be the hypothesis by which the largest number of legitimate requirements are met. (James 1961, 405)

While the intellectual climate of opinion is perhaps no longer quite as anxiously conservative as it was in James's time, his comment is not entirely out of place today.

PUNARJANMAN

Cyclic existence (*samsāra*) can be defined as the inevitability of an unenlightened, individuated being undergoing continuous "recycling," or rebirth.

This is understood differently in Hinduism/Jainism and Buddhism. Their views stand in sharp contrast to mainstream Christianity, which teaches that a person has but one chance at heaven, and if he or she fails to attain it, that person faces the terrifying prospect of eternal damnation.

Before I discuss the two former cultures, I want to quote from one of the American-Czech psychiatrist Stanislav Grof's books:

> We can now summarize the objective evidence that forms the basis of the widespread "belief" in reincarnation and karma. The term *belief* is actually inappropriate when applied to this area. Properly understood, it is a theoretical system of thought, a conceptual framework that is trying to provide explanation for a large number of unusual experiences and observations. (Grof 1993, 177)

As with all theories, this one is also frail. As Grof (1993, 183) admits, "Neither a categorical denial of the possibility of reincarnation, nor the belief in its objective existence are true in an absolute sense."

We could say that reincarnation holds true for us as long as we are subject to *samsāra* (the world of change) but not when we realize that we are the ultimate Reality.

In Hinduism, the idea of rebirth made its first definite appearance simultaneously with the idea of karma in the *Brihadāranyaka-Upanishad* (3.2.13). Here, the sage Yājnavalkya explains that when a person's body drops away at death—the eye goes to the sun, the ear to the cardinal directions, and so on—karma remains and is responsible for the next embodiment. What this means is explained in two subsequent passages (4.3.36; 4.1–4.5). The second passage will be explored in conjunction with my discussion of the death process, but here is my rendering of the first passage:

> This [body] becomes frail, whether one grows frail from old age or disease. Just as a mango or a fig or a peepal fruit detaches itself from its stalk, even so this person releases himself from these limbs and rushes along the same path and through the same opening (*yoni*) to return once again to a [new] life.

To paraphrase this passage, in death, the "person" (*purusha*) withdraws from the slowly disintegrating body, but who is that person? In his commentary, the great Vedānta teacher Shankara understands *purusha* as the Self.

But since the Self is transcendental, it cannot truly be an agent within the phenomenal world, and we must therefore assume that the surviving part is a subtle form of the living being (*jīva*), that is, of the mind. The karmic seeds are contained within that residual mind and then attract, or are drawn to, the next body in the womb of a woman, starting out as an ovum and then growing into an embryo, fetus, neonate, infant, adolescent, and adult.

The popular belief that this rebirth process somehow occurs to the same individual is clearly not the case. Nothing with a sense of identity travels, or transmigrates, from one body to another. The transcendental Self merely becomes seemingly and temporarily associated with successive bodies. It is the same in all beings and is present as the perennial backdrop of all rebirths. We can, however, speak of a certain (mental) continuum that extends from one lifetime to the next. Apart from the idea of a permanent transcendental Self in the background, the Hindu notion of rebirth is rather close to its Buddhist counterpart.

Since Buddhism does not accept that there is an ultimate essence (*ātman*) of anything, it also does not accept that an individuated being is reborn in the conventional sense. Rather, the factors constituting one being give rise to related factors, eventually including the sense of individuality.

Strictly speaking, what links one rebirth to another are the unconscious activators (*samskāra*) giving rise to corresponding mental complexes. In the early scriptures of the Pāli canon (see, for example, *Majjhīma-Nikāya* 1.265–266), there is mention of a *gandhabba* (Skt.: *gandharva*), or an odor (*gandha*)-consuming spirit-entity that is in proximity during coitus (though not necessarily observing the act). When the conditions are right, this entity descends into the womb to assume a new life. Later accounts speak of the rebirth process in terms of the cluster of personality factors called *skandhas*. These are: (1) body (*rūpa*, literally "form"); (2) sensation (*vedanā*), or sense impression; (3) perception (*samjnā*), which is a sense impression when interpreted by the brain; (4) intention (*samskāra*), which can be an idea, sentiment, intention, and so on; and (5) consciousness (*vijnāna*), which is consciousness dependent on an object (be it coarse or subtle). It is the last factor that survives after death and triggers the next life (or rebirth). From the perspective of the reborn, we could argue that *vijnāna*'s object is the embryo.

We can understand this as the factors *aaabbbcccddd* giving rise to *aaabb-bccddde,* which in turn give rise to *aaabbccddddee* and so on. Because there is a certain mental continuum (without an accompanying sense of conscious identity, or ego), it is possible—according to the Tibetan Buddhist tradition—to determine whether a person is a *tulku* or not. A *tulku* is the consciously engineered rebirth by a highly evolved adept (lama). This engineering is thought to be made possible by the peculiar mind of an advanced adept who has consciously navigated the death process and entered the after-death state with the subtle mind intact.

The formal identification of a *tulku* (Tib.; pron. *sprul.sku*) is not accomplished by purely intellectual means; rather, advanced practitioners use their extended set of paranormal abilities to look into the assumed *tulku*'s past to detect the postmortem trajectory between one rebirth and another. Only a fully enlightened being, or buddha, is said to be able to see all rebirths, at least in theory. Gautama the Buddha, the founder of historical Buddhism, is remembered to have seen his former lives over a period of ninty-one *kalpas* (or eons). A similar claim is made of some Hindu Yoga masters in the *Mahābharata*.[8] A *kalpa* is a day and night in the life of Brahma, whose total life span of one hundred cosmic eons is estimated to be 311.04 trillion years. The Buddha wisely did not give any figure but came up with this beautiful simile: Imagine a huge rock and you use soft cloth to strike it every day. The cloth will be shredded long before the *kalpa* comes to an end.

At the end of a *yuga,* the material cosmos collapses until the next cosmic day, when it arises again. At the end of a *mahā-yuga,* or great eon, the multidimensional world—with all the subtle levels—vanishes along with the creator-deity Brahma. After an interval of latency, the world, Brahma, and all nonliberated beings come into existence once more. What a remarkable, breathtaking vision!

A gifted clairvoyant, such as Edgar Cayce (1877–1945), allegedly can relate one's present life to its precursor on the basis of the karmic connections he or she is able to see. The possibility of this is guaranteed by the fact that, as the *Yoga-Sūtra* (4.8) explains, no one experiences the ripening of someone else's karma.[9] In the West, it has become popular to regress people under hypnosis back to the time before their present birth. Interesting stories often emerge, but these are liable to be mere fantasies of the hypnotized, perhaps under the suggestive influence of the hypnotist when he or she is not careful enough. Traditionally, it is understood that only an advanced adept can sift the wheat from the chaff in such matters.

According to the wisdom traditions of India, rebirth can take place in all conceivable realms, but Westerners often find the idea of being reborn as an animal or other nonhuman creature abhorrent. When we understand that at death, most of the mental faculties that we hold dear are dismantled and only the karmic propensities survive along with whatever subtle "vehicle" is required in the postmortem state, rebirth in nonhuman bodies is perhaps easier to imagine.

Kyabje Pabongka Rinpoche, a great Tibetan master of the twentieth century, gave an inspiring twenty-four-day teaching in 1921 that was attended by some seven hundred monastics and laypeople. Early on in his first talk, he said pointedly,

> As long as we remain uncritical, we will never suspect that we might be going to the lower realms [such as the animal realm].... The trouble is we have not looked into things properly. We should think it over in detail, then we would see that we are not free to choose whether we go to the lower realms or not. This is determined by our karma. We have a mixture of virtuous and non-virtuous karma in our mental streams. The stronger of these two will be triggered by craving and cling when we die. When we look into which of these two is the stronger in our mental streams, we will see it is non-virtue. (Pabongka 1991, 28)

Realizing that the topic of karma and rebirth tends to evoke strong emotional reactions either for or against, I will leave the discussion here and merely refer open-minded readers to Ian Stevenson's multivolume series of investigative empirical studies of so-called reincarnation cases that are scattered throughout the world. By no means do all of them have probative value, but some are nonetheless remarkable. There are also the many cases of Tibetan *tulkus* who, as advanced practitioners, are unlikely to be subject to self-delusion or plain lying. The same could be said of the Buddha himself. Any in-depth consideration of the psychology of Yoga needs to take these matters into account.

While the concept of suffering undeniably has its place in modern psychology, notably in the various psychotherapeutic approaches, karma and rebirth do not. They are generally rejected as mere religious or metaphysical beliefs that have no place in "scientific" investigation. Even though traditional Yoga can be, and at times has been, practiced without reference to these twin notions, it makes more sense to regard them as bona fide axioms. Few scientists are willing to accept this, however, because they presume there is no empirical evidence to support it and because they think this would open the door to other "irrational" beliefs. But these so-called beliefs need not be dismissed as irrational. In any case, a scientist could accept them as working hypotheses without forfeiting the scientific method. For a phenomenologist, they are happenings to be investigated rather than prejudged. In this connection, the following observation by Sri Aurobindo is pertinent:

> Even men who consider vigilance against error an intellectual or a practical duty are yet content with the most careless stumbling when they get upon higher and more difficult ground. Where precision and subtle thinking are most needed, there they are most impatient of it and averse to the labour demanded of them.... It is not surprising then that men should be content to think crudely about such a matter as rebirth. (Aurobindo 1991, 13)

One final point I wish to broach here concerns the modern objection to rebirth on mathematical grounds. It is sometimes argued that not enough people have existed in the past to account for today's rate of rebirthing humans. This objection does not take into account the argument that, according to Indian traditions, humans can take rebirth from beings of other realms (such as the animal kingdom). It also does not consider that beings could come from other planetary systems.

CHAPTER 3

Psychocosmological Matters

> Know then thyself! Presume not God to scan!
> The proper study of mankind is man.
>
> —ALEXANDER POPE (Cary 2006, 225–26)

As the neologism *psychocosmology* suggests, cosmology has psychological implications and psychology is relevant to cosmology. Here I will explore this relevance according to Sāmkhya, whose ontology underlies the classical branch schools of Yoga.

CLASSICAL YOGA AND CLASSICAL SĀMKHYA

We cannot understand the psychology of Yoga without having a clear idea about the ontology (science of being) given preference in some of the most preeminent branches and schools of Yoga. This ontological teaching is closely allied with Yoga's sister tradition, namely Sāmkhya.

Classical Sāmkhya, as articulated in Īshvara Krishna's *Sāmkhya-Kārikā* in about 400 C.E., postulates two ultimate principles: (1) the beginningless, eternal, and immutable transcendental Self (*purusha*) of karma-free, pure Consciousness/Awareness; and (2) the beginningless, ever-self-modifying, karma-driven Cosmos (*prakriti*) that lacks pure Consciousness/Awareness but includes the multilayered mind. Kashmiri Shaivism, the Shaiva Siddhānta system of South India, and Hindu Tantra all adopted the basic ontological schema of Sāmkhya but expanded it to include more principles (*tattvas*), integrating this innovative framework with the metaphysics of either nondualism or dualism.

Classical Sāmkhya differentiates twenty-four psychocosmic principles that are contrasted against primordial Consciousness/Awareness, the twenty-fifth principle of this system. The twenty-four *tattvas* that make up the scaffolding of *prakriti* are as follows:

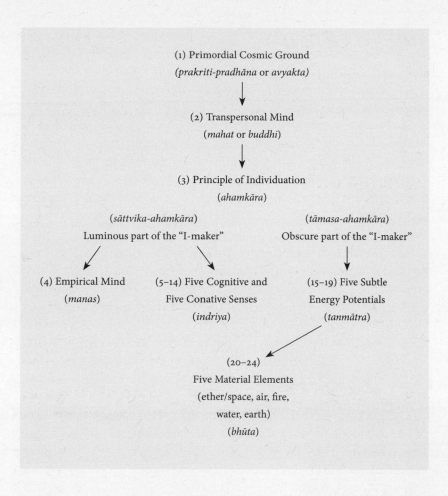

(1) Primordial Cosmic Ground
(*prakriti-pradhāna* or *avyakta*)

(2) Transpersonal Mind
(*mahat* or *buddhi*)

(3) Principle of Individuation
(*ahamkāra*)

(*sāttvika-ahamkāra*)
Luminous part of the "I-maker"

(*tāmasa-ahamkāra*)
Obscure part of the "I-maker"

(4) Empirical Mind
(*manas*)

(5–14) Five Cognitive and
Five Conative Senses
(*indriya*)

(15–19) Five Subtle
Energy Potentials
(*tanmātra*)

(20–24)
Five Material Elements
(ether/space, air, fire,
water, earth)
(*bhūta*)

Other similar models are proffered in various schools of thought. Sometimes, the ten senses are conceived as emerging out of the empirical mind. Basically, however, the various models are extremely similar to each other. One model, which is prominent in Kashmir and South India, has thirty-six *tattvas*. Following is the thirty-six-principle version. The first twelve principles belong entirely to the ultimate Reality, or Godhead, and hence they are marked with *T* for "transcendence."

Perhaps the most confusing part of this schema concerns the presence of "illusion" within the ultimate Reality. But for anything to be complete, it must contain its own antithesis. The inclusion of *māyā* in the ultimate Reality in principle allows for the effective concealment of the real nature of Reality at the finite level. It is at the finite, or empirical, level that we understand things only partially (*kalā*), have only limited knowledge (*vidyā*), have our attachment (*rāga*) to the finite rather than the Infinite, are subject to linear time (*kāla*) and to destiny or karma (*niyati*).

The Sāmkhya thinkers came up with a battery of reasons for the preceding frameworks. In the present context, I do not discuss these and other similar philosophical matters relating to Sāmkhya but confine myself to their psychological relevance. Sāmkhya philosophy has been ably mapped out by Gerald J. Larson (1969) in his excellent monograph *Classical Sāmkhya*. There is also the outstanding anthology edited by Gerald Larson and Ram Shankar Bhattacharya (1987) that covers the entire developmental history of the Sāmkhya tradition and pays exhaustive attention to its classical form.

Each category of existence modifies itself to give rise to the next category in hierarchical order just by recombination of the *gunas,* or "qualities." The *gunas*—which are of three types (*sattva, rajas,* and *tamas*)—are the ultimate building blocks of the cosmos. This evolutionary model starts with the unmanifest ground of the world, goes through what can be called the "higher mind" (*buddhi*) and the principle of individuation, and then bifurcates into a psychological and cosmological line. The former terminates in the senses; the latter, in the material elements. These two lines are obviously uniquely correlated so that sensory perception of the material world is made possible.

The Sāmkhya- and Sāmkhya-derived ontologies are neither purely rationalist schemas, as some scholars maintain, nor purely a creation of yogic imagination or (more benevolently) of yogic or paranormal perception, as others postulate. Perhaps they are best seen as rationally constructed schemas that have been enriched by what is called "yogic perception" (*yogi-pratyaksha*), which is one of the paranormal capacities of Yoga.

The purpose of each and every one of the ontological principles, or categories, is to provide a road map for the spiritual practitioner on his or her inward journey to liberation. This inner pilgrimage is rendered possible only by traversing the diverse realms, or levels of existence, that make up the phenomenal world (*samsāra*). If the ontological schemas were utterly useless, they would have been abandoned long ago by *yogins,* who are experientially minded.

Beyond the material level, then, there are many subtle or psychic levels, because the psyche or mind is considered an integral part of existence as a whole in all these ontological schemas. What this effectively means is that the mind, which is proportionally the "larger" aspect of the insentient

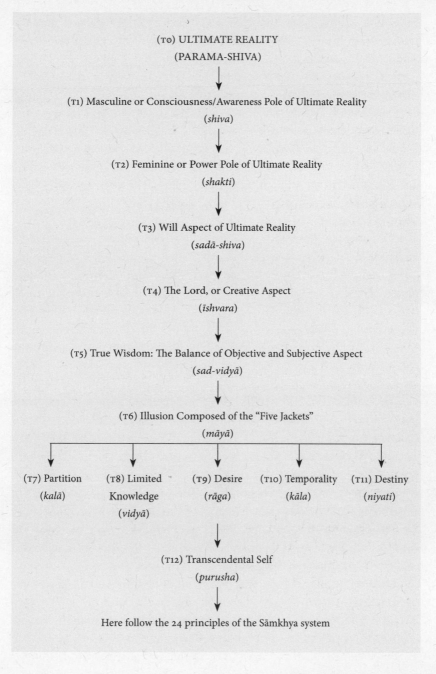

(T0) ULTIMATE REALITY

(PARAMA-SHIVA)

(T1) Masculine or Consciousness/Awareness Pole of Ultimate Reality

(*shiva*)

(T2) Feminine or Power Pole of Ultimate Reality

(*shakti*)

(T3) Will Aspect of Ultimate Reality

(*sadā-shiva*)

(T4) The Lord, or Creative Aspect

(*īshvara*)

(T5) True Wisdom: The Balance of Objective and Subjective Aspect

(*sad-vidyā*)

(T6) Illusion Composed of the "Five Jackets"

(*māyā*)

(T7) Partition	(T8) Limited	(T9) Desire	(T10) Temporality	(T11) Destiny
(*kalā*)	Knowledge	(*rāga*)	(*kāla*)	(*niyati*)
	(*vidyā*)			

(T12) Transcendental Self

(*purusha*)

Here follow the 24 principles of the Sāmkhya system

Cosmos (*prakriti*), is actually a "material" structure in the sense that it is distinct from immaterial primordial Consciousness/Awareness (*cit*). Here our language is evidently too limiting, and it makes more sense to talk about "subtle" (*sūkshma*) and "coarse" (*sthūla*) features of cosmic existence.

Sāmkhya and Sāmkhya-dependent philosophies understand the spectrum of ontological levels as hierarchically nested structures. They represent aspects of the mind as well as their respective "environments." To distinguish them from the material world, these inner levels are called subtle and coarse.

What all ontological structures have in common is that they are constituted, in different proportions, of three primary qualities called *gunas*. This transempirical triad is made up of *sattva* (the factor of lucidity or lightness), *rajas* (the factor of dynamism), and *tamas* (the factor of obscurity or heaviness). In his early essay on Yoga psychology, published in his book *Philosophical Essays,* the renowned historian of Indian philosophy S. N. Dasgupta (1990, 181) explains these factors as "intelligence-stuff," "energy-stuff," and "mass-stuff," respectively. In other words, similar to modern notions, the mind is material, and there would be no objection from Sāmkhya to the idea that mental processes are neurological.

It is probably best to understand these qualities in the broad sense as phenotypes. Only in the sixteenth century did the Yoga-oriented Vedānta authority Vijnāna Bhikshu propose an "atomistic" explanation, namely that innumerable *gunas* underlie everything, including the material atoms (*anu*) and the mind (*manas*). But this raises more questions than it solves. The perceptible difference between phenomena is due to the proportion in which these three *guna* types are present in each thing. Thus, the mind has a predominance of *sattva* in it, while the body is preeminently composed of *tamas* with just a little *rajas* and *tamas*. The presence of all three *gunas* in any given phenomenon is essential, and one could say that if all three were not present, nothing could exist. We have a parallel in the material world at the atomic level where, according to one model, an atom is made up of a core of protons and neutrons, with electrons swirling around that nucleus. Of course, in modern terms, the *gunas* would be irreducible "subsubsubatomic" reals. At their unmanifest level, the *gunas* could be compared to the physicist's quantum foam or quantum soup, which is thought to be the ultimate substratum of everything in manifestation.

Yoga can be understood as a voluntary process for which I have elsewhere coined the expression "sattvification,"[1] that is, the progressive refinement of one's being by increasing the high-octane *sattva* content of the mind. As the

Yoga-Sūtra (3.55) states, "When the [mind's] *sattva* [attains] equal purity with the Self, 'aloneness' [is established]." As I will discuss in chapter 15, this is one of Patanjali's two definitions of the state of liberation.

In Jainism, we find an ontological schema comparable to but quite distinct from the Sāmkhya system. Like Patanjali, the Jaina philosophers subscribe to a sharp dualism between sentient beings (*jīva*) and insentient matter (*pudgala*). The sentient beings can be either (1) bound, or obscured by karmic matter, to cyclic existence (*samsāra*) or (2) free from it and thereby experiencing the *jīva's* innate consciousness, bliss, and energy. In addition, Jainism acknowledges the existence of a third ontological category that comprises four insentient but formless "substances" (*dravya*)—space, time, the quality of motion, and the quality of immobility. None of these conceptual structures are easy to comprehend. The last two substances are particularly difficult to grasp; they are understood as the efficient causes of movement and immobility, respectively. All kinds of logical difficulties are associated with these three ontological categories, but this is not our problem or our field of investigation here.

Buddhism differs markedly from the ontologies of both Hinduism and Jainism. Historically, it rejected this kind of naive philosophizing, preferring the notion of process in the form of the doctrine of dependent origination. Sāmkhya came under heavy criticism at the hands of Buddhist philosophers, especially subsequent to Nāgārjuna (second century C.E.) who, like Kant fifteen hundred years later, sought to refute the idea that the mind can know Reality as it is in itself.

Nāgārjuna's apophatic (or negative) method did not take firm root in all branches of Buddhism. Thus, the Yogācāra branch of Mahāyāna Buddhism, founded by Asanga (fourth century C.E.), reformulated the idealism found in the early Mahāyāna scriptures. Similar to the later school of the *Yoga-Vāsishtha*, Asanga affirmed that everything in existence is "mind only" (*citta-mātra*). Thus, the world is a true phantom; mind perceives only mind, and the objects of the world do not exist per se. Neither does the cognitive subject. When obscured, the Ultimate (*nishpanna*), which is empty (*shūnya*), appears either as the "storehouse consciousness" (*ālaya-vijnāna*) or as the empirical consciousness (*pravritti-vijnāna*) that is further differentiated into the mind consciousness (*mano-vijnāna*). The storehouse consciousness, which has often been equated with the Western concept of the unconscious, contains all the karmic seeds in the form of "traits" (*vāsanā*). I will discuss this further in chapter 8.

In regard to *nishpanna*, Hans Wolfgang Schumann (1973, 152) states, "As the Absolute, as being in itself and immutable, it is often compared to the ocean." Yet this image gives Mind a substantiality that it does not possess. On a different note, Sangharakshita remarked in his brilliant *Survey of Buddhism* (1980, 265n1), "It is a great mistake to describe the Yogācāra as Subjective Idealism when it explicitly declares the subject to be an illusion." We can realize the Ultimate, or Absolute Mind, by turning away (*parāvritti*) from mentation.

Asanga's younger brother, Vasubandhu, created the closely related system of Vijñānavāda, which I will not discuss separately. The idealist position within Buddhism, as articulated in the Mahāyana Sutras, in the schools of Yogācāra, and Vijñānavāda, is criticized in the *Yoga-Sūtra* (4.16). Without a doubt, Patanjali espoused a realist philosophy affirming two ontological realities—*purusha* on the one hand and *prakriti* with its multiple products, or emergents, on the other. Since Vyāsa, the fifth-century author of the *Yoga-Bhāshya* commentary, based his observations on an intact version of the *Yoga-Sūtra*, we may assume that Patanjali's criticism referred to an earlier idealist school, unless we speculate that the Yogācāra masters and also Patanjali lived in the early fourth century C.E. Patanjali is, however, usually assigned to the second century and earlier, while the original Yogācāra preceptors lived in the third century C.E. (see Sangharakshita 1980, 354).

CHAPTER 4

Of Paradigms, Models, and Participatory Reality

> Concepts, hypotheses, and theories are
> not eternally valid—they are fallible.
>
> —ERVIN LASZLO (2007, 14)

What is Reality, or Truth? Kant, like the towering Buddhist philosopher Nāgārjuna before him, thought that we could never *know* Reality. The Kantian "thing in itself" is beyond the pale of the senses and the mind. Many Hindu scriptures give us a similar message. Thus, we can read in the *Brihadāranyaka-Upanishad* (4.4.22):

> This Self is neither this nor that (*neti neti*). It is ungraspable, for it cannot be grasped. It is undecaying, for it does not decay. It is unattached, for it does not attach itself. It is unfettered, for it does not tremble and is not injured.

The *Kena-Upanishad* (1.3), which belongs to the early post-Buddhist era, pronounces thus: "It cannot be reached through speech, not by the mind, and not by the eye."

For Buddhism, there is not just one ultimate Thing but a process of interlocking "things" that disappear as individual things as soon as we begin to analyze them. Because of this, Buddhism has often been compared to the late Ludwig Wittgenstein, but on closer inspection, the two are apparently incompatible.

Despite all these caveats, the philosophical literature of both Hinduism/Jainism and Buddhism is replete with statements that offer conventional descriptions of the Ultimate. These pronouncements are to be understood as concessions to the ordinary mind that clings to something concrete or tangible. Buddhism has perhaps been more consistently apophatic (descriptively negative) than other traditions, but even here we see occasional references to *nirvāna* as indicative of "an unborn, an unbecome, an unmade, an uncompounded" (*Udāna* 8.3).

We must bear the most advanced understanding of each tradition in mind so as not to be misled by conventional accounts. In a similar vein, if we were to interpret the Christian concepts of heaven and hell literally, we would succumb to fundamentalism, which is a parochial orientation that has no anchor in reality.

Modern psychology is guilty of a similar laxity when major concepts are reified and a given theory or model is treated as Reality itself. In this regard, systems theory, which is more process-oriented, recommends itself. Similarly, Henryk Skolimowski's participatory model could prove useful in steering clear of reification.

PARADIGM

This brings me to the notion of paradigm. In science, this term generally stands for the dominant way of seeing things, which shapes theorizing and research. This has been true ever since Thomas S. Kuhn's epochal work *The Structure of Scientific Revolutions*. The concept of paradigm suggests that even supposedly value-neutral science proceeds in ways that are governed by the interests of what is accepted as "normal" science. But as Kuhn (1962, 5) pointed out, normal science "often suppresses fundamental novelties because they are necessarily subversive of its basic commitments." We can think of Copernicus, Isaac Newton, Charles Darwin, Max Planck, and Albert Einstein as innovators or paradigm shifters whose findings were at first resisted and rejected, if not ridiculed. The scientific community has a strong commitment to keeping the reigning paradigm on the throne. Thus, so-called anomalies pile up and increasingly demand an explanation. More than a century ago, William James offered this graphic description:

> Round about the accredited and orderly facts of every science there ever floats a sort of dust-cloud of exceptional observations, of occurrences minute and irregular and seldom met with, which it always proves more easy to ignore than to attend to. The ideal of every science is that of a closed and completed system of truth.... No alternative, whether to whole or parts, can any longer be conceived as possible. Phenomena unclassifiable within

the system are therefore paradoxical absurdities, and must be held untrue. (James 1909)[1]

These "paradoxical absurdities," or anomalies, ultimately lead to the overthrow of the prevailing scientific paradigm and the establishment of a new paradigm with its favored theories and models. This is a brief and simplistic description of Kuhn's sociological ideas, which have been ably critiqued and extended, for instance, by the learned contributors to the anthology *Criticism and the Growth of Knowledge* (1970), edited by Imre Lakatos and Alan Musgrave. The most striking example of a scientific paradigm is Newtonianism, which is applied in most scientific disciplines. The most prominent exceptions are quantum physics and parapsychology, which can be considered heralds of a likely new paradigm. In our own time, these two disciplines offer the greatest and most serious challenge to the Newtonian paradigm.

MODELS AND REALITY

A scientific model is a conceptual representation of reality, which is as close to the actual situation as science can make it. Many models form a system, which is also a close-to-reality approximation, and many systems may be subsumed under a paradigm. Sometimes scientists forget that their models, systems, and adopted paradigm are only conceptual approximations, and they defend these artifacts as if they were reality itself. For example, a physicist might insist that unless parapsychological research follows the rules and models of physics, it can never yield anything but invalid findings. A parapsychologist, in turn, might insist that only quantum theory or something like it is equipped to understand his field of investigation. A Buddhist, struck by the processual nature of existence, may insist on dismissing ontological systems like that of Sāmkhya. A Sāmkhya philosopher may insist on dismissing Buddhism because he denies that the postulated momentary nature of things can adequately explain the observed continuity of existence. And so on.

Most commonly, scientists and thinkers accept the idea, which originated with Aristotle, that truth *corresponds* to reality. As the Polish philosopher Henryk Skolimowski noted in his book *The Participatory Mind* (Skolimowski 1994, 199), this notion of "objective" truth entails several presuppositions that are not normally stated. One of them is that objective reality is necessarily unchanging or static and that, yet another presupposition, each person can apprehend this unchanging reality equally. The correspondence theory of truth, as this is called, also presupposes that language can describe reality adequately.

These are big ifs. They have seldom been questioned, never mind challenged. As Skolimowski (1994, 199) rightly states, only the mystics have seriously disputed or simply defied this widespread theory. Mystics, however, have not commanded enough respect to be taken seriously in their conclusion that Reality is transconceptual and cannot be objectively measured or even described.

The Greek philosopher-sage Plato, who learned at the feet of Socrates and tutored the empirically minded Aristotle, would have understood the mystics very well. It was Plato who also put forward an alternative to the correspondence theory of truth, namely what has come to be known as the coherence theory of truth: if we cannot know Reality, at least we can make our ideas about it as consistent, or coherent, within themselves as possible. This theory was never very popular, though some renowned philosophers—like Gottfried W. Leibniz, Benedict de Spinoza, Georg W. F. Hegel, and the eighteenth-century physicist and philosopher Ernst Mach—proposed it as a valid approach. There are various logical and epistemological difficulties with this theory, but most important, it seems to be a form of intellectual escapism and a defeatist attitude in regard to the issue of truth or reality.

This is why Skolimowski's notion of participatory truth is a better and important alternative to the two traditional theories. He explains it as follows: "[T]ruth is intersubjective and in a sense universal, but not objective or absolute" (1994, 309). He describes participatory truth as having the following characteristics:

- Species specific
- Culture specific
- Evolving
- Determined by what he calls the "spiral of understanding," which is the peculiar fit between the cosmos and the mind whereby the former reveals itself increasingly as the mind comprehends it, or vice versa
- Processual, which implies that participatory truth is always partial or fragmentary

The fulcrum of Skolimowski's theory of truth is that we participate in truth, or reality, in various ways and in an evolving manner (which, according to Skolimowski, is tied into geological, biological, and even epistemological evolution). The evolution of knowledge involves, as he understands it, "noetic monism," which "maintains that things *become* what our consciousness makes out of them through the active participation of our mind" (1994, 27–28). This is another way of saying that "Nous [or *buddhi*] pervades the universe" (312). Reality is of necessity always our cultural reality. Because our understanding changes and grows, reality is participatory, whatever it may be by itself.

This participatory theory may be viewed as a possible candidate for the next paradigm in science, which is plainly in the offing. Something like it is called for if we want to extricate ourselves from the dilemma in which the hard and most soft sciences find themselves today. Skolimowski supplements his theory of truth with a "philosophy of hope" that overlaps with the profound insights of Abraham Maslow (1971), other transpersonal psychologists, and Mahāyāna Buddhism. Although I personally have a problem with the Christian language of hope, I concur with what it stands for. As is evident from Skolimowski's treatment, he includes introspection, intuition, and feelings like compassion in his epistemological arsenal. This represents a major break with much of the current paradigmatic thinking.

PART TWO   Mind and Beyond

CHAPTER 5

Mind and Its Layers, States, Structures, and Functions

> As we look at consciousness closely, we see
> that it can be analyzed into many parts.
>
> —CHARLES T. TART (1975a, 3)

THE MIND'S LAYERS

Contrary to the popular use of the term *mind,* our mental life is not a feature-less landscape. Depth psychology, which has given the structure of the mind most careful attention, distinguishes several salient facets: the conscious, the preconscious, the personal unconscious, the collective unconscious, the ego, the shadow, and the superego. Some approaches, such as Roberto Assa-gioli's psychosynthesis or Ken Wilber's integral psychology, make further distinctions that bring them into close proximity to the Indian spiritual tra-ditions. Assagioli (1993), for instance, admits a "higher self" and a "higher unconscious," which is superconscious, and the *fons et origo* for creativity and altruistic love, as well as ecstasy. Wilber (2000a, 287–325) distinguishes between the psychic level, the subtle level, the causal, and the nondual.

These features of the mind can usefully be called categories or layers, providing we are careful not to reify them into spatial arrangements. The mind is immaterial and therefore can be talked about meaningfully only in metaphorical terms. The categories mentioned here are all shorthand for very complex processes.

The same is true of the psycho-ontological categories, or principles (*tat-tvas*), identified in Classical Sāmkhya and the other Indian traditions. In his *Sāmkhya-Kārikā* (33), Īshvara Krishna speaks of the threefold "inner instru-ment" (*antahkarana*) comprising the higher mind (*buddhi*), the "I-maker" (*ahamkāra*), and the lower mind (*manas*). We have encountered these prin-ciples already in chapter 3. They constitute what in stanza 35 is called the "doorkeeper" (*dvārin*), who guards the ten "doors" (*dvāra*), that is, the five cognitive and the five conative senses (*indriya*).

The *buddhi* (a feminine noun meaning "awakened") is defined in stanza 23 as consisting at best of ascertainment (*adhyavasāya*), virtue (*dharma*), knowledge (*jnāna*), dispassion (*virāga*), and lordship (*aishvarya*). The qualifier "at best" stands for "sattvic" (*sāttvika*), which means "primarily consisting of *sattva*." This stanza also specifies that in its "tamasic" (*tāmasa*), or inertial, feature, the *buddhi* is the opposite of its sattvic qualities. The attitude of dispassion is assigned to the higher mind, because it entails the kind of neutrality that goes with the quality of *sattva,* as do virtue, knowledge, and lordship. Their tamasic opposites are dullness, attachment/passion, vice, ignorance, and powerlessness.

Ontologically rather than psychologically, the *buddhi* is called *mahat* ("great principle") or *mahān* ("great one"), which is explained as "mere beingness" (*sattā-mātra*) in the *Yoga-Bhāshya* (2.19). Being or beingness is all that can be predicated about it. Ontogenetically, it is the direct or indirect source of all subsequent principles. Only the I-maker evolves out of it directly.

Psychologically, it is the storehouse of the beginningless unconscious activators (*samskāra*), or subliminal impressions, corresponding to the unconscious of modern psychology. It is clear, however, that it is a transpersonal principle or function, being the seat of the karmic deposit, which is the totality of the unconscious activators relating to a particular mental continuum (persisting from lifetime to lifetime). At the same time, the *buddhi* corresponds to what Assagioli (1993) labelled the "superconscious," because it is inherently bright.

In the Vedānta tradition, the *buddhi* in its macrocosmic aspect also bears the designations of "golden germ" (*hiranya-garbha*) and "lord of creatures" (*prajā-pati*); both correspond to the Greek (Neoplatonic) notion of nous and are often personalized. But in Vedānta, the *buddhi* also designates the higher mind, or reason. It knows things only by virtue of having the Self's Awareness illuminating it, whereas in reality it is an insentient principle evolving out of the ground of *prakriti*. This illumination is often explained as the Self being mirrored in the higher mind (see, for example, *Upadesha-Sāhasrī* 18.70). It is this reflected consciousness that wrongly presents itself as true Self-Awareness.

In the *Yoga-Sūtra,* the technical term *buddhi* is used in the sense of "cognition," which is also its meaning in the context of Buddhism, which inspired

Patanjali. In Classical Yoga, the term *citta* can be translated as "mind" in general. Thus, it is *citta* that (according to *Yoga-Sūtra* 4.24) is speckled with countless traits (*vāsanā*) that are chains of related *samskāras*. This is discussed in more detail in chapter 8.

In contrast to Sāmkhya and Sāmkhya-based ontologies, Buddhism does not propose a hierarchy of *tattvas*. The central Buddhist notion is that everything is in flux. There is no monolithic transcendental essence, or Absolute. In a very few places in the Pāli canonical scriptures (*Udāna* 8.1), *nirvāna* is admittedly explained in absolutist terms: "There is, O monks, a place where there is neither earth nor water...."

This is nothing but a concession to popular understanding. It is contradicted by many other passages that, as far as we know, are true to the doctrine of early Buddhism. The Buddha's own disciples found this teaching puzzling. He classified the state of enlightenment among the "undetermined" (*avyākrita*) matters. When Upasiva asked him whether a buddha is nonexistent or established in everlasting bliss, the master responded that nothing meaningful can be affirmed or denied about enlightenment (see *Sutta-Nipāta* 1076). Mahāyāna and Vajrayāna teachers have insisted on the same truth.

Because Gautama the Buddha refused to commit to a particular metaphysical stance, his teaching has often been decried as nihilistic. But the Buddha actually favored a middle path between nihilism and eternalism (as mirrored in the *ātman* doctrine of Vedānta).

Jainism, which goes along with Buddhism in that it does not recognize the Sāmkhya *tattvas*, distinguishes four levels of spiritual maturation and, hence, layers of conscious intensity:

1. *mati-jnāna,* the level on which a sentient being is endowed with one or more sensory capacities and the mind (*manas*), serving as a rallying point for the senses (*sensus communis*). For the Jainas, *manas* is only a quasi sense (*anindriya*). This level is characterized by the absence of language.
2. *shruta-jnāna,* "heard," or received knowledge; the level of reasoning that represents a greater sensitivity than level 1.
3. *avadhi-jnāna,* the level of suprasensory capacity that occurs either naturally (as with deities or hell beings) or by means of yogic cultivation; the term *avadhi-darshana* indicates not so much perception as mental awareness.

4. *manah-paryaya-jnāna*, the level of clairvoyant awareness of the contents of another's mind. It emerges at the tenth level of the fourteen-step path of Jainism (see chapter 15).
5. *kevala-jnāna*, the level of omniscience relative to every existing being or thing. The phrase *kevala-darshana*, or absolute knowledge, is used metaphorically to indicate a state of immediate knowing.

In each case, the corresponding type of perception—whether literal or figurative—involves a karmic limitation of the *jnāna-āvaranīya-karma* variety that obscures knowledge in one way or another. The knowledge occurring at the first level is called indirect (*paroksha*), because it is mediated by the senses. The other forms of knowledge originate within consciousness and are direct. All forms, except omniscience, are liable to error.

Suprasensory capacity (level 3) is said to have six forms:

- *anugami:* "accompanying" *avadhi,* which is never lost, regardless of where we move, even from one life to another
- *ananugami:* "nonaccompanying" *avadhi,* which is lost when we move from one place to another
- *vardhamana:* "growing," or increasing, *avadhi*
- *hiyamana:* "decreasing" *avadhi*
- *avasthita:* "stable" *avadhi,* which remains the same
- *anavasthita:* "unstable" *avadhi,* which is subject to increase or decrease

Omniscience is the highest evolutionary state and upon attaining it, the Jaina adept no longer experiences the other types of knowledge, because he is free from karma. This is not an experience but the natural state of the *jīva.*

THE FOUR STATES OF CONSCIOUSNESS

The Vedānta tradition has an old teaching going back to the *Māndukya-Upanishad.* According to this, consciousness has four states (*avasthā*) or modalities: waking (*jāgrat*), dreaming (*svapna*), sleeping (*sushupti*), and the Fourth (*turīya*). Another word used for "waking" is *vaishvānara,* meaning "relating to all (*vishva*) humans (*nara*)"—a phrase that can be explained by the fact that all humans experience the same world. In distinction, we know that we are dreaming when the experienced world is our own personal version of it. Dreaming is also known as *taijasa,* or "relating to *tejas,*" because, as the *Brihadāranyaka-Upanishad* (4.3.6) explains, in our dreams, we are our own "light" (*tejas*, literally "glow"). We create the dream world through imagination rather than perception. We know from EEG studies that the rapid eye movement (REM) state associated with dreaming is exceptionally busy. Graphs show amplitudes of up to 8–12 hertz.

Deep sleep is far more quiet but patently still involves brain activity of up to 3 hertz (delta waves). The opinion expressed in some Vedānta texts that we can remember "we slept well" because the Self is always awake is questionable. First of all, the Self is utterly transcendental; therefore, we cannot retrieve any information from it. The wakeful faculty would have to be the *buddhi*. Also, there is an EEG pattern showing that the mind is not disabled in deep sleep. Even though the conscious mind is in abeyance in this phase, a simple physical scan might tell us at once whether we slept well or not. In his *Panca-Dashī* (8.20), Vidyāranya likens deep sleep to fainting (*mūrchā*) and ecstasy (*samādhi*), emphasizing that there is no mental activity (*vritti*) in any of these states.[1] In the next verse, he argues that the interval between the disappearance of mental activity and its reappearance is witnessed by the "summit-abiding" (*kuta-stha*) Self. According to Vidyāranya (*Panca-Dashī* 8.23),[2] the *buddhi* cannot cognize itself. He is articulating the Vedānta position on this. But Buddhists assert just the opposite. Since the *buddhi* is the storehouse for all the unconscious activators, we could argue that the higher mind somehow knows its own contents, even if this is accomplished—as Shankara thought—by the reflection (*ābhāsa*) of the Self in the mind.

The Fourth state is thought to be transcendental Reality beyond all mental states. Strictly speaking, it should not be considered a *state* of consciousness at all but pure Awareness (*cin-mātra*) itself.

The Waking State

Of the four states of consciousness, the waking state would seem to be ideally suited for spiritual practice, and traditionally much of spiritual practice occurred in this state. In our busy modern life, however, we are facing a surfeit of diversions that stand in the way of the steady pursuit of yogic practices in daytime hours. As Tenzin Wangyal Rinpoche articulates so well,

> The waking part of the day is around sixteen hours, and the mind is busy the whole time. Often, it seems there is not enough time, and so much of

what time there is, is spent in distraction and unpleasant experience. The modern world seems constantly to be making demands—to take care of job and family, to watch movies, to look in store windows, to wait in traffic, to talk to friends—a thousand things to grab attention and carry it off, until the day is a blur leading to exhaustion and the hunger for even greater distraction that offers escape. (Wangyal 1998, 134)

Also, as we have seen in the discussion of Tart's (1987) notion of consensus trance (see page 142), much of the time we cannot consider ourselves fully awake and alert. We could also point to depth psychology and its prominent concept of the unconscious, which is responsible for such diverse phenomena as slips of the tongue, daydreaming, compulsive behavior, mass hysteria or delusions, and so on. Wakefulness is, therefore, not a defining characteristic of the waking state. It would probably be more reliable to define it neurologically as the condition in which the brain generates predominantly beta waves (15–50 hertz).

DREAMING EAST AND WEST

Ever since Freud's classic monograph *Die Traumdeutung* (The Interpretation of Dreams) (1900), depth psychologists have paid close attention to the symbolic content of dreams in their efforts to heal the ailing psyche. Also, since the 1980s, parapsychologists have made dreams a target of their research, and it was found that ordinary people can have significant precognitive or clairvoyant dreams (see, for example, Broughton 1991, 89ff.). Most premodern cultures had a lively interest in the messages coming from dreams and took them seriously enough to allow them to regulate waking life. We find this also in the cultures of Hinduism, Jainism, and Buddhism. In particular, Jainism has a rich lore of dream interpretation.

There is obviously a fine line between dream divination and the psychotherapeutic use of dreams. In either case, the dream symbols are both personally and culturally conditioned. In bygone ages, the dreams of rulers were regarded with utmost interest, because the mind of, say, a king was held to determine the destiny of the population at large. Their personal dreams might refer to larger social issues. That there is some truth to this can be gauged by the personal dreams of dictators like Adolf Hitler or Saddam Hussein. In democratic governments, the effect of one politician on the destiny of the country is more diluted because of the checks and balances that tend to be in place and make autocratic decisions somewhat less compelling than in a dictatorship.

The earliest Indian reference to dreaming can be found in the *Brihadāra-nyaka-Upanishad* (2.1.18):

> Wherever (*yatra*) he moves about in a dream, these are [his] realms, and he becomes as it were a great king, and [he becomes] as it were a great Brahmin. And he enters as it were high and low [states]. Even as a great king, taking [his] people, moves about at will in his country, so likewise this [dreamer], taking the breaths, moves about at will in his body.

We all are familiar with slipping into various identities and roles in the dream state. The unusual part of this vivid description is the distinct involvement of the life breaths (*prāna*). This is probably a reference to the five main breaths, as hinted at in the *Brihadāranyaka-Upanishad* (3.4.1). The subtle airs called breaths play a central role in mental activity in the waking state and are also instrumental to dream sleep. As stated in passage 4.3.10 of the same text, anything can be exploited in one's dream imagery, and the dreamer is the creator. These breaths are necessary for drawing the energy away from the senses and into the psyche. For Shankara, the creations of the dream state are illusory, because they can always be refuted by means of space, time, and causality, as experienced in the waking state. And yet, Shankara notes, dreams are not entirely illusory, because some of them do point to events that come true.

While the senses governed by the mind (*manas*) are active in the waking state, the senses are more or less disabled in the dream state, but the mind remains active. According to Vedānta, the mind generates dreams by roaming in the subtle channels (*nādī*) of the body and by assembling the memories inscribed in the unconscious (or depth mind). Some of these assemblages can be quite fanciful (such as a centaur-like creature) or flying bodily to the moon in an instant. The mechanics of the dream state, as we will see, are important in the death process.

Dreams play an important role in Buddhism, especially in the hagiographical literature, as Serinity Young has shown in her outstanding book *Dreaming in the Lotus* (1999). Dreams are looked on as essential signs of divination. Buddhism also treats dreams simply as memories of events that occurred in the waking state, perhaps just before falling asleep. It is admitted, however, that dreams can also result from an imbalance of the humors (*dosha*) or from the influence of the unconscious, that is, from meritorious or demeritorious karma. The *Milinda-Panha,* an extracanonical Pāli text that records a dialogue between the Buddhist teacher Nāgasena and the Bactrian king Milinda (or Menander, c. 200 B.C.E.), describes six kinds of dreams: those due to the three types of temperament; those originating with the deities; those arising from habit; and those that are prophetic. It is thought that while each person has the key to understanding a dream, a dream interpreter—as in depth psychology—is necessary to uncover its meaning.

In Vajrayāna (Tibetan) Buddhism, Dream Yoga (Tib.: *rmi lam,* pron. *milam*) figures as one of the six Yogas of the eleventh-century Indian Buddhist master Nāropa. These six teachings, which are part of Tibet's Unexcelled Yoga (*anuttara-yoga*), also include the Yoga of Psychophysical Heat (Tib.: *gtum mo,* pron. *tummo*); the Yoga of the Illusory Body (Tib.: *sgyu lus,* pron. *gyulu*); the Yoga of the Clear Light (Tib.: '*od gsal,* pron. *ösel*); the Yoga of the Transitional Realm (pron. *bardo*); and the Yoga of Consciousness Transference (Tib.: '*pho ba,* pron. *phowa*). *Svapna-Yoga,* or *milam* as it is called in Tibetan, essentially consists of remaining aware during the dream state—a possibility that became well-known in the West with Stephen LaBerge's (1986) research on "lucid dreaming." In a helpful appendix on this topic, Young (1999) makes it clear that LaBerge's approach and Dream Yoga differ in significant ways (context, content, method, and aim).

Tibetan Dream Yoga is based on the recognition that we spend about one-third of our lives in the sleeping state, and much of this time is given to dreaming. In comparison with the waking state, and not unreasonably, we consider our dreams "unreal." On closer inspection, however, our waking state is just as unreal. From the perspective of Tibetan Buddhism, both states of consciousness are unreal, or illusory, in relation to enlightenment. They are unreal only insofar as our true nature (called *dharma-kāya*) is obscured in them.

The purpose of Dream Yoga is to use dreams as an opportunity for spiritual practice, that is, the practice of mindfulness. As Wangyal Rinpoche (1998) explains in his highly readable book *The Tibetan Yogas of Dream and Sleep*, this consists in a mental attitude that emotionally steers the middle path between attraction (or desire) and aversion, both of which merely create karmic deposits (unconscious activators, or *samskāra*) and thus bind the mind to the never-ending cycle of phenomenal existence, or *samsāra*. These karmic deposits, or impressions, in the mind are at least partially activated during sleep. They emerge in the form of dreams in which our semiconscious sleep identity (that is, the subconscious) plays an active role.

As we learn to become aware during sleep that our dreams are projections of our mind, we can also gradually see the same process at work during waking consciousness. The karmic deposits in the unconscious are never idle, and unless we practice mindfulness, our daytime consciousness is just as reactive as our consciousness in the dream state. The occurrences in the dream state are, however, in some ways more accessible than those of the waking state. Often we confront the forces of the unconscious more directly, which is why psychotherapists are curious about our dreams. The unconscious seems to be able to express itself more readily when our mind is not directly preoccupied with the business of daily life. Somehow our conscious mind is buffered against the contents of our dreams, though in Dream Yoga we make use of this relative desensitization to see our karmically driven unconscious at work.

Dream Yoga affords us the opportunity to control our dreams and open ourselves to their messages from the unconscious or from the transpersonal dimension of the personality. Additionally and importantly, it can serve more advanced Yoga practitioners as a platform for deepening their yogic practice. Thus, we may become receptive to teachings given by a teacher in the dream state, or we may even experience the phenomenon of Clear Light, which is thought to present itself automatically in the after-death state. When the latter happens, we can regard Dream Yoga as a means of preparing for the appearance of Clear Light in the postmortem condition.

In all forms of Yoga, dreams are recognized as possibly having symbolic value as "omens" (*arishta*). Patanjali makes a point of mentioning this in aphorism 3.22. Dreams forewarning about one's own or another person's death have special importance. This lore is particularly developed in Tantra, which has integrated many folk traditions.

The encyclopedic Jaina work *Trishashti-Shalākāpurusha-Carita* (The Life of the Thirty-Six Distinguished Persons [in Jainism]), compiled by Hemacandra in the twelfth century, contains the vivid but stereotypical dreams of the mothers of these culture heroes. Mahāvīra's mother, Trishalā, is said to have dreamed of the following fourteen items on the day the founder of Jainism was conceived: an elephant, a bull, a lion, the goddess Shrī, a garland, the moon, the sun, a banner, a vase, a lotus lake, the ocean, a celestial palace, a heap of jewels, and a flame. These items are all symbolic of a great individual—a spiritual conqueror—destined to make his mark in the world.

The mothers of fourteen *jinas* all had dreams containing these fourteen symbols. Personages of lesser importance are said to be heralded by their conceiving mothers dreaming a selection (but not all) of these symbols.

DEEP SLEEP IN YOGA AND VEDĀNTA

In the philosophical system of Vedānta, which rests on the Upanishads, we find the perplexing teaching that associates dreamless deep sleep (*sushupti*) with a condition in which the ego-personality is immersed in profound ignorance (*ajnāna*). Yet, according to Vedānta, the ever-witnessing Self is present, allowing upon waking the knowledge that "I slept well." This appears to be a fallacious argument, because the Self is, by definition, transcendental and hence cannot be a source of information or in any way involved in the process of knowledge.

Some Vedānta authorities regard the state of unconsciousness, or swoon (*mūrccha*), as similar enough to deep sleep to be disregarded. Others distinguish it from deep sleep by arguing that the level of ignorance is still more abysmal. By and large, however, the state of unconsciousness is ignored, presumably because it is thought to have no practical importance. When it is mentioned in Hatha-Yoga, it has a technical significance in connection with the technique of breath control (see, for example, *Hatha-Yoga-Pradīpikā* 4.60).

The *Yoga-Vāsishtha* (3.117.1ff.), a ninth-century Sanskrit text comprising nearly thirty thousand stanzas, teaches that there are seven levels of ignorance, disregarding swoon: seed state of wakefulness (*bīja-jāgrat*), wakefulness (*jāgrat*), great wakefulness (*mahā-jāgrat*), wakeful dream (*jāgrat-svapna*), dream (*svapna*), dream wakefulness (*svapna-jāgrat*), and deep sleep (*sushuptaka*). This list is in descending order and starts with the potential of wakefulness as present in pure Awareness, in which the mind (*manas*) and psyche (*jīva*) exist only nominally. The second level corresponds to the emergence of "I" and its numerous distinct objects that may be equated with Kashmiri Shaivism's transcendental, or at least transpersonal, *tattva* (principle of existence) called "I/That" (*aham-idam*). The third level is interspersed with the karmic propensities of previous lifetimes, which are just as illusory as any other experience. The ordinary waking state is called "wakeful dream," which corresponds to Tart's (1987) "consensus trance." The *Yoga-Vāsishtha* makes much of the dreamlike nature of the waking state. Dream wakefulness, the sixth level, stands for the confusing recall of past experiences as if they were happening in the present (or what we would call "hallucination"). The least realistic level or state of consciousness is deep sleep (*nidrā*). We could add the state of unconsciousness, or complete torpor, as an eighth level.

The *Yoga-Vāsishtha* (3.118.1ff.) also expounds on the sevenfold path of knowledge (*jnāna*) that leads from abject spiritual ignorance to enlightenment and represents the reverse of the preceding seven levels of ignorance.

In Buddhism, the mind immersed in deep sleep is thought to have entered the state of *bhavanga*. This is a state in which life flows along without the up-and-down experience of pleasure or pain but which nonetheless is a type of consciousness.

THE FOURTH

The Vedāntic designation "the Fourth" (*caturtha* or *turīya*) denotes transcendental Awareness, or *cit*, which is the the Self (*ātman*). The Fourth, therefore, does not rightly qualify as a state of consciousness, though it is often talked about loosely in this way in the literature.

THE GEBSERIAN STRUCTURES OF CONSCIOUSNESS

In his monumental work *Ursprung und Gegenwart* (translated as *The Ever-Present Origin* in 1985), the Swiss cultural historian and poet Jean Gebser (1949 and 1953) introduced the concept of "structures of consciousness," by which he meant four basic modalities that are detectable in the progressive evolution of consciousness since the Paleolithic era: the archaic, magical, mythical, and mental modality, or frequency. His work inspired Ken Wilber's spectrum approach; Wilber's cultural-historical dimension is articulated in the 1996 edition of *Up from Eden*.

Gebser also postulated an emerging fifth structure, which he called integral, corresponding roughly to Wilber's "vision-logic." It is perhaps best to understand these structures as psychohistorical configurations. Psychohistory is a subdiscipline of history that applies psychological, especially depth-psychological, insights to historical circumstances and figures. Although Gebser's model is somewhat more static, his structures are definitely interpretative frameworks that allow us to better understand the inner dynamics of a given cultural type or era.

THE YUGA DOCTRINE

Gebser and Wilber's cultural-historical models were somewhat anticipated in ancient India by the *yuga* doctrine. In Hinduism, a *yuga* is a span of time characterized by certain psychological and cultural specifics. Four such *yugas,* or world ages, are recognized. They form a set that indicates progressive spiritual, social, and cultural decline: *krita-* (or *satya-*), *dvāpara-, tretā-,* and *kali-yuga.* The designations are adopted from the favorite Vedic game of dice, with *kali* standing for the least advantageous throw; this term is, by the way, unrelated to the fierce goddess Kālī. Tradition assigns one, five, one hundred, or one thousand years to a *yuga.* In the *Mahābharata* epic and the Purānas, the *yugas* are assigned much longer spans of time, namely, hundreds of thousands of years in human terms.

The *yuga* teaching, which was already present in a late hymn of the *Rig-Veda* (10.10.10), came to be associated with important astronomical-astrological shifts arising from the rotation of the polar axis, which does a full turn every 25,800 years; the Indian tradition gives the idealized number of 24,000 years. Generally, the set of four *yugas* is thought to span 10,000 years, with the *yugas* extending 4,000, 3,000, 2,000, and 1,000 years respectively, each with a transitional period of 10 percent. Also, these are understood as "divine" years corresponding to a total of 4,320,000 human years, which is a *kalpa,* or one day and night in the life of the creator-deity Brahma.

According to the Puranic literature (from perhaps 500 C.E. on), the most recent *kali-yuga* commenced on February 18, 3102 B.C.E., which supposedly coincides with the eighteen-day Bharata war between the Pāndava heroes (fighting on Arjuna's side) and the opposing armies of the Kauravas. Other authorities have the beginning of the *kali-yuga* coincide with the death of Krishna thirty-six years after the war. Yet other estimates exist as well, and the available astronomical-astrological evidence (of star positions and eclipses) is thoroughly confusing. The war, whenever it occurred (if it is not merely allegorical), was devastating, ending in the death of almost all the fighters on both sides. It ushered in a new era attendant with most undesirable psychological and cultural features but giving the surviving world the spiritual teachings of the *Bhagavad-Gītā* imparted on the day after the first battle. Using the long count for the *yugas,* we are still at the very beginning of the *kali-yuga.*

The *yuga* doctrine gained special momentum in conjunction with the Vaishnava divine incarnations (*avatāra,* literally "descent"); each *avatāra* is thought of as a full or partial embodiment of God himself descending into the empirical universe for the spiritual regeneration of all beings. This is best explained in the *Bhagavad-Gītā* (4.6–4.8) by the God-man Krishna:

> Although [I am] unborn, the immutable Self, [and] although being the Lord of [all] beings—[yet] by governing My own nature (*prakriti*), I come-to-be through the creative-power (*māyā*) of Myself. (4.6)

> For, whenever there is a diminution of the law, O descendant-of-Bharata [that is, Prince Arjuna], and an upswing of lawlessness, then I create Myself [in manifest form]. (4.7)

> For the protection of good [beings], for the destruction of wrong-doers, for the sake of establishing the law, I come-into-being from age to age (*yuge yuge*). (4.8)

The *yugas*—similar to the world ages (*aiōns*) of ancient Greece—are psychohistorical structures of diminishing vibrancy and integrity. Gebser's structural model does not have this historical bias. His monumental work, *The Ever-Present Origin,* is an outstanding contribution toward the archeology of consciousness. Basically, using a wealth of cultural-historical data, Gebser illustrated first that our human species has undergone a series of cognitive leaps, or restructurings of consciousness, and second that we are currently witnesses to and participants in a fifth major reorganization of our cognitive field—the emergent "arational structure of consciousness." (The arational-integral structure, which he thought was trying to constellate itself in our epoch, is an integrating type of consciousness that transcends all preceding but still copresent structures of consciousness.) Gebser further argued that the modern psyche is the aggregate of *all* historically preceding structures and that these must be lived according to their own particular valence and in integrated harmony.

The following is a slightly modified portion of an article that was originally published in *Investigations: A Research Bulletin of the Institute of Noetic Sciences.*

THE MENTAL STRUCTURE

The *mental structure of consciousness,* as the name suggests, is the domain of *mens,* the thinking mind, of reasoning in its different forms. It is a cognitive style that operates on the principle of duality, of either/or. It implies a conscious subject that experiences itself as standing apart from the objects, or contents, of awareness. According to Gebser and other historians, this style of cognition is a relative latecomer in the noetic evolution of humankind. It made its appearance around the middle of the first millennium B.C.E.—the age of Pythagoras, Socrates, Aristotle, and Plato in Greece, Gautama the Buddha and Mahāvīra in India, and Lao-Tzu and Confucius in China. What we see in all these thinkers is an astounding ability to reason, though without sacrificing the mythical dimension of existence, which pertains to values and feelings.

Only with the European Renaissance do we see the seedlings of a new rationality that is at once more egocentric and demythologizing—the kind of rationality that has led us into the cul-de-sac of the nuclear arms race and the ecological devastation of our planet.

THE MYTHICAL STRUCTURE

Representing a kind of consciousness (and of subjectivity) that is less focused and more diffuse than the *mental structure* is the *mythical structure of consciousness*. It is a cognitive style that operates with polarity rather than duality and unfolds through symbol rather than calculus, myth rather than hypothesis, feeling or intuition rather than abstract thinking, and value-creation rather than fact-finding, as well as interpersonal sensitivity and compassion rather than interpersonal (egoic) conflict. It is the type of consciousness that has been and still is responsible for the world's immense variety of religious traditions, art, and literature.

THE MAGICAL STRUCTURE

A still more diffuse (pre-egoic) awareness is represented by the *magical structure of consciousness*. It operates on the principle of identity, as it is expressed in analogical "thinking." This is the kind of mental activity that, through a gut-level (archetypal) response, relates apparently disjointed elements into a whole—but a whole that does not necessarily make sense from a rational, logical point of view. We see this style of cognition in action in the marvelous hunting scenes depicted in Paleolithic cave paintings. These early works of art are really signposts of a primitive hunting ritual: They anticipate the death of the animal to be slain, its heart pierced by an infallible (magically guided) spear or arrow.

THE ARCHAIC STRUCTURE

The simplest and earliest identifiable cognitive style is that of the *archaic structure of consciousness*. It has the least degree of self-awareness and is almost completely instinctual. Historically, it predates the Neanderthals and Cro-Magnons. For Gebser, the archaic consciousness represents a consciousness of maximum latency and minimum transparency. That is to say, it contains the possibility of further evolution but is itself dim. Gebser referred to a cryptic remark by Chuang Tzu (c. 350 B.C.E.) who said that the "true men" of earlier times slept dreamlessly. This suggests that they had no self-awareness sufficient to generate dreams. While the statement is mythological and probably wrong (since apparently apes and even dogs dream), it nevertheless contains a significant clue to the general psychic condition of pre-Neanderthal humanity. For Gebser, the archaic structure of consciousness is closest to the "ever-present Origin." Indeed, we may postulate that it has certain features—such as synchronicity—of the trans-spatial/transtemporal Origin itself. (*Investigations* 1988, 22–26)

Each structure represents a distinct "interpretational" platform. An earlier generation of anthropologists distinguished between a logical and a pre-logical mentality. This was a simplistic distinction that deservedly courted criticism and also suffered from a great deal of misunderstanding. Gebser's differentiation into an archaic, a magical, a mythical, and a mental structure of consciousness is appealing, because it actually does justice to the complex data about premodern mentalities and also makes sense from the perspective of the psychology of the individual.

Each structure is thought to have both a flourishing ("efficient") and a declining ("deficient") phase, as is clear from the table at the back of Gebser's book. Thus, the efficient aspect of the magical structure is spell casting, while its deficient aspect is witchcraft. Similarly, the efficient side of the mythical structure is envisioned myth, while its deficient side is mythology. In the case of the mental structure, which is dominant nowadays, *logos* is on the efficient and ratio on the deficient side.

Gebser believed that a new structure of consciousness is trying to emerge out of the mental-rational structure, which he called the arational-integral structure. As already mentioned, this structure is called vision-logic in Wilber's (2000a) spectrum model. It is not entirely clear why the structure bears this name. In terms of Gebser's framework, vision belongs to the mythical and logic to the mental type of consciousness.

From the vantage point of several decades of development since Gebser formulated his work, Wilber has endeavored to differentiate this structure further by distinguishing early, middle, and late phases. He qualifies the early phase as Erik Erikson's "centaur" (see Erikson 1950), which consists of mature body-mind integration; the middle phase is associated, for example, with Lawrence Kohlberg's "universal ethics" (see Kohlberg 1984); and the late phase with globalism. Beyond these three phases of vision-logic, Wilber sees development in the "postformal," transpersonal dimension at the psychic, subtle, causal, and nondual levels.

As I have shown in my book *Wholeness or Transcendence?* (1992), Gebser's model is relevant to Yoga. The four structures of consciousness that are particularly pertinent are the archaic, magical, mythical, and mental structure. The archaic structure seems to be activated in the conscious forms of ecstasy (*samprajñāta-samādhi*), which are based on a *unio mystica* with the object of contemplation, perhaps what Freud (1961, 12–13) called the "oceanic feeling," which he admitted he could not discover within himself and which he therefore understood as an intellectual perception with a certain feeling tone. For Freud, sadly, the melting of the boundary of the ego in the mystical state necessarily spells pathology. The testimony of the *yogins* and the world's mystical connoisseurs is otherwise. This matter is, in the final analysis, a question of theory versus experience.

The magical structure is helpful in understanding the shamanic elements of Yoga, such as asceticism (*tapas*) and certain paranormal abilities (*siddhi*). The mythical structure is relevant to understanding yogic introversion and meditation, the striving for immortality, or the insistence on silence, and so on. The mental structure is advantageous to bear in mind when seeking to comprehend the intellectual elaborations of Yoga, such as Patanjali's system, the Buddhist *Abhidharma,* or the teachings of Shankara. The more integral aspects of Yoga—as, for instance, in the medieval teaching about *sahaja,* usually translated as "spontaneity"—can be better understood in light of Gebser's arational-integral structure, which he associates with transparency, openness, integrality, a perspectival viewpoint, and ego-freedom (rather than egolessness or egocentricity).

Taking a panoramic view of human developmental history (and future history), Ken Wilber postulates four additional structures of consciousness beyond Gebser's configuration, or what he calls vision-logic: psychic, subtle, causal, and nondual. Wilber (2000a, 221n5) readily admits that "the higher levels are still evolving themselves, and thus they are great potentials, not pregiven absolutes." While his suggested super levels are indeed plausible stages of spiritual unfolding, they cannot easily be considered psychohistorical structures. It is difficult to imagine a sociocultural framework informed chiefly by psychic, subtle, causal, or nondual development. In this sense, Wilber's higher levels differ significantly from the Gebserian structures and their various equivalents selected by Wilber from Huston Smith and Plotinus to Stanislav Grof, Sri Aurobindo, William Tiller, Lawrence Kohlberg, and Jürgen Habermas, and so on.

While it makes sense to divide Gebser's integral structure into several substructures, how Wilber's postintegral levels relate to the integral structure is not immediately obvious. We can develop psychic and subtle capacities without the integral structure. In fact, many *yogins* do just that and never get to the integral structure of consciousness. Many more never fully develop the mental structure but remain caught up in the archaic, magical, and mythical structures. The causal structure consists of realizing the all-identity, the formless ground behind all other mental contents. That this realization is not dependent on the prior actualization of the arational-integral consciousness is suggested by the fact that it was apparently already known to the thirteenth- and early fourteenth-century German mystic Meister Eckhart. The nondual structure, again, is marked by the realization that it is nondual in an all-inclusive sense: it is not just the *ātman* (the core Self) that is realized to be identical with the *brahman* (the universal ground), but also the phenomenal world that was previously renounced and therefore segregated.

In *Integral Psychology* (2000a, 156–57), Wilber makes the point that these postformal structures were realized by a select few in the past and that they will be the "common" or "average" mode of consciousness in the future. This is, of course, mere speculation, which Wilber seeks to soften by speaking of a "gentle persuasion" that aligns the multitudes to what otherwise looks very much like a historical inevitability. Gebser, who was clearly friendly toward Eastern nondualism and himself experienced a *satori* state apparently confirmed by D. T. Suzuki, would presumably not have known what to do with this part of Wilber's speculative psychology.

From a psychohistorical point of view, the emigration of Yoga out of the Indian subcontinent is a significant development, because Yoga encounters the full brunt of the mental structure and is thus challenged to respond differently to its adaptation within India. The emergence of Western Yoga can be understood from all kinds of perspectives. It has seldom been considered in the context of the pronounced mental structure of the Occident, much less in the context of the arational-integral structure. Sri Aurobindo pointed toward something like this in his critique of traditional Yoga, but his understanding of the West was incomplete, and he did not know of the work done by Gebser and others like him. His critique of traditional Yoga therefore can be said to have remained unfinished and to have stayed too close to the Hindu prototype.

Unfortunately, much of Western Yoga has come under the influence of what Gebser would regard as the deficient form of the mental structure of consciousness, which is articulated, among other things, in the commodification of Yoga and the ideology behind it. The commodification of Western Yoga has been ably addressed by John Philp in his probing book *Yoga, Inc.* (2009). The investigation of its psychohistorical potential is an urgent desideratum, which must take Carl Jung's astute counsel and early caveat into careful account.

CHAPTER 6

Mind and Brain

> If the brain were just electrical, if its only language
> were the binary code of the action potential, we might
> really be deterministic, computerlike machines. But
> the chemical brain is more slippery.... At each synapse
> the impulse can either be duplicated exactly, reduced,
> increased, or delayed.... Maybe all this uncertainty
> makes for a subtle, fluid, and unpredictable mental life.
>
> —JUDITH HOOPER and DICK TERESI (1986, 72)

This chapter looks at the mind from both a Western and an Indian perspective. Without wanting to anticipate too much of chapter 9, I will say that the relationship between the immaterial mind and the material brain is extraordinarily complex and that the two are somehow coupled via the network of *prānic* currents. This intricate connection between the mind and the brain is only imperfectly understood scientifically, but the explanations found in the Yoga scriptures are highly suggestive.

As far as the Indian spiritual traditions are concerned, the general idea is that the mind is senior to the brain and that the brain acts similar to a filter to the mind. This contradicts the materialism of modern psychology, which insists that consciousness is an effect of the brain and nervous system and that, therefore, the mind has no independent existence. This was most forcibly argued by the British philosopher Gilbert Ryle (1949), who stated that one can and ought to restate all mentalistic statements in terms of physicalistic ones. Thus, in Ryle's opinion, it would be as meaningless to say, "I feel elated," or "I feel bored," as for the magician to say, "Abracadabra."

Most philosophers and psychologists have found Ryle's solution to the body-mind problem unconvincing. Other theories have been proposed, but none of them has been any more acceptable. Neuropsychology, a discipline that arose sometime in the mid-twentieth century, has given us both new data and new theories. In light of Indian traditions like Yoga, Sāmkhya, Vedānta, and so on, as well as parapsychological and thanatological evidence, we are irresistibly steered toward the kind of interactive dualism, or dualist interactionism, espoused by the neuroscientists Sir John C. Eccles (who received the Nobel Prize in Medicine) and Daniel N. Robinson (1985), as well as by the renowned philosopher Sir Karl Popper (1977).

Alternatively, we might gravitate toward a panpsychistic theory, as favored, for example, by the German biologist Bernhard Rensch (1968), the American biochemist and Nobel Laureate George Wald (1980), the Polish philosopher and systems theorist Ervin Laszlo (2007), the British philosopher Alfred North Whitehead (1919), the Australian philosopher David John Chalmers (2002), and the Dutch cardiologist and near-death researcher Pim van Lommel (2010), who has written one of the more thought-provoking books of recent years.

Panpsychism assumes that both psyche (mind) and matter are copresent in the universe; they complement each other. A panpsychistic theory meshes well with J. J. Poortman's psychohylism, or hylic pluralism, which he explains as follows:

> This implies the view, not that matter paradoxically also has lasting consciousness—this is known as hylozoism—but that consciousness constantly has a material and corporeal aspect. (Poortman 1978, 1:14)

THE BRAIN/MIND QUESTION

The question of the relationship between the cerebrum and the mind has plagued psychologists and philosophers alike ever since Hippocrates, who accepted the brain as the seat of intelligence. Socrates agreed with this belief.

A century or so later, Plato also agreed, but his pupil Aristotle did not; instead, Aristotle located mental processes in the heart. This view was discarded by subsequent researchers. Recently, matters were made far more complex when neuroscientists discovered that the heart does, in fact, have a nerve plexus composed of neurons that are remarkably similar to those in the brain. The heart emits strong electromagnetic waves that, when it is functioning optimally, synchronize with the brain. So the heart is equipped to do some brainy work after all. The HeartMath Institute in Northern California has studied the "emotional waves" of the heart for many years and has sought to educate the public about cultivating the right kinds of emotions, which we would consider positive, not only for nourishing the physical heart but also for supporting the work of the brain.

The brain/mind question became particularly prominent with the rise of neuroscience in the twentieth century. How can the immaterial thought to raise one's arm, for instance, translate into the actual movement? How do we move our body as a whole? This type of question led to the discovery of many physiological processes, such as the transmission of nerve impulses across synapses connecting one neural cell to another. This is accomplished by means of neurotransmitters—messenger chemicals (hormones) like glutamate and gamma-aminobutyric acid and the less common norepinephrine and histamine that send a buzz of electrical communications among the brain's 15 to 33 billion neurons. The brain also has about four times that number of glial cells, which lend the brain structural and metabolic support, as well as insulation and so on, but they are not equipped to send neural messages to each other. In summary, the brain is a rather complex configuration, which our ancestors intuited.

Most of the body's processes happen automatically. Remarkably, even our internal command to raise an arm takes effect neurochemically 350 milliseconds *before* we send the mental signal. In other words, there are energy processes occurring in the nerves that suggest an immediate intention *before* the mental command is issued. Thus, we could argue that there is no free will: we are willing something for which the body is already preparing. With paradoxical findings like this, it is not surprising that thinkers have found it extremely difficult to explain the relationship between the body (brain) and the mind. Most physicians, who are educated in (or, more correctly, indoctrinated into) the current materialistic paradigm of science, regard consciousness as an epiphenomenon of the brain. But the optimistic quest of the 1950s and 1960s for straightforward neurochemical correlations of mental phenomena did not pan out. Instead of matters becoming simpler and clearer, they have become, if anything, more complicated and more obscure.

The good news is that the brain is far more plastic than was earlier assumed. In other words, contrary to popular belief, the brain is constantly changing throughout a person's life and can even repair itself in unexpected ways—and relatively quickly at that (see Doidge 2007).

THE PRĀNA/MIND QUESTION

If the brain/mind question has been a prominent issue in the modern psychological disciplines, then the *prāna*/mind question has been given comparable priority in the spiritual disciplines of India. Speculations about this topic go back to the *Atharva-Veda* (11.4, 15.15) well over three thousand years ago. The Vedic knowledge about *prāna* was carried over into the early Upanishads. Thus, the *Brihadāranyaka-Upanishad* (4.2.3) mentions the 101 conduits (*nādīs*), of which only one leads to immortality. The *Taittirīya-Upanishad* (2.8–2.9) mentions the five sheaths (*kosha*), which are important in later Vedānta. One of these sheaths is the *prāna-maya-kosha*, the sheath made of *prāna*. The *nādīs* are part of the "subtle" architecture. This topic is best considered from the perspective of India's naturopathic system of Āyurveda that is said to derive from the *Atharva-Veda* and distinguishes between the veins and arteries of the physical body and the *nādī* network of the subtle sheath.

According to the *panca-kosha* model, the *prāna-maya-kosha* is wedged between the "food body"—that is, the body made of flesh and bones—and the lower mind (*manas*). This arrangement suggests that the *prānic* body is coarser than the mind but subtler than the physical body.

The reason for this is not hard to see. Every successive *kosha* requires an intermediate structure (or field) that allows for the hierarchically higher body to communicate with the lower vehicle and vice versa. The *prānic* body performs this task for the lower mind on one side and the physical body on the other.

This brings us to the *ākāsha* problem. The *ākāsha*, or ether-space, which the Indian sages assume to exist, is the environment of *prāna*. It is a subtle field that has many unexpected properties. The Michelson-Morley experiment conducted in the late 1890s is thought to have disproved the notion of a physical ether once and for all. Albert Michelson and Edward Morley used a light beam to measure the speed of the earth. A physical ether would have interfered with the speed of the split light beam, which did not happen. This may be so, but *ākāsha* is the subtle ether that could not have been measured that way.

In recent years, the *ākāsha* has raised its head again. It was carefully studied by Ervin Laszlo. He writes,

The Akashic experience comes in many sizes, forms, and flavors, to all kinds of people, and all its varieties convey information on the real world—the world beyond the brain and the body. The experience ranges from artistic visualizations and creative insights to nonlocal healings, near-death experiences, after-death communications, and personal past life recollections. (Laszlo 2009, 1)

CHAPTER 7

The Sensory Apparatus

Perception is not direct. It is a *construction*.

—KARL PRIBRAM
(Hooper and Teresi
1986, 338)

Our human body is equipped with sense organs that give us sensory information about our body (the kinesthetic sense) and our environment, which allows us to navigate in the so-called outside world. Without sensation, we would be locked in our mind and unable to sustain our body. As we are taught, we have five principal sense organs: the eyes, the ears, the nose, the taste buds of the mouth, and the skin. These organs have sensory receptors (or nerve cells) that yield information like the position of the body and outside objects, sounds, smells, tastes, and warmth/touch.

Sensory functions, notably sight, have been speculated about since the time of the ancient Greeks. Plato fancifully thought that the eyes send out emanations to objects and actively gather information about them, which is then relayed to the eye and the brain. His pupil, Aristotle, in *De Anima* (book 2, chapter 7), begged to differ. Wrongly disagreeing with Empedocles that light travels, he assumed instead that the transparent medium of air made things visible by a kind of perturbation that reached the eyes.

About two thousand years later, the German astronomer Johannes Kepler recognized that the eye acts like a lens and casts an (upside-down) image of the object on the retina. Not until the nineteenth century, however, were the senses scientifically investigated. In 1802, Thomas Young—a British physician—deduced that three types of light receptor in the eye are involved in color vision. (More than 90 percent of research on sensory perception focuses on vision.) This was further studied in the nineteenth century by the German physicist Hermann Helmholtz (1862) and is now known as the trichromatic theory. By the middle of the twentieth century, perception research had amassed an incredible amount of data, and interest shifted increasingly to the mental component of perception, which is colossal. This coincided with the introduction of computers and artificial intelligence (AI) models that significantly shaped our thinking about the brain.

If we imagine that our senses give us a photographic image of the world, then we forget that the brain is involved in perception, and the brain interprets and colors. Self-conscious perception is inevitably interpretive. Take visual perception. Light hits the retina and, via millions of cones and rods, creates a highly fragmented image of objects in the outer world. The retina itself is responsible for the first level of reconstructing a patchy image. The optic nerve conveys this first synthesis in the form of nerve impulses to the lateral geniculate nucleus in the thalamus. Here, a further synthesis occurs that is relayed to the prefrontal lobes of the cortex via seven million nerve fibers like oceanic cables.

Further interpretation happens, not least through input from the limbic system, which is lodged in the interior of the brain. The limbic system, consisting of a complex system of nerve fibers, infuses basic emotions into the perceptual construction. Another area of the brain, one that is involved in language, also furnishes a link between the senses and presents an even more interpretive picture, allowing us to pin a name on a given thing. In the end, the interpreted object is no more than a simulation (or simulacrum) of the real object, which can be quite wrong. A dramatic example, often used in the Indian literature, is that of a rope that is mistaken for a snake. In one one-hundredth of a second, the brain interprets the rope as a snake.

Clearly, if we were to act/react to this false or distorted image, we would be caught up in equally wrong or unproductive action. Much of our life is made up of such interpretations and actions. This is obviously important. While we can move about in the environment with relative dexterity, many people arguably find it difficult to move through life with adequate skill.

Much of this has to do with how we conceptualize, which happens at the level of the cortex. In other words, right view (*samyag-darshana*) is critical, as many Indian schools of thought acknowledge by placing it at the head of other factors of the spiritual path. The management of anger and fear (which belong to the limbic system) is also crucial. There is no yogic-type system that does not seek to intervene in the prevention of these two demonstrably destructive emotions.

The five senses (*indriya*) have unsurpassed importance in the yogic systems, because we invest a considerable amount of time and energy in them. It would not be wrong to say that the life of the unenlightened individual revolves around the material world as conveyed by the senses and the mind. Only when we have stepped onto the spiritual path do higher faculties (*indriya*) come into play—notably, as Buddhism has it, faith (*shraddhā*), energy (*vīrya*), mindfulness (*smṛti*), concentration (*samādhi*), and wisdom (*prajnā*).[1]

HINDU YOGA: THE ELEVEN SENSES

In the era of the Vedas many millennia ago, there was nothing resembling the Yoga-Sāmkhya theory of sensory functioning. In keeping with the myth-ological-symbolic tone of the four Vedas, there is an obscure accounting of the senses as "seers" (*rishi*). This correlation is explicitly affirmed in the *Bri-hadāranyaka-Upanishad* (2.2.4), which was composed (not written!) much later but undoubtedly drew on Vedic wisdom. According to this passage, the two ears are the seers Gotama and Bharadvāja; the two eyes are Vishvāmitra and Jamadagni; the two nostrils are Vasishtha and Kashyapa; speech—that is, the tongue—is Atri. These seven seers are also found as seven kinds of breath (*prāna*) and as stars in the constellation of Pleiades in the celestial vault. This kind of macrocosmic-microcosmic parallelism is typical of the early Hindu oral "literature."

Also in the *Brihadāranyaka-Upanishad* (2.4.11), we encounter the earliest known reference to more than five senses. Here is the whole passage:

> As the ocean is the single resting-place (*eka-ayana*) of all waters; so the skin is the single resting-place of all contacts; so the nostrils are the single rest-ing-place of all smells; so the tongue is the single resting-place of all tastes; so the eye is the single resting-place of all forms; so the ear is the single resting-place of all sounds; as the mind (*manas*) is the single resting-place of all concepts; so the ear is the single resting-place of all insights; so the hands are the single resting-place of all actions; so the penis is the single resting-place of all [ephemeral] joys; so the anus is the single resting-place of all [bodily] evacuations; so the feet are the single resting-place of all movements; so speech is the single resting-place of all the "knowledges" (*veda*).

It is obvious that this Upanishad has been assembled from transmitted wisdom of varying age. Behind the seers are the gods (*deva*), who represent higher cognitive centers. They were apparently envisioned as fundamental structures of the mind, though they have not yet been studied from this perspective.[2] In the preceding passage, we have the eleven senses, or sensory capacities (*indriya*), known to the Sāmkhya tradition of later times, including the lower mind (*manas*), which acts as the *sensus communis* for all sensory input. This archaic model takes note of all the main functions of the human body. These functions comprise perceptual, conative, and conceptual tasks. The reference to the "knowledges" is probably a reference to the sacred Vedic hymnodies that are thought to represent the culmination of knowledge. The five cognitive senses (*jnānendriya*) furnish information about the outside world; the five conative senses (*karmendriya*) allow us to interact with the outside world; and the conceptual activity of the lower mind orchestrates the input from the sense organs and presents it in a meaningful way to the brain-mind (*citta* or *buddhi*). It is conceivable that we have here one of the sources of later Sāmkhya psycho-ontology.

All the senses entangle us in the world of objects and thereby—rather as the name *indriya* ("capacity") suggests—incapacitate us, or drive us away from the transcendental core of our personality.

In late Vedānta scriptures, such as the *Viveka-Cūdāmani* (77), the objects (*vishaya*) of the world are called poisons (*visha*), because they pervert the mind by distracting it from the spiritual path. Renunciation (*samnyāsa*) is the recommended avenue for dealing with the objective world. Nearly two thousand years earlier, the *Mahābharata* epic (12.194.58) declared,

The Self (*ātman*) cannot be perceived with the senses, which, disunited, are scattered and difficult to restrain for those whose self [personality] is not prepared.

The *Bhagavad-Gītā* (3.34, 3.40), which is roughly contemporaneous, states,

Passion and hatred are [ordinarily] directed toward the objects of the senses [corresponding to their respective] senses. Let none come under their power, for both are way-layers on his [path].

The senses, the lower mind (*manas*) and the higher mind (*buddhi*) are called the hiding-places of this [enemy of wisdom]. Through these, it fools the body-essence (*dehin*), concealing knowledge.

In the *Yoga-Sūtra* (1.7), Patanjali designates sensory perception (*pratyaksha*) as the leading means of valid cognition (*pramāna*), together with inference (*anumāna*) and testimony (*āgama*). That he admitted the possibility of error (*viparyaya*) indicates that he did not necessarily regard perceptual knowledge as infallible. We can err in many ways. Contemporary research on so-called optical illusions has driven home the point of just how much our mind distorts what we perceive. Clearly, we must begin our spiritual journey from a correct point of view, and we can ensure this by relying on the testimony (*āgama*) of the illumined sages in the form of their spiritual teachings. We can assume that they perceived appropriately (that is, without distortion) and also communicated the truth, as they realized it, without distortion.

PERCEPTION IN JAINISM AND BUDDHISM

Seeing (*darshana*) can happen at various levels of sensitivity. At the lowest level, *mati* ("intelligent perception"), sensation occurs by means of one or more sensory capacities, including the *manas*. At a somewhat higher level, *shruta* ("heard," involving reasoning), seeing is suffused with conceptualization. At both the *mati* and *shruta* levels, perception can be either visual (*cakshur-darshana*), that is, by means of the eyes, or nonvisual, that is, through the other sensory capacities. The *shruta* level presupposes the *mati* level, but the latter is not based on the former. Some authorities disagree and assume that *mati* and *shruta* are interdependent.

The third level of sensitivity accessible to the sentient being (*jīva*) is known as *avadhi*. In Hinduism, this Sanskrit word means "limit," but in Jainism, it denotes "limited nonsensory knowledge," or intuition, of forms. It does not extend to formless things, such as souls, space itself, and time. This capacity is natural to the godlings in heaven and the infernal beings (*nāraka*) in hell; it is variable, depending on their spiritual maturity. Humans can also acquire various degrees of *avadhi*, depending on the elimination of specific karmas.

The fourth level is *manah-paryaya* or *-paryāya*, which denotes direct "access to [another's] mind," or natural clairvoyance. It is possible only for those who have overcome "insight-deluding" (*darshana-mohanīya*) karmas. Only at the last rung of the fourteen-rung ladder to perfection are all karmas eliminated, which coincides with death. The fifth and final level of perception, or spiritual intensity, is omniscience, or absolute knowledge (*kevala-*

jnāna), which is total knowledge of all beings and things. At this level, the *jīva* freely perceives itself, or has perfect self-knowledge, and also perfectly perceives all others.

In the *Bhāgavatī-Sūtra* (5.3), sensory perception (*pratyaksha*) is listed as the leading source of knowledge, along with inference (*anumāna*), analogy (*aupamya*), and testimony (*āgama*), which shows the importance of the senses.

During its protracted history, Buddhism has repeatedly addressed the question of sense-derived and other forms of knowledge. It grants sensory perception as significant a role as the other traditions. But most important, it understands it as a source of distraction. Thus, according to the *Sabbāsava-Sutta* of the *Majjhīma-Nikāya* (2), the Buddha himself explained that some things are unfit for attention yet are generally given prominence in life and some things that are fit for attention are ignored. The monastic, however, is said to practice wisdom by paying attention to what is fit and ignoring what is unfit.

In particular, the monastic restrains the faculties of the eye, ear, nose, tongue, and body (skin). In this way, he also controls his own mind. The sense functions are understood as specific types of consciousness. The mind gives rise to mental consciousness. Understanding this is the first step. The next step is to realize that these six consciousnesses are not the "I" (see the *Channovāda-Sutta* of the *Majjhīma-Nikāya* 144.9).

The I-function is something we superimpose on all mental processes, including perception. In Yoga, this is not acceptable, since the conventional self-sense is destructive to the spiritual process and seeks to reidentify with the Self or its equivalent.

CHAPTER 8

The Unconscious and Its Mechanisms

> Many things happen semi-consciously, and an
> incalculable number of occurrences may even be
> entirely unconscious.
>
> —CARL G. JUNG (1939, 4)

THE UNCONSCIOUS IN MODERN DEPTH PSYCHOLOGY

The now-familiar concept of the unconscious was not invented by Sigmund Freud. He stands on the shoulders of other philosophers and psychologists. One of the earliest references to the concept of the unconscious can be found in the philosophical work of the late-seventeenth-/early-eighteenth-century German philosopher-mathematician-physicist-historian-diplomat Gottfried Wilhelm Leibniz. In his posthumously published *Nouveaux essays sur l'entendement humain,* in which he discusses chapter by chapter John Locke's similarly titled 1690 book, he speaks of the *petites perceptions,* or the "little perceptions." These are perceptions of which we are never aware, as when we hear a single thundering sound for a multitude of waves crashing into the shore, each of which produces its own distinct sound. This was Leibniz's way of going beyond Cartesianism, which insisted that consciousness alone governs our inner life. Decades later, in 1777, Goethe used the term *unbewusst* ("unconscious") in one of his poems, and this idea was subsequently taken over and expanded by the German Romantics in the eighteenth century.

Thus, via the Romantic philosopher Friedrich Wilhelm Schelling, the idea influenced the maverick German philosopher Eduard von Hartmann, who attempted to synthesize the systems of Hegel and Schopenhauer. He made the notion of the unconscious into a mainstay of his own philosophizing. Hartmann, whose rambling three-volume work achieved great popularity, believed that the purpose of the unconscious is to release us from the suffering involved in striving after the fulfillment of our will. If this sounds Buddhist, it is—thanks to the work of Arthur Schopenhauer. As the nineteenth-century German physician and writer Max Nordau (1883) acerbically expressed it, "Schopenhauer is God, and Hartmann is his prophet" (see also Ford 1999; Barnes 1994; Callahan 2004). An important link in the chain that spans from Leibniz to Freud was C. G. Carus (royal physician, philosopher, painter, natural scientist, and psychologist), who articulated a comprehensive theory of the unconscious for the first time.

Freud and his colleagues modeled their concept of the unconscious primarily on the work of those who—like the German physician Anton Mesmer, the founder of dynamic psychiatry; the French neurologist Jean-Martin Charcot at the famous Hôpital Salpêtrière in Paris; the French pharmacist Émile Coué; and the French professor of philosophy and psychotherapist Pierre Janet, the founder of the "new system of dynamic psychiatry"— used hypnosis or suggestion to treat various neuroses (before they were so named). By placing their patients—or clients—under hypnosis, these popular physicians were able to demonstrate certain unconscious processes, especially those of hysteria.

Far from inventing ex nihilo the concept of the unconscious, Freud refined existing notions. Thus, he also adapted Georg Groddeck's idea of *Das Es* (the It), turning it into the psychoanalytical concept of the id. This It is composed of inborn drives and instincts and is entirely unconscious. For Freud, the unconscious is something of an overspilling garbage can–containing material that the conscious individual would find difficult to live with and therefore represses. Because something is unconscious, however, does not mean it is ineffective. Repressed or suppressed impulses continue to have their undesirable effect "underground," emerging in the form of neuroses and psychoses, as well as psychosomatic illness. Through psychoanalytical intervention—comprising the methods of free association and dream analysis— the unconscious content is brought to full consciousness, which supposedly dissolves the underlying psychological problem between the id and the ego.

Carl Jung, a student of Freud, considered this notion too limited, and he expanded the concept of the unconscious to include what he called the "collective unconscious." Jung saw this part of the unconscious as the storehouse of archetypes like anima (the image of the feminine); animus (the image of the masculine); the shadow (consisting of socially undesirable, repressed character traits); the old sage (male or female); and, not least, the Self (as a prime symbol of wholeness and integration). This is also the psychic location where we find the rich imagery of mythology and religion. (See Odajnyk 1993 for a critique of Wilber.)

The notion of the unconscious received a further significant revision at the hands of the Austrian psychiatrist Viktor E. Frankl (1997, 31). Where Freud, as he put it, "saw only unconscious instinctuality," Frankl also attributed a *spiritual* side to the unconscious, which he felt ought to be sharply separated from the instinctual part. It is this spiritual force present in the unconscious that makes a person a "meaning-seeking" creature—the pivotal theme of Frankl's system of logotherapy.

Another important contribution to the Freudian concept of the unconscious was made by the French psychoanalyst Jacques Lacan, who, applying a structuralist approach, drew attention to the homology between the unconscious and language.

The concept of the unconscious in whatever guise has repeatedly come under scholarly and scientific scrutiny, and there are many specialists—who are mostly strongly committed to the materialist-behaviorist paradigm—who question one or the other aspect of it or who even dismiss it as altogether improbable (which in itself is improbable). While the psychological notion of the unconscious includes aspects that are subject to criticism, depth psychology has amassed sufficient clinical evidence to place the existence of the unconscious beyond reasonable doubt. We should also bear in mind the experiential evidence accumulated in the Indian spiritual traditions to which we will turn next.

THE UNCONSCIOUS IN YOGA
AND OTHER INDIAN TRADITIONS

Because Sanskrit and Tamil, the two great languages of traditional India, have no term for the unconscious, Western psychologists have long thought that they also lack the underlying concept. This is not so. We need only study the *Yoga-Sūtra* of Patanjali (for Hindu Yoga) and the Yogācāra school of Mahāyāna Buddhism, as well as the early Pāli literature of Buddhism, to see evidence to the contrary.

The *Brihadāranyaka-Upanishad* (4.4.1ff.) describes the mental process of a dying person, who is "sinking," that is, whose sensory functions are slowly fading out. The mind, so the text states, draws inward to the heart. Next the top of the heart become luminous, then the self, that light, and the life force (*prāna*) exit the body. Exiting usually occurs through one of the portals in the head—if the person is fortunate, through the crown.

An important part of the postmortem process is when "learning and rites, as well as memory, take hold of him [or her]" (4.4.2). Here "memory" (smṛti) likely stands for at least one aspect of the unconscious. From later teachings, we know that the unconscious mind is the seat of the unconscious activators (samskāra). Put differently, the unconscious is the place where a person's desires (kāma) are stored. These desires—or the will—prompt him or her to seek renewed embodiment in the phenomenal world (samsāra). By contrast, according to the Upanishadic teachings, the person who comes to know—or realize—the Self has all desires fulfilled, and rebirth becomes unnecessary. Unfortunately, in the extant Sanskrit literature of that early period, the concept of memory is not developed further along these metaphysical lines.

The next stage of conceptual development in the early Buddhist literature is written in Pāli. Here we find the problematic concept of bhavanga, which has been ably discussed by Peter Harvey (2004, 155ff.). In her path-making book The Birth of Indian Psychology and Its Development in Buddhism, Caroline Rhys Davids (1936, 378) suggested long ago, contrary to the Pāli commentators, that the word is a corruption of the abstract term bhavangya, or "becomingness." The term bhavanga, which is not constructed by joining bhāva ("becoming") to anga ("factor, limb"), occurs only once in the Pāli canon itself (namely, Anguttara-Nikāya 2.79). As Rhys Davids noted, however, it is common in the later (post-Ashokan) literature, where it is generally understood to mean the resting state of the mind. What precisely this means has to be teethed out from the Pāli sutras, the commentaries, and the Abhidhamma texts.

The problem about this notion is that it may suggest a static state, whereas Buddhism is intrinsically what could be called "process philosophy." Rhys Davids (1936, 379) perceptively remarked, "They needed this word 'potential.' They have no Aristotle and did not find it. But they found bhavanga." Apparently, the term was imported into the Anguttara-Nikāya from the later literature. Bhavanga needs to be appreciated as signifying "mental flux," which is present in latent form between the other flickerings of consciousness. As Peter Harvey (2004, 260) has shown, the early Pāli sutra literature contains concepts that prepared the ground for the idea of bhavanga; therefore, there is no need to assume that bhavanga is alien to the Buddha's teaching, though some Theravādins feel ill at ease with this concept.

According to the Buddhist scriptures, the bhavanga is in the nature of discernment, that is, mentation that is not turned toward the senses but is a natural resting state of the mind. It forms a category of the mental process all its own. It is a type of dynamic continuum that focuses on the mental contents carried over from one's last life. It is a critical factor in nonkarmic living and the remains of the mind in deep sleep. It exists in the gap between one meditation level and another. In the later Buddhist literature, the *bhavanga* is equated with the "radiant mind" (*pabhassara-citta*). Cleared of all obstructions, the radiant mind makes for an optimal facilitator to nirvāna.

The term *bhavanga* has been variously translated as "unconscious continuum" (Sarachchandra 1958, 49); "infra-consciousness" (Saddhatissa 1970, 42); "dynamic unconscious" (Jayatilleke 1975, 226); "life continuum" (Ñānamoli and Bodhi 1995); "factor of life" (van Gorkom 1997); "subconsciousness" (online Dhammawiki 2008); "ground of becoming" (Wikipedia 2010); "stream of being" ("Abhidhamma Papers," http://samatha.org 2011); and "life-stream" ("Glossary of Buddhist Terms," http://dharma.ncf.ca 2011).

The early Pāli texts are sufficiently ambiguous to allow for various interpretations according to the Hīnayāna and Mahāyāna schools. In the latter, *bhavanga* came to stand for the "Buddha potential," the *tathāgata-bīja*, or "seed" of enlightenment present in everyone. This is our spiritual potential. In the Yogācāra school of Buddhism, we meet with the concept of *ālaya-vijñāna*, or "storehouse consciousness," which is similar (as discussed earlier).

Switching to Hinduism, Patanjali and Sāmkhya assumed the existence of a most refined part of the mind, similar to the *bhavanga*, called *lingamātra* ("sign only"), which is the same as *buddhi* ("cognition, intellect, will"). This principle is thought to be both luminous (similar in nature to the transcendental Self) and at the same time the receptacle (*āshaya*) of all karmic seeds, or unconscious activators. The *buddhi* is primarily composed of *sattva-guna,* the principle of lucidity at the base of the mind that is normally obscured in the ordinary person. The obscurations spring from our karmas and make us look at ourselves as an ego rather than the Self, as bound rather than free. According to Gaudapāda's *Bhāshya* on Īshvara Krishna's *Sāmkhya-Kārikā* (23), which is the classical text on Sāmkhya philosophy, the *buddhi*—also known as *mahat* ("great [principle]")—has a natural predisposition toward virtue (*dharma*), knowledge (*jnāna*), dispassion (*virāga*), and mastery, or lordship (*aishvarya*).

The higher mind is thus the *yogin*'s greatest ally on the spiritual path. It negotiates between the Self and our empirical nature, that is, our occluded mind. It is the ontogenetic principle (*tattva*) that gives rise to the other twenty-two categories of mental and physical existence that belong to the dimension of insentient materiality (*prakriti*).

This is a fundamental concept of Sāmkhya metaphysics, which we also encounter in the Vedānta tradition. Thus, in his brilliant *Upadesha-Sāhasrī* (2.16.23), Shankara explains that the *buddhi* has the function of ascertainment (*adhyavasāya*), which he probably adopted from the Sāmkhya tradition. In the fourteenth century, the renowned swami Vidyāranya explained in his *Panca-Dashī* (1.20) that the higher mind is in the nature of determination (*nishcaya*). This corresponds to our will. A couple of centuries later, Sadānanda Yogendra offered the same explanation in his *Vedānta-Sāra* (65), and the same elucidation is given in other Vedānta works.

While the *buddhi* is, from a certain perspective, the "higher" mind, it is also the repository (*āshaya*) of all unconscious activators (*samskāra*) or traits (*vāsanā*). They are the particles of which the *buddhi* is made. This is touched on in the *Yoga-Sūtra*, which was composed under the inspiration of Buddhism's process philosophy. Thus, the idea of transformation (*parināma*) is central to Patanjali's psychology-cum-philosophy (see 3.18). He mentioned an ecstatic practice (called *samyama*, or "constraint") through which the *samskāras* can be made conscious.

In particular, he sought to make conscious that activator (or those activators) that were responsible for the calm flow of the mind (see 3.10) at the advanced level of the *nirvicāra-vaishāradya* ecstasy. Thus, everything—even ecstasy—involves the unconscious. In the end, all unconscious processes must be transcended. Freedom lies beyond the impulses of the unconscious, that is, beyond the history and historically conditioned forces of the individual. This is made clear in aphorism 2.10, which states that the subtle form of the causes of affliction (*klesha*)—namely, the unconscious activators—are to be overcome by the involutionary process (*pratiprasava*), which is the backward flow of the *gunas* into the cosmic matrix (*prakriti-pradhāna* = *alinga*).

In the special state of *nirvicāra-vaishāradya* ecstasy, an unconscious activator is created that opposes and gobbles up all other unconscious activators and leads to the "seedless" (*nirbija*) ecstasy (see *Yoga-Sutra* 1.50–51), which is an elevated condition also known as *asamprajnāta-samādhi*.

In Jainism, what we call "mind" is a lower gradation of the conscious principle, or soul (*jīva*), which is obscured by karmic matter to one degree or another. The Jainas do not acknowledge a specific category of existence like the *buddhi* or the *abhanga*. They think that the *jīva* simply functions at various levels, depending on the influx of karmic material.

They think of space as being completely filled by matter (*pudgala*) that consists of numberless, indivisible atoms (*paramānu*). As it goes about its business, the soul picks up matter particles, which are then automatically converted to karma. Although the soul is inherently omniscient, eternal, and of unlimited energy, it manifests empirically with opposite qualities because of the obscuration of karma. This and the 148 forms of karma recognized in Jainism have been ably explained by Helmuth von Glasenapp (1991).

Thus, the souls have different shades (*leshya*) of karma and are accordingly color coded from black to white. This is connected with the fourteen stages of spiritual development. The twelfth stage is free from the passions (*kashāya*)—anger, pride, deceitfulness, and greed—and without attachment (*rāga*). A practitioner apparently remains at this level for less than forty-five minutes (*muhūrta*) before he or she becomes an omniscient adept. At this stage, we can assume that the mind functions similarly to the *buddhi*.

THE UNCONSCIOUS, THE SUBCONSCIOUS, AND THE CONSCIOUS

For most of his life, Freud distinguished three major functional levels of the personality: the unconscious, the preconscious, and the conscious. He saw the unconscious as that part of the mind that contains features that are not ordinarily known to the conscious ego. The unconscious material has been repressed and is primarily inferred from its effects (such as a neurosis). In his book *Die Traumdeutung* (1900), he views the preconscious as a screen between the unconscious and the conscious. The content of the preconscious, consisting of urges or desires that have been pushed into the unconscious mind, is capable of reaching consciousness by various means, notably dream analysis. In later years, Freud made a distinction between the id, the ego, and the superego. The id ("It") is at the core of the unconscious, while the ego is synonymous with consciousness. The superego is that part of the "psychic apparatus" that censors what we do based on how our parents and educators have taught us to behave.

The *Yoga-Sūtra* mentions the term *smṛti* six times. It literally means "memory," but on closer examination, the word is used once to stand for "mindfulness" (see 1.20) and at least three times to stand for something more comprehensive than ordinary memory or remembering (see 1.43, 4.9, and 4.21)—that is, depth memory, or what we would call the unconscious. In other words, in the latter three text passages, the term *smṛti* represents the *buddhi,* which is considered the storehouse of the unconscious activators, though it is difficult to find a place in the Sāmkhya literature where this doctrine is specifically discussed.

CHAPTER 9

The Emotive Side of Yoga

> Yoga practice brings us to a state of ripeness....
> The psychological and emotional obstacles
> get flushed to the surface.
>
> —LAMA PALDEN DROLMA
> (Weintraub 2004, 201–2)

Emotions are slippery and not easy to conceptualize. Yet they are also essential to human life. *Yogins* and *yoginīs* are no strangers to experiencing affects. If anything, they must pay special attention to them and have done so. It is, therefore, especially curious that Yoga has generally been stripped of emotional content, and the practitioners of the yogic traditions are confused with emotionless automatons. Reality is far from this widespread misconception. In his book *The Heyapaksha of Yoga*, P. V. Pathak states,

> In Indian philosophical thought, we find a very meagre treatment of emotions. Its point of view is that of Yoga which includes Ethics. Emotions on account of their opposition to the final goal posited by such a system were never treated except negatively, so that in general an absolute freedom from emotions was enjoined upon anyone aspiring after spiritual attainments. (Pathak 1932, 192)

"Freedom from emotions" has often been misconstrued to mean "without emotions," whereas the position of Yoga is that the adept is simply free in relationship to the affects that arise in the mind. By contrast, the average individual compulsively goes with the emotions and behaves as if he or she were identical to them: "I am joyous," "I am sad," "I am angry," and so forth.

Over the years, the American psychiatrist Mark Epstein, who is also a long-time practitioner of Buddhism, has addressed the problem that spiritual practitioners tend to have with emotion. He notes,

There exists in most of us the desire to be free from the pressures of our emotions.... We assume that the only way to be free of suffering is to be completely rid of it.

This longing for a realm of emotional quiescence has had an important impact on the way we practice Buddhism....

This desire to destroy the offending emotions is also one that is very common in people seeking psychotherapy. (Epstein 2007, 155)

Epstein argues that we ought not to negate, or transcend, our affects or suppress them in meditation but allow them to surface fully while witnessing them through the practice of mindfulness. We should treat them like the itch that sometimes manifests when we want to sit still. We don't scratch it; we simply let it be.

Jack Engler makes much the same point when he says,

We did find a path and a liberation in Buddha-dharma that we have not found anywhere else.... But as time has gone on, we have discovered something else about practice: it is not immune from our personal history, our character, our inner conflicts, and our defensive styles. (Engler 2006, 17)

Because we approach spiritual practice with our emotional baggage, we must not expect to free ourselves from suffering. This was ably discussed by Harvey Aronson (2004). Engler (2006, 25–27) has a list of ten "unhealthy motivations" that Westerners tend to bring to their spiritual practice:

- A quest for perfection and invulnerability
- A fear of individuation
- Avoidance of responsibility and accountability
- Fear of intimacy and closeness
- A substitute for grief and mourning
- Avoidance of feelings (As Engler acknowledges, "Western practioners often have a problem with anger and its derivatives.")
- Passivity and dependence
- Self-punitive guilt
- Devaluing of reason and intellect
- Escape from intrapsychic experience (As Engler states, "States of samādhi that have the power to suppress perception, thinking, imagery, and aversive emotions can be used to keep the mind relatively free of unwanted thoughts and feelings, substituting 'bliss' instead.")

These are the classic "sins" of an ascetic and ways to avoid engaging in life. Clearly, those aspiring to true liberation must do the exact opposite. If necessary, we ought to contemplate seeking help from a sympathetic therapist.

Looking at Tantra, the American psychotherapist Rob Preece, who has spent many years on intensive retreat in the Himalayas, uses Jungian ideas to make the position of Tantric practice intelligible and to correctly understand this tradition as a means of transformation. Rejecting the "sanitized" Tantra in the West, he argues that authentic Tantric practice "is not designed to make our lives safe by providing a neat system" (Preece 2006, 11). Psychological transformation can get messy, and we must be courageous to engage in Tantra.

Preece says, "Even spiritual practices such as meditation can be used to avoid feelings, responsibilities, relationships, and even living fully in our bodies" (13). To engage Tantra squarely, we must be willing "to abandon the habitual disposition of avoiding facing ourselves" (14).

Ever since the *Rig-Veda* appeared, so-called negative emotions like anger, greed, and lust have been singled out as obstructions on the spiritual path. What is negative about them is that they automatically limit awareness to a narrow position. So-called positive emotions have been recommended for conscious cultivation, and they are positive because they do not bind consciousness. Whether or not one recognizes the Vedic teachings as an archaic form of Yoga, they were definitely antecedent even to Buddhism and would have had to contribute to the evolution of the yogic teachings.

EMOTIONS IN PRECLASSICAL YOGA

Preclassical Yoga is a Western-made historiographic category that refers to the spiritual teachings in the ancient, pre-Patanjali Sanskrit and Pāli literature, including the Vedic Samhitās, the Brāhmanas, the Āranyakas, the Upanishads, and the early *dharma-shāstras,* as well as the *Mahābharata* epic (including the *Bhagavad-Gītā*), the *Rāmāyana* epic, and a few other select works.

In the *Bhagavad-Gītā* (16.5), the divine character or fate (*sampad*)—which is contrasted with the demonic character, or fate—is attributed with positive emotions like fearlessness, purity of mind, generosity, self-control, rectitude, nonharming, truthfulness, freedom from anger, peacefulness, noncovetousness, gentleness, modesty, and absence of fickleness. These qualities are said to lead to freedom. By contrast, the undesirable qualities associated with the demonic character are said to lead to bondage, the exact opposite of freedom.

The *Bhagavad-Gītā* (17.1ff.) also has a tripartite scheme that depends on the three *gunas*—*sattva* (the principle of lucidity), *rajas* (the principle of dynamism), and *tamas* (the principle of inertia). These principles shape individuals' character, which can be good, passionate, or dull. Accordingly, they worship the deities, the demigods and demons, or the ancestors or host of elemental spirits. They also turn to scripturally correct asceticism, violent asceticism, or oppressive physical asceticism, and so on. Clearly, those marked by *sattva* are, in Abraham Maslow's (1971) terms, metamotivated. In other words, they have their instincts (or physiologically rooted drives) under firm control.

In the *Rig-Veda*, qualities like (spiritual) heroism or manliness, worshipfulness, respect, contentment, generosity, control, and devotedness are highly valued. This is also true in the Brāhmanas, the Āranyakas, the Upanishads, and the later Yoga literature. How could it be otherwise when we are looking at an ideal human life sub specie aeternitatis?

EMOTIONS IN CLASSICAL YOGA

The historiographic category of Classical Yoga invented by Western scholars refers to the teachings of Patanjali encoded in the *Yoga-Sūtra* (c. 200 C.E.) and the dependent commentarial literature (notably the fifth-century *Yoga-Bhāshya* of Vyāsa and the ninth-century *Tattva-Vaishāradī* of Vācaspati Mishra). The rational flavor of Classical Yoga has misled scholars and students to largely ignore the emotional content of Patanjali's work. Western students—in particular those pouring over Patanjali's *Yoga-Sūtra*—often inquire about Yoga's perspective on emotionality. It is true that Patanjali is curiously silent about major affects such as envy, fear, grief, guilt, hope, humility, jealousy, love, pride, remorse, resentment, shame, and so on. Contrary to popular opinion, however, he does not altogether ignore our affective life, as is evident from the following list of affects mentioned in his *Yoga-Sūtra*:

POSITIVE AFFECTS

· *ānanda*, or "joy/bliss" (1.17)
· *karunā*, or "compassion" (1.33)

- *muditā,* or "gladness" (1.33)
- *sukha,* or "joy/pleasure" (1.33, 2.5, 2.7, 2.46)
- *upekshā,* or "equanimity" (1.33)
- *vishoka,* or "nongrieving" (1.36)
- *hlāda,* or "delight" (2.14)
- *aparigraha,* or "greedlessness" (2.30, 2.39)
- *samtosha,* or "contentment" (2.32, 2.42)
- *saumanasya,* or "gladness" (2.41)

NEGATIVE AFFECTS

- *duhkha,* or "pain/suffering/displeasure" (1.30, 1.33, 2.5, 2.8, 2.16, 2.34)
- *ālasya,* or "sloth" (1.30)
- *styāna,* or "languor" (1.30)
- *daurmanasya,* or "depression/dejection" (1.31)
- *paritāpa,* or "distress" (2.14)
- *tāpa,* or "anguish/distress" (2.15)
- *krodha,* or "anger" (2.34)
- *lobha,* or "greed" (2.34)
- *vaira,* or "enmity/hostility" (2.35)

This binary arrangement of the affects corresponds to the dual nature of the human personality taught in the preclassical Yoga literature.

The affective side is especially addressed in the *kriyā-yoga* text[1] of the *Yoga-Sūtra.* There, we find the set of the five *kleshas,* or causes of suffering, which roughly correspond to the psychological drives. This is most obvious in the disciplined regulation of the sex drive through the virtue of *brahmacarya* or the disciplined regulation of the intake of food through the virtue of moderate eating (*mitāhāra*). The root cause of suffering is spiritual ignorance (*avidyā*), which is tied into "I-am-ness" (*ātmatā*), that is, our misidentification with a particular body, a particular mind, and a particular social identity (role or status). This, in turn, produces attachment (*rāga*) or aversion (*dvesha*). The fifth cause of suffering is the will to live (*abhinivesha*), which Patanjali states in the *Yoga-Sūtra* (2.9) is entrenched even in a sage. We can explain this as the ingrained drive for self-preservation. The affects are interwoven into this drive system.

Before proceeding, a terminological clarification is in order. Affects are composed of temperament, moods, attitudes, feelings, and emotions. Temperament is an individual's basic affective disposition. Thus, a person may be even-tempered, taciturn, quick to anger, and so on. Attitudes are fairly stable predispositions by which we react in a more or less predictable way to stimuli from the environment (people, organizations, material objects, or ideas). Emotions are intense affects, whereas feelings carry a much milder charge. The following table shows a number of affects arranged by degree of intensity, starting on the left with the least intense and ending on the right with the most intense:

relief	pleasure	delight	happiness	joy	bliss
uneasiness	apprehension	fear	panic		terror
sadness	gloominess	dejection	sorrow		grief
liking	infatuation	fondness	passion		love
dislike	disgust	contempt	hatred		loathing
annoyance	irritation	anger	fury		rage
concern	caring	compassion	pity		sympathy
hankering	longing	yearning	coveting		greed
desire	itch	lust	concupiscence		lechery
surprise	amazement	astonishment	wonder		awe

It is possible to argue about the relative assignment of some of these affects, because we tend to use terms differently and also because cultures may place different values on a given affect. There are many more affective states that we animate in our interpersonal behavior but that are not mentioned in this list.

In composing his Sanskrit work, Patanjali adopted an aphoristic (*sūtra*) style that forced him to be incredibly succinct, but this does not explain why he did not discuss the affects in any detail.

Patanjali leaves most of the positive (desirable) and negative (undesirable) affects unexplained, and their exact meaning is not obvious from the context in which they appear. In the case of the negative affects, the lack of explanation is not an immediate handicap, with the notable exception of *duhkha*. In Sanskrit, this term has numerous connotations—unease, discomfort, sorrow, pain, suffering—though all imply strong unpleasantness and undesirability. Patanjali (2.16) tells us that what is to be overcome is future suffering. We may not be able to stop our present experience of *duh-kha,* which is the result of corresponding past actions in either this or an earlier lifetime. But we can always lay the groundwork for better conditions in the near or distant future, including another lifetime.

However, the absence of a clear explanation of the positive affects is, in at least some cases, problematic. It matters, for instance, whether *saumanasya* stands for "gladness," as typically translated, or "positive mind-set," which is closer to the original meaning of "good mentation" (from *su* denoting "good" and *manas* denoting "mind").

Here we must recall that the *Yoga-Sūtra* was intended as a *vade mecum* for Yoga ascetics, so it appropriately focuses on the higher processes of Yoga, especially meditation and the various levels of ecstatic unification (*samādhi*). Patanjali simply took it for granted that anyone attempting the eightfold path, as he mapped it out, was emotionally stable and ready for the practice of sensory inhibition, concentration, meditation, and ecstasy. In other words, he showed no interest in the psychopathology of ordinary individuals and mentioned negative affects only insofar as they might arise as obstacles on the spiritual path.

Patanjali deals with affects summarily via the previously mentioned categories of attachment (*rāga,* 1.37, 2.3, 2.7) and aversion (*dvesha,* 2.3, 2.8), explaining the former as "that which rests on pleasure" and the latter as "that which rests on pain/suffering." From his perspective, neither pleasure nor pain is deemed worthy of cultivation. Rather, the *yogin* seeks to promote a mental state in which the seesaw play of pleasure and pain is transcended in favor of a condition in which mental activity is controlled (*niruddha*). For the yogic process to be ultimately fruitful, control has to happen at three levels:

1. *vritti-nirodha,* or "control of the fluctuations" through the cultivation of meditation.
2. *pratyaya-nirodha,* or "control of (higher) ideation" in the state of ecstasy through the cultivation of formless ecstasy (*asamprajnāta-samādhi*). The concept of *pratyaya* extends to the emotions.
3. *samskāra-nirodha,* or "control of the subconscious activators" through the event of the seedless ecstasy (*nirbīja-samādhi*).

These three levels of control indicate a progressive deconditioning of the mind through ever higher levels of mental control to the point of actual enlightenment, or *kaivalya*. For Patanjali, this state apparently coincided with the recovery of our transcendental Identity (as the Self, or *purusha*)— that aspect of our being that is free from all conditioning because it is devoid of the mind itself. The *purusha,* or ultimate Awareness monad, is utterly transcendental and thus, strictly speaking, nonhuman.

According to Patanjali's opening definition in aphorism 1.2, Yoga consists of the control (*nirodha*) of the whirls of the mind, the *citta-vrittis.* But these are very specific types of mental activity, namely correct perception (*pramāna*), misperception (*viparyaya*), imagination (*vikalpa*), sleep (*nidrā*), and memory (*smṛti*). To the consternation of many Western students of Yoga, emotions are simply not included in the *vritti* category.

Even when Patanjali talks about the motivating forces, he refers only to the five *kleshas,* or causes of affliction, which, as stated earlier, comprise ignorance, I-am-ness, attachment, aversion, and the will to live (or survival instinct). Attachment/attraction and aversion are, in contemporary terms, "like" and "dislike." This dualism represents a simplistic model of affective/ motivational behavior. Some psychologists, therefore, speak of three basic response patterns: "going toward" (love), "going against" (hate), and "going away" (withdrawal). Ordinarily, we never seem to be in a completely neutral disposition, and Patanjali appears to agree with this. We always experience shades of either attraction or aversion. Neutrality comes into play only when the yogic process of self-transcendence is involved, leading to a profound and persistent mood of equanimity (*upekshā*), or calm indifference.

Until we attain this state of even-temperedness, however, we must expect varyingly strong emotions to arise, particularly in our interpersonal activities. Patanjali acknowledged this by insisting that spiritual practitioners begin by harmonizing their social interactions through the five moral disciplines (*yama*)—nonharming, truthfulness, nonstealing, chastity, and greedlessness. These are supposed to be practiced under any circumstance and without exception, which is easier said than done. In fact, the moral disciplines are very demanding and involve a complete retraining of our motivations. Because of the great popularity of Hatha-Yoga postures, many Western practitioners completely bypass the moral disciplines and thus the spiritual process itself, for the five *yamas* are not merely moral rules but cornerstones of spiritual life.

Patanjali tells us clearly in aphorism 2.33 that if our practice of the moral disciplines is threatened by undesirable mental states (*vitarka*) based in negative affects, we should immediately cultivate their opposites—a practice known as *pratipaksha-bhāvana*. Thus, when our heart is filled with anger and we are on the verge of breaking the virtue of nonharming (either in deed, word, or thought), then we should at once engender thoughts of kindness and love toward the object of our anger. Unfortunately, the *Yoga-Sūtra* is not specific about how to do this. Positive psychology, as developed by Barbara L. Fredrickson, follows a similar principle and may help us out. Fredrickson (2009, 21, 25) writes, "Positivity opens us. The first core truth about positive emotions is that they open our hearts and our minds, making us more receptive and more creative"; and, "Positivity broadens and builds. It transforms people and helps them become their best. And when at their best, people live longer."

We can imagine that Patanjali might have advised his disciples to remember that they are the transcendental Awareness and mistakenly identify with the arising emotion of anger. Next he might have asked them to sit still, take a few deep breaths, and use the energy of anger by converting it into a powerful visualization of radiating positive energy and thoughts toward the person or persons who are the object of that anger. Of course, this approach presupposes a certain level of emotional control. An individual who is subject to fits of rage is incapable of assuming the position of the transcendental Witness. But then, Patanjali and other Yoga masters like him were probably not interested in teaching unqualified disciples.

What can we do when an intense emotional response is triggered in us? Yoga is clear that we must not just "let it rip." Unchecked expression of intense emotions—especially anger—is manifestly disruptive, harmful, and also physically and psychologically debilitating. But neither do the Yoga masters expect us to repress anything, which is unproductive and damaging. They would not quarrel with our using a psychological technique for managing strong emotions until regular Yoga practice has brought more balance to our mental life. Once a certain measure of emotional stability and inner witnessing has been achieved, the technique of *pratipaksha-bhāvana,* or cultivating the opposite, works well.

Emotions are an integral part of human existence. In their pursuit of enlightenment, Yoga practitioners are not expected to excise all emotionality. Rather they must, step by step, transcend the false identity of the ego-personality and thereby overcome negative emotions and refine or ennoble their emotional life. In this way, they also effectively contribute to greater social harmony and world peace.

THE NINE SENTIMENTS OF BHAKTI-YOGA

An important branch of post-Classical Yoga is Bhakti-Yoga. It was first enunciated in the *Bhagavad-Gītā* (c. 400 B.C.E.) and then in the *Bhāgavata-Purāna* (c. 900 C.E.); the *Hari-Vamsha* (c. 1000 C.E.); the *Bhakti-Sūtra* of Nārada (c. 1100 C.E.); the *Shrī-Bhāshya* (1200 C.E.), which is Rāmānuja's sagacious commentary on the *Brahma-Sūtra;* and the late medieval *Bhakti-Sūtra* of Shāndilya (see Marchand 2006).

According to the *Bhāgavata-Purāna* or *Shrīmad-Bhāgavata,* Bhakti-Yoga is associated with the nine sentiments. These are also found in the theory of aesthetics:

- *shringāra,* or "love"
- *hāsya,* or "laughter"
- *karuna,* or "pathos"
- *raudra,* or "wrath"
- *vīra,* or "heroism"
- *bhayānaka,* or "fear"
- *vibhatsa,* or "disgust"
- *adbhuta,* or "wonder"
- *shānta,* or "tranquillity"

It is clear that these sentiments were borrowed from aesthetics. They fall into two broad categories: love, laughter, pathos, heroism, wonder, and tranquillity are desirable; wrath, fear, and disgust are undesirable. These are also known as the *sthāyi-bhāvas,* or "permanent dispositions." Each sentiment (*rasa,* or "taste") has various secondary moods (*vibhāva*):

- *shringāra,* or "love": devotion, appreciation
- *hāsya,* or "laughter": joy, humor
- *karuna,* or "pathos": compassion, sympathy
- *raudra,* or "wrath": irritation, violence
- *vīra,* or "heroism": courage, determination
- *bhayānaka,* or "fear": anxiety, nervousness
- *vibhatsa,* or "disgust": depression, dissatisfaction
- *adbhuta,* or "wonder": astonishment, curiosity
- *shānta,* or "tranquillity": peacefulness, relaxation

EMOTIONAL ASPECTS IN BUDDHIST AND JAINA YOGA

In ancient times, the ideal of spiritual discipline—as upheld, for instance, by the Buddha—required such intense focus that it was typically pursued in solitude, away from the distracted and distracting crowds. It is all the more surprising that the four dwellings of Brahma (*brahma-vihāra*) were known not only in Buddhism but also in other traditions. In *Buddhist Thought in India*, Edward Conze (1967, 80) notes that they "are not specifically Buddhistic, occur in the *Yoga Sūtras* of Patañjali [see 1.33], and may have been borrowed from other Indian religious systems.... For centuries they lay outside the core of the Buddhist effort, and the orthodox élite considered them as subordinate practices, rather incongruous with the remainder of the training which insisted on the unreality of beings and persons,... and in the Mahāyāna became sufficiently prominent to alter the entire structure of the doctrine."

The emotions may originally have lain "outside the core of the Buddhist effort," but they were certainly not entirely absent. That the four *brahma-vihāras* were so readily assimilated is a sign that the conceptual ground was ready for them. I would go further and say that the Buddha's teaching was eminently moral, so the art of taming the mind necessarily involved the control of the emotions. To test my opinion, I once again started to read the *Dīgha-Nikāya* discourses and encountered an abundance of references to our emotional life; I needed no further convincing.

The *Majjhīma-Nikāya* (59.3ff.) contains the story of the carpenter Pancakanga, who asked the venerable Udāyin how many kinds of feeling (*vedanā*) the Buddha had taught. The two started to argue. Udāyin stated three, and Pancakanga insisted on two. When Ananda, who had overheard the dispute, went to the Buddha for clarification, the Buddha said that he had mentioned 2, 3, 5, 6, 18, 36, and 108 kinds of feeling in various discourses. This goes to show the importance of feeling.

Feeling is one of the five *skandhas* ("heaps," or "piles"): *rūpa* ("form," meaning the body); *vedanā* (also translated as "sensation," which I think is wrong); *samjnā* (perception); *samskāra* ("formation," meaning the unconscious motivators); and *vijnāna* (consciousness). These are something like Weberian ideal types. The first is shorthand for the body, and the others are aspects of the various mental factors. The idea is to provide summary labels for our diverse somatic and mental processes to drive home the point that they are all *anātman*, that is, lacking a substantial essence.

The Mahāyāna teachers added to this the cultivation of positive emotions like friendliness (*maitrī*), compassion (*karunā*), joy (*muditā*), and impartiality (*upekshā*), or what in Hindu Yoga is known as *sama-darshana* ("same vision")—that is, the attitude of being friendly toward everyone and having no expectations of them. These emotions are to be practiced against the backdrop of the grand ideal of emptiness: Although the ego/self is a chimera, the social emotions are to be practiced, but there will be no one wanting acknowledgment or approval, because the ego has been transcended. The reason including friendliness is that the ordinary person's egocentricism is a function of his or her unenlightenment, whereas the enlightened being, who is fully settled, has a surfeit of energy and attention to address the suffering of others.

In the *Trimshikāvijnapti-Bhāshya* (38), Sthiramati, who lived in the sixth century, made the following point:

Karma and the emotions are the reason for the way of the world, and among them the emotions are the principal condition.... But when the power of the emotions has been exhausted then the world will cease to exist. (Guenther 1976, 9)

Arthur J. Deikman, whose views on the witnessing Self were quoted earlier, has this pertinent comment to make about the role of feelings in psychotherapy:

Anxiety, joy, anger, sadness ... constitute ... the emotional self. At times this aspect seems closest to the core of our being, for nothing seems to be more completely our self than our emotion. (Deikman 1983, 93)

In other scriptures of Hindu, Buddhist, and Jaina Yoga, many more affects are mentioned. As a rule, however, we are seldom given precise instructions on how to deal with affects, particularly strong emotions.

Jainism, because of its ascetic tenor, is more in harmony with Classical Yoga than with Mahāyāna Buddhism. The virtues, which are grouped into "vows" (*vrata*), give us the best clue about the numerous vices recognized in Jainism. Thus, under the vow of nonharming, the wrong behaviors of keeping a being in captivity, beating, mutilating, overloading, and depriving of food and drink are mentioned. Under the vow of truthfulness, we find the wrong behaviors of telling the untruth about a virgin; of telling the untruth about a cow, a piece of land, or a valuable piece of property in one's custody; bearing false witness; using speech that is tactless, insulting, and harmful; and so on. Such behaviors are associated with ignoble emotions and are not conducive to spiritual liberation. Through proper moral conduct, the influx of karma is gradually reduced and the way to liberation is prepared.

CHAPTER 10

The Subtle Body
Its Structures and Functions

> *Eì estin sōma psuchikon estin kai pneumatikón.*
> [There is an enlivened (natural) body,
> and there is a spiritual/breathing body.]
>
> —1 Cor. 15:44

Yoga is unthinkable without the subtle body. The question is, how should we understand it? In the broadest sense, we can take it to be a nonmaterial to semimaterial medium that couples the physical body with the immaterial mind. In Sāmkhya-based Yoga and other Hindu systems, it is analogous to the role of the higher mind (*buddhi*), which mediates between the brain-dependent mind (*manas*) and the Self.

The idea of a subtle body is found in many traditional cultures of the world—both primitive and more advanced. This has been explored by the Dutch philosopher and scholar J. J. Poortman in his four-volume study entitled *Vehicles of Consciousness,* which has a foreword by the well-known parapsychologist Wilhelm H. C. Tenhaeff. The idea that the soul is closely attached to or in tandem with the body, and that it can occasionally and must at death separate itself, belongs to both folklore and occultism. This is known by the German word *doppelgänger,* which literally means "double-goer."

On the basis of his materials, Poortman (1978) distinguished six metaphysical perspectives, or what he called "standpoints," within hylic pluralism, which is one of the more interesting conclusions of his research:

1. *Alpha standpoint.*
   This position, also known as monistic materialism, is defined by the interrelated ideas that all of reality is material in the ordinary sense of the term, that consciousness is an epiphenomenon of matter, and that the human being is machinelike. This perspective characterizes the dominant scientific paradigm.

2. *Beta standpoint.*

This opinion revolves around the idea that there are two kinds of matter—one ordinary and the other more subtle and invisible to the senses under normal circumstances. Poortman referred to the philosophy of Democritus, Epicurus, Lucretius, Panaetius, Tertullian, and Thomas Hobbes, as well as that of the Dutch parapsychologist K. H. E. de Jong, as expressed in the book *Die andere Seite des Materialismus* (The Other Side of Materialism, 1932).

3. *Gamma standpoint.*

This perspective assumes that God is immaterial but the soul is made of fine matter. Poortman cited Bernard of Clairvaux, Saint Ambrose, and the *Bhagavad-Gītā*, as well as theosophy as examples of this view. Although Buddhism does not acknowledge God, Poortman places most of its schools here, but it may deserve a standpoint of its own. He wrestled with the various Buddhist philosophies over many pages that make illuminating reading.

4. *Delta standpoint.*

This position, which accepts a clear, threefold division of existence (coarse matter, fine matter, immateriality), insists on the immateriality of the soul and God and the corporeality, or materiality, of everything else. Poortman detected this view in the works of Plotinus, Sāmkhya and Vedānta, Saint Augustine, Francis Bacon, Paracelsus, Jakob Böhme, the Romantics, and Gustav Fechner. Because Jainism does not affirm God, Poortman did not include it here.

5. *Epsilon standpoint.*

This viewpoint represents strict dualism, which we find in the writings of Saint Thomas Aquinas, René Descartes, and Benedict de Spinoza.

6. *Zeta standpoint.*

This standpoint, which could also be called monistic spirituality, is the kind of idealism that marks the beliefs of Bishop George Berkeley and a few others.

I will not argue over the assignment of representative systems and individual thinkers to these six categories or whether the six categories are sufficient to cover all actualities, but together these systems and individuals stand for a spectrum of metaphysical possibilities ranging from sheer materialism to pure spiritualism. In this book, we are mostly looking at systems representing the delta standpoint, to which I would also assign the *Bhagavad-Gītā*, because it clearly assumes that God and the soul are immaterial and that there is a realm of subtle matter in addition to the material world.

NINETEENTH- TO TWENTIETH-CENTURY RESEARCH

Aspects, or functions, of the subtle body first aroused interest among scientists in the late eighteenth century with the invention of mesmerism by Franz Anton Mesmer, a German physician. He attempted to heal physical and mental diseases by means of what he called "animal magnetism," the forerunner of hypnosis. Mesmer, who drew considerable crowds in Paris, sought to heal by making "magnetic passes" around a patient's body. He speculated that everything is suspended in a "universal fluid" that could be projected through the hands. A government-appointed commission of renowned scientists investigated Mesmer and concluded that his magnetic fluid was a myth. It did not help that Mesmer was typically dressed in a magician's gown, complete with wand. Mesmer found the commission's charge preposterous and insisted that his method worked and was helping people. In 1789, he left Paris to escape the French Revolution.

In 1831, a second French government commission concluded that mesmerism, which was by then quite widespread, could not be rejected out of hand. While Mesmer and his many students and imitators healed and no doubt regaled the masses by "massaging" the fluidic medium, the Romantics, partly via Western hermetism and partly via Eastern teachings, promoted the idea of a subtle body.

In 1842, the Scottish surgeon James Braid interpreted the effects of mesmerism in terms of hypnotic suggestion, which was the explanation and method taken over by depth psychology at the end of the century. An important figure around that time was the German industrialist-chemist Karl Freiherr von Reichenbach. In the 1840s, he started to experiment with magnetic induction, using photography, to document the existence of a luminous force that he named *od,* the equivalent of *prāna.*

To this period also belongs one of the great heroes of conventional psychology: Gustav Theodor Fechner, who is celebrated as the father of experimental psychology. After what seemed to amount to a spiritual crisis during which he completely lost his eyesight and apparently went insane, Fechner recovered and burst into print with a book called *Nanna: Über das Seelenleben der Pflanzen* (Nanna: The Soul Life of Plants, 1848). He also enthusiastically participated in séances, which supposedly put the mediums in touch with departed spirits; the events were made popular by the psychically gifted Fox sisters of Hydesville, New York. This trio inadvertently turned a "pastime" into the hugely fashionable movement of spiritualism.

Toward the end of the nineteenth century, the Theosophical Society entered this popular arena, warning against "psychism" versus genuine spirituality. The society's many pioneering publications were on Indian wisdom, not least the first translations of classic texts on Yoga.[1] The twentieth century opened with the seminal works on Tantra by Sir John Woodroffe (see Taylor 2001), who acquired his knowledge about Indian philosophy while serving as a high-court judge in Calcutta, and K. Nārayānaswami Aiyar's *Thirty Minor Upanishads* (1980). Woodroffe's book *The Serpent Power* (1919), written under the pseudonym Arthur Avalon, included a lengthy and knowledgeable treatment of the subtle body and its structures according to the Hindu yogic teachings.

The early decades of that century also witnessed the East-West miscellany of Ramacharaka (a pseudonym for William Walker Atkinson); Pierre Bernard (dubbed "Oom the Omnipotent" by the American press); Swami Mukerji; and others. At any rate, by approximately the mid-1920s, when Carl Jung (1929), Oscar A. H. Schmitz (1923), and others delved deeply into Indian and Far Eastern wisdom, the yogic idea of a subtle duplicate of the physical body was no longer revolutionary.

New Thought, which originated in America around the terminal decades of the nineteenth century, was the first religious (Christian-derived) mass movement based on mental healing ("mind cure"). This movement, which was carried chiefly by women and became increasingly concerned with lifestyle issues, was originally influenced by Immanuel Swedenborg and Jakob Böhme. It flowed into the so-called New Age movement that emerged in the late 1960s and was a mixture of psychedelic thought; shamanism; secular, quasi-religious, fringe methodologies (for example, Erhard seminars, Silva Mind Control, and Scientology); and Eastern spiritual teachings (such as Zen, Sufism, Hare Krishna, and Transcendental Meditation). With so many New Age writers enthusiastically plunging into the subject of Hinduism, it seems imperative to allow India's yogic traditions to speak for themselves, which I will do next.

PRĀNA AND PRĀNIC STRUCTURES

Prāna is cosmic energy, which is everywhere and in everything. The subtle body is structured life energy, as are its "wheels" (*cakra*) and conduits (*nādī*). The former are concentric concentrations of layered life energy, and the latter are transport lines of *prāna*. *Nādī* are *prānic* arcs in the subtle body but are generally thought of as conduits.

In the late 1980s, Beverly Rubik, who earned a PhD in biophysics, and her collaborators worked on promising research in the area of the interconnection of mind and matter. Proceedings of an international conference hosted by her Center for Frontier Sciences, which was established in 1987, contained a series of promising contributions. Rubik (1989) herself reported on a fascinating experiment with the bona fide healer Olga Worrall in which Worrall did "laying on of hands" on normal, chemically inhibited, or nutritionally starved cultures of *Salmonella typhimurium* with significant results. Unfortunately, Rubik's center was short-lived at Temple University in Philadelphia, Pennsylvania, and her research there has been all but forgotten.

Seven years after Frederic William Henry Myers's death in 1908, the subtle body—or a part of it, the aura—came under scientific scrutiny. Walter J. Kilner, MD, a physician at St. Thomas's Hospital in London, stumbled on this phenomenon while doing electrical experiments with a viewing filter stained with dicyanin dye.

HINDU YOGA

The first time we hear about the subtle body in the Indian literature is in post-Vedic times, though we may assume that it existed from the Paleolithic era on, wherever ocher burial practices were known. Hence in the Vedas, the departed spirit, whose human body has been burned on the funeral pyre, is enjoined to unite with an immaterial body (*tanū*). As Jeanine Miller (1974, 138) conjectured in her excellent book *The Vedas: Harmony, Meditation and Fulfilment,* we may equate this with the later *linga-sharīra* ("sign body"). The subtle body is explained in the *Sāmkhya-Kārikā* (40) as follows:

> The sign [body] previously arisen [that is, in a former incarnation], unbound, unrestrained, inclusive of the subtle elements, the great one (*mahat,* or *buddhi*), etc., transmigrates endowed with conditions [but exists] without enjoyment.

The sign body has no self-enjoyment because it is the Spirit (*purusha*) that enjoys all experiences. These are merely presented to the sign body. It extends from the *mahat* down to the ego principle, the lower mind (*manas*), the subtle elements, and the ten sense capacities. The conditions (*bhāva*) total fifty (see *Sāmkhya-Kārikā* 46–51), and this section has been marked as a later interpolation.

The Vedic *tanū* was apparently subject to the departed's desire or will, as is suggested by the prayers invoking Agni or Yama. The Vedic hymns also indicate that this postmortem body is made of light, as are the heavenly regions. This ancient tradition survived into the era of the Upanishads. Here, we find a more differentiated treatment in the *Brihadāranyaka-Upanishad* (4.3.19), which is a pre-Buddhist text. Even more vivid accounts can be found in the early post-Buddhist texts, notably the *Katha-Upanishad* (2.1.13; 2.3.16).

BUDDHIST AND JAINA YOGA

In Buddhist Yoga, the subtle body receives close attention in the Tantric schools (see Dasgupta 1974). Many of the ideas and practices are the same as in Hindu Yoga. Vajrayāna Buddhism also knows of the *kundalinī* process and regards it as central to Tantric work. As in Hindu Tantra, the body is viewed as the abode of reality and epitomizes the cosmos at large. The body is recognized as the medium for realizing truth. According to the eighth-century *Hevajra-Tantra* (1.12), "great knowledge is located in the body."

The major difference from Hindu Yoga is that there are four instead of the usual seven *cakras*. This is connected with the four varieties of bliss, or the four seals (*mudrā*): *karma-, dharma, mahā-,* and *samaya-mudrā* and, in ascending order, the goddesses Locanā, Māmakī, Pāndarā, and Tārā. The four *cakras* (and the crown *cakra*) are as follows:

1. Lumbar plexus at the level of the navel, corresponding to the Hindu *manipura cakra*
2. Cardiac plexus at the base of the heart corresponding to the Hindu *anāhata cakra*
3. Laryngeal plexus at the level of the throat corresponding to the Hindu *vishuddha cakra*
4. Pharyngeal plexus behind the nose and corresponding to the Hindu *ājnā cakra*

5. Protuberance on the crown of the head (*ushnīsha-kamala*) corresponding to the Hindu *sahasrāra cakra*

Even in Hindu Tantra, the *kundalinī* is often described as being generated somewhere near the navel. Thus, the Buddhist Tantra model is not entirely peculiar. The two are also different regarding the number of petals associated with each *cakra*.

The Buddhists furthermore acknowledge the existence of numerous *nādī*—the figure seventy-two thousand is mentioned—of which thirty-two are individually named; this corresponds to Hindu Tantra. In addition, there are innumerable secondary conduits (*upanādī*). Of the thirty-two conduits, only three are considered important: the central conduit (*avadhutī*), through which flows the *bodhicitta*[2] that corresponds to the *sushumnā;* the left conduit (*lalanā*), which is associated with wisdom (*prajñā*) and corresponds to the *idā;* and the right conduit (*rasanā*), which is associated with skillful means (*upāya,* meaning compassion) and corresponds to the *pingalā.* The *kanda* ("bulb"), in which the seventy-two thousand *nādī* originate, is said to be situated below the center of the navel.

Uniquely Buddhist is the association of the three *kāyas—nirmāna-kāya, sambhoga-kāya,* and *dharma-kāya*—with the *cakras* (at the navel, the throat, and the heart, respectively). Also, the *sahaja-kāya* is naturally associated with the crown center.

CHAPTER 11

The Serpent Power
The Goddess in the Body

Kundalinī Yoga is of great scientific, parapsychic, and metaphysical interest.

—Sir John Woodroffe
(Rele 1927, ix)

A concept central to many schools of Tantra and Hatha-Yoga, which is an offshoot of the Tantric tradition, is that of "serpent power," or "coiled power" (*kundalinī-shakti*). Metaphysically, this fundamental spiritual energy (*shakti*) is the microcosmic replica of the macrocosmic *devī*, or the goddess, who is the divine partner of Shiva. We have no Western equivalent of this psychocosmic energy, though the concept of libido in depth psychology or that of élan vital in Henri Bergson's philosophy is analogous to it.

We know that Sigmund Freud sexualized the libido, which, strictly speaking, represents just a slice of our total life—even if it is an important slice. The concept of élan vital has more to recommend itself, even though we must understand it as a metaphysical speculation. Bergson intended for it to mean a "current of consciousness" that has inserted itself into matter to create countless bodily forms shaped by evolution. In his later years, Bergson saw the élan vital as God understood as pure dynamics.

The goddess—or female pole of the masculine Shiva—is thought to be responsible for all aspects of creation. Whereas Shiva represents transcendental Awareness (which does not evolve), Shakti stands for the core power that is behind every evolving thing and makes existence possible. Shiva and Shakti are inseparable, and their strict differentiation happens only at the empirical level.

In Tantric biopsychology, the dynamic *shakti* pole is to be found at the base of the bodily axis (corresponding to the spine), while the static *shiva* pole is conceptualized at the crown of the head. Some scholars interpret the Vedic *kunamnamā*—mentioned only once in the *Rig-Veda* (10.136.7)—as an early expression for the *kundalī*, or *kundalinī* (see also Miller 1980, 17–30). Most proceed more conservatively and prefer to associate the emergence of the coiled energy with the early Tantric goddess Kubjikā (Crooked One)[1] perhaps about 700 C.E. Because of the prominent Vedic bipolar ideology and ritualism, a much earlier introduction of the *kundalinī* idea in the Vedic era is conceivable but not likely.[2] To my knowledge, the concept is not referred to in the *Mahābharata* (200 B.C.E.–400 C.E.) nor does it appear in Patanjali's *Yoga-Sūtra* (c. 200 C.E.).

The polarization between Shiva and Shakti in the human body has immediate practical psychological consequences. Freud formulated his libido theory in the years following 1892, adopting the concept of libido as "sexual drive" from sexologist Alfred Moll. In keeping with his theoretical edifice, he was endeavoring to quantify (and measure) this drive. He believed that when a person amassed a certain quantity of libido, which he thought was produced by the seminal vesicles, it rose to the brain where it was converted into psychic libido. When this conversion failed, it manifested in anxiety neuroses. Freud felt that the libido was a fundamental energy that fed both the conscious and the unconscious.

The French philosopher Henri Bergson's idea of élan vital is similarly problematic. This life energy dwells and mobilizes the whole universe, pushing it into continuous developmental differentiation. This concept is intuitive and must be understood intuitively. Ultimately, élan vital is God working in and through Nature (which is purposive).

GOPI KRISHNA AND MODERN RESEARCH[3]

The *kundalinī* was first introduced to the Western world in the early years of the twentieth century by the work of Sir John Woodroffe, notably in his book *The Serpent Power* (1919), which stimulated Carl Jung's interest in this phenomenon.

Vasant G. Rele, in his prominent book *The Mysterious Kundalini* (1927), applied Western anatomy and physiology to this Eastern phenomenon. In an opinion printed in the front of the book, C. H. L. Meyer, MD, who was a professor of physiology at Grant Medical College in Bombay, states,

> I have read this work of my old pupil ... with the deepest interest. His views ... are of fascinating interest. The work has involved much study and thought and has been carried out with great ability. (Rele 1927, vii)

In his foreword to the 1927 edition, Woodroffe (ix–xi), a superior court judge in India and an intrepid researcher of Tantra, admits that he may have underrated "the value of some adverse criticism of this Yoga" in his original edition. He goes on to say that "Kundalini Yoga is of great scientific, parapsychic, and metaphysical interest" and that Rele's book is a "conscientious and valuable enquiry." At the same time, he disagrees with him that the *kundalini* is the right vagus nerve. Instead, he correctly proposes that it is a form of *shakti* (divine power). But he admits that "if I am right in this, that is not to say that the Author's theory is without value" and that "he has made out a case for examination." Woodroffe's vacillating tone suggests that he wanted to cover all bets.

In 1932, Jung held a seminar on the *kundalini* in which he explored some of its psychological aspects (see Shamdasani 1996). The *kundalini* was reintroduced and made popular in the West through the autobiography of the Kashmiri pundit Gopi Krishna, a government official.[4] In 1937, Krishna, a meditator for seventeen years, experienced an unexpected, sudden, and cataclysmic awakening (*bodhana*) of the *kundalini* that caused havoc in his body and mind for a long time and, in the end, positively revolutionized his physiological and mental life. James Hillman's psychological commentary probably opened important doors for Gopi Krishna in Western scientific circles.

In a subsequent book titled *The Real Nature of Mystical Experience,* Krishna had this to say about the final state he had achieved:

> I do not claim to see God, but I am conscious of a Living Radiance both within and outside myself.... It persists even in my dreams. (Krishna 1979, 28)

Not surprisingly, he was so mesmerized by this experience that he not only wrote a compelling autobiography but also sought to understand it from a scientific point of view. In the late 1960s, he managed to enlist the interest of the prominent German scientist Carl Friedrich von Weizsäcker in this extraordinary phenomenon. In his introduction to *The Biological Basis of Religion and Genius,* Weizsäcker, the then-director of the Max Planck Institute in Munich, says about Gopi Krishna,

> He answered precise questions precisely, and in a sometimes surprising way and with a deeply human sincerity, which was often enhanced by a smile. His presence was good for me. (Weizsäcker 1972, 42–43)

He also addresses an issue that looms large in Krishna's presentation of the role of sexual energy in the *kundalinī* process and evolution:

> It has been a thesis of European science since the nineteenth century that the development of animals occurs through lines of physical descent, a thesis which Gopi Krishna as well as other evolutionist Indian thinkers (especially Shri Aurobindo) simply have adopted. But the notion that there is a special "force of evolution" contradicts a dominant doctrine in contemporary biology, the Darwinian theory of natural selection. (Weizsäcker 1972, 25)

Weizsäcker goes on to explain that there is an enormous contrast between Krishna's almost Reichian physiology of *prānic* energy from the sexual center to the brain (the main evolutionary organ) and Freud's psychological idea of sublimation of libido. The problem, according to Weizsäcker, lay in the fact that the natural scientist has no idea what *prāna* is. In the meantime, the concept of *prāna* has become more familiar but not necessarily lost its tenuous quality. Perhaps Weizsäcker would not have been so confounded if Krishna had written about the process of *ūrdhva-retas,* or "upward[-streaming] semen," in terms of nervous impulses going from the sacroiliac plexus—which is correlated but not identical with the *mūlādhara-cakra*—to the cerebrum (the "thousand-petalled lotus").

Gopi Krishna looked on the *kundalinī* both as an evolutionary (biological) mechanism and as the great goddess. Not fully conversant with modern advances in biology and anthropological thought, he used expressions and metaphors that meant very little to specialists unless, like Weizsäcker, they were sensitive to different styles of thinking and able to translate "strange" notions into current scientific jargon. Thus, the pundit's concept of an evolutionary energy could readily have been couched in terms of the transmission of chromosomal patterns through the reproductive process (although possibly at the cost of the spiritual dimension of the *kundalinī* phenomenon). But the really problematic issue is that the agent, or direct medium, of this evolutionary change—the *prāna,* which according to Krishna (1979, 107) is "an intelligent vital medium that, using the elements and compounds of the material world as bricks and mortar, acts as the architect of organic structures"—is so far not observable. For this reason, Weizsäcker (1972, 29) recommended the translation of the subjective physical sensations into physiological concepts, contending that "this may at least become a prolegomenon to a physiological classification of Prana."

This is always possible, but again to avoid mere speculation, we would have to retranslate those physiological concepts into subjective experiences, which, at the present stage of physiology, does not look very promising. Not all scientists are as skeptical about the *prāna* concept as Weizsäcker, and in recent years, sophisticated electronic equipment has been used to verify *prānic* currents in the body (see, for example, Motoyama 1978a). It is not clear, however, whether these currents are identical to the *nādī* of *prāna* as conceptualized in Yoga and Tantra. Nor is it evident whether the "bioplasma" studied by some avant-garde researchers is synonymous with *prāna*. The field is wide open for interpretation and speculation, and obviously more investigations are necessary to throw light on this highly interesting and important but obscure phenomenon. At any rate, Krishna's experience, in some sense, supplies an explanation for Freud's abstract notion of sublimation.

Krishna's account (1971, 117) is confusing, because he interpreted the *kundalinī* as entirely biological in nature but failed to explain how a biological force can "transcend the normal limits of the human brain." One may ask how this admittedly "psychic" energy can rise in the axial channel (*sushumnā-nādī*) of the body, which the author wrongly and explicitly equates with the spinal cord. It is also perplexing that, in the book *Kundalini: The Secret of Yoga*, he called the *kundalinī* "a divine power center in man designed to lead him to a knowledge of his own immortal, superearthly nature" (Krishna 1972, 175). Unfortunately, he freely shuttled between traditional (metaphoric) and biological levels of discourse, which leaves his explanations unclear and ultimately powerless.

Perhaps the most bewildering aspect of Krishna's exposition concerns the relationship between the *kundalinī* and *prāna*. In his book *The Dawn of a New Science*, he states,

> In its cosmic form Prana is a highly diffused, intelligent energy spread everywhere. But in the individual it takes a specific form as the bio-plasma or individual Prana composed of an extremely subtle organic essence drawn from the elements and compounds of the body. (Krishna 1978, 216)

The latter explanation matches his understanding of the *kundalinī*. In fact, in his autobiography (1971, 108), he states, "In dealing with Kundalini we are concerned only with Prana or Prana-Shakti." And yet he is highly critical of the traditional view that regards the *cakras* and *nāḍīs* as being composed of *prāṇa,* though he often claims just that.

My criticisms notwithstanding, Krishna's publications—especially his exacting autobiography—are seminal and vitally important.

THE PHYSIO-KUNDALINĪ

In the 1970s, the American psychiatrist and ophthalmologist Lee Sannella became interested in the *kundalinī* crises that some of his patients were reporting. In association with Harold Streitfeld and Gabriel Cousens, MD, he founded the Kundalini Clinic in 1975–76 with the mission to reassure, advise, and treat those suffering from what were really atypical *kundalinī* symptoms (or *kundalinī* gone awry). The treatment modalities included mainly Reichian breathwork, Yoga, and psychotherapy. The clinic was taken over in 1983 by the psychotherapist Stuart Sovatsky (see Sovatsky 1998), who has since then operated it in Berkeley, California.

Sannella was primarily concerned with the neurological symptoms associated with this phenomenon, and he coined the term "physio-kundalinī" to describe them. In his book *The Kundalinī Experience,* first published in 1976 and released in a revised edition in 1987, he observed,

> As for the present book, two interconnected theses are strongly argued. The first is that a process of psychophysiological transmutation, most usefully viewed as the "awakening of the kundalini," is indeed a reality. The second is that this process is part of an evolutionary mechanism and that as such it must not be viewed as a pathological development. Rather, I will strongly propose that the kundalini process is an aspect of human psychospiritual unfolding that is intrinsically desirable. (Sannella 1987, 11)

Sannella availed himself of a physicist model of micromotion formulated by the maverick Czech-born researcher Itzhak Bentov. The model, which Bentov explains in *Stalking the Wild Pendulum* (see Bentov 1988), seeks to explain that the universe is a composite of many oscillating and interacting fields. These fields all pulsate in harmony. At the personal and impersonal level, disease is an out-of-tune rhythm in a component of the body that can be restored through a strong, harmonious pulse. Bentov demonstrated experimentally that the cerebrospinal fluid has a fine micromovement that is measurable with magnetometers and can be correlated with a feeling of ecstasy induced by the brain core.

In his book, Sannella also drew attention to comparable phenomena in other cultures, such as the *n/um* energy known among the !Kung Bushmen of the Kalahari Desert.

HINDU YOGA

The best traditional explanation of the *kundalinī* process can be found in the *Shat-Cakra-Nirūpana*, a sixteenth-century Sanskrit text first translated by Arthur Avalon (alias Sir John Woodroffe) in 1919 (Avalon 1974, 317–479). The first thing we notice is that the *kundalinī*, contrary to statements in much of the Western literature, is not simply equated with *prāna*. While the former can be seen as a psycho*spiritual* force, the latter is a psycho*energetic* agent. It does, however, require the bombardment of the axial pathway by *prāna* before the *kundalinī-shakti* is roused. This can be compared to an A-bomb triggering an H-bomb. But the *kundalinī* process is somewhat less predictable (and is traditionally dependent on grace).

It also becomes clear from this authoritative Hindu text that what has been dubbed the physio-kundalini has little in common with the description of regular *kundalinī* awakenings. The symptoms described by Gopi Krishna and others in recent times have all the characteristics of irregular (spontaneous and pathological) awakenings or mere *prānic* flows rather than proper awakenings of the serpent power. In other words, they are best regarded as examples of *kundalinī* "failures."

It is also evident from a perusal of the *Shat-Cakra-Nirūpana* and other similar Sanskrit texts that the *cakras* and *nādīs* are not located in the physical body and that the *kundalinī* process must not be confused with nervous excitation. The opposite was strongly argued by the theosophist Vasant Rele in his 1927 book, *The Mysterious Kundalinī*. Rele argued that the entire *kundalinī* process can be interpreted along physiological lines, and many recent discussions have followed his suggestion. Thus, it is frequently maintained that the *cakras* are identical to the nerve plexuses. Following the seven *cakras* model, Rele gives the correspondence as follows:

> *mūlādhāra cakra* = pelvic plexus
> *svādhishthāna cakra* = hypogastric plexus
> *manipura cakra* = solar plexus

anāhata cakra = cardiac plexus
vishuddha (or *vishuddhi*) *cakra* = pharyngeal plexus
ājnā cakra = nasociliary nerve plexus
sahasrāra cakra = brain
kundalinī = right vagus nerve

Others have made the following physical correlations:

mūlādhāra cakra = sacrococcygeal plexus
svādhishthāna cakra = sacral plexus
manipura cakra = solar plexus
anāhata cakra = cardiac plexus
vishuddha cakra = cervical plexus
ājnā cakra = pituitary plexus
sahasrāra cakra = cerebrum

That a connection exists between the *cakras* and the nerve plexuses should not be doubted, but it would be a grievous mistake to equate them. The *cakras* belong to the subtle and not the physical body.

THE BUDDHIST DOMBĪ

The *kundalinī* is known in Buddhist Tantra as the *bodhicitta* and as the goddess Candālī, Yoginī, or Dombī. The latter term means "washerwoman" and refers to the fact that just as the washerwoman cleans clothes, the *kundalinī* purifies the body's *nādīs*.

THE SERPENT POWER IN JAINISM

In Jainism, *yoga* generally stands for "activity." As a discipline, Yoga is primarily connected with the eighth-century Haribhadra Sūri, a prolific scholar-practitioner to whom more than one thousand texts are attributed. His finest work is the *Yoga-Bindu,* and no mention is made of the *kundalinī* in this text. Although Haribhadra Sūri writes about seven kinds of Yoga that deal with the body, he seems to be unacquainted with Hatha-Yoga.

CHAPTER 12

Knowledge, Wisdom, Gnosis

> Wisdom is superior to action.
>
> —GEORG FEUERSTEIN (2011a, 3.1)

In conventional terms, *knowledge* is the intellectual comprehension of information about a subject and, according to the ideology of materialism, is derived from sensory input. By contrast, as I explained in an essay written for Roger Walsh's anthology on wisdom,[1] *wisdom* "grows, transforms, and deepens a person; intellectual ideas at best broaden his or her intellectual horizon. Intellectual ideas are tied into other intellectual ideas to make a web of models or systems. Wisdom organically relates to other living values, which uplift and make whole. Intellectual ideas increase information, knowledge. Wisdom enhances the quality of life and is healing."

At the highest level of wisdom, we find *gnosis*. The term stems from the Greek wisdom traditions and suggests liberating knowledge, or wisdom that frees the soul from the "prison" of the body. This is not merely doctrinal knowledge or gray theory, but actual, living wisdom that frees the soul from the chains of the physical realm.

Wisdom became of interest as a research topic only in the 1970s (see Sternberg 1990). All three concepts are present in the schools of Hindu, Buddhist, and Jaina Yoga and are often captured in the Sanskrit term *jñāna*, though the second and third connotations—wisdom and gnosis—are often expressed as *vidyā*, implying a higher form of knowing.

HINDU YOGA

In Vedic times, the common term for knowledge was *veda*, while wisdom was captured in the Sanskrit word *madhira*, and gnosis was generally expressed by *dhī* ("vision"). The most detailed analysis of the last term is offered by the Dutch Indologist Jan Gonda, who observes,

By "vision" is...to be understood the exceptional and supranormal faculty, proper to "seers," of "seeing," in the mind, things, causes, connections as they really are, in the faculty of acquiring a sudden knowledge of the truth of the functions and influence of the divine powers, of man's relation to them, etc. (Gonda, 1963, 68–69)

Vision, then, is higher insight, a divine knowing (or gnosis). The boundaries between knowledge, wisdom, and gnosis were somewhat fuzzy.

BUDDHIST YOGA

In Buddhism, especially the Mahāyāna branch, the principal Sanskrit term for wisdom and its result (gnosis) is *prajñā*. This is best captured in the preeminent literary genre of the *Prajñā-Pāramitā* scriptures. Sangharakshita explains *prajñā* as follows:

Prajñā is not just knowledge; it is supreme or even superlative knowledge ...What is the object of this supreme knowledge? The answer to this, throughout all Buddhist literature...is quite unambiguous. *Prajñā* means knowledge of reality; it means knowledge of things as they really are. (Sangharakshita 2000, 11)

In Mahāyāna Buddhism, wisdom is the means whereby the practitioner penetrates emptiness, which stands for all beings' lack of an essence. The *Abhisamāya-Alankāra* (1.2.7) section of the *Pancasāhasrikā-Prajñā-Paramitā* (Conze 1975), distinguishes a bodhisattva's five sets of eyes. The first set is the fleshly eye, the second is the heavenly eye, and the third is the pure wisdom eye. Higher than these are the pure dharma eye and the pure buddha eye. The fleshly eye can see across the physical universe; the heavenly eye knows about the death and rebirth of all species; the pure wisdom eye recognizes wherever a person may dwell (whether in the physical world or some other *loka*); the pure dharma eye is connected with the attainment of the five cardinal virtues and arhatship;[2] and the pure buddha eye, which comes with full enlightenment, has knowledge of the spiritual status and destiny of a bodhisattva.

Tibetan Buddhism recognizes five kinds of wisdom, which are supported by the five meditation buddhas—Vairocana, Amoghasiddhi, Ratnasambhava, Amitābha, and Akshobhya. These buddhas are consecutively associated with the following highest wisdoms:

- The wisdom of the basic space of phenomena (*chos dbyings ye shes*): takes on many forms and is still of "a single taste" and is ineffable
- All-accomplishing wisdom (*bya grub ye shes*): the acts of enlightened beings seeking to accomplish the welfare of sentient beings
- The wisdom of equality (*mnyam nyid ye shes*): the understanding of the sameness of phenomena
- Discerning wisdom (*so sor rtogs pa'iye shes*): knowledge of each transcendental quality
- Mirrorlike wisdom (*me long lta bu'i ye shes*): effortless omniscience

JAINA YOGA

Jainism, which culminates in omniscience (*kevala-jnāna*), also has separate words for knowledge (*jnāna*), wisdom (*prajnā*), and gnosis (*samyag-darshana*). The latter term denotes liberation, which is understood as a state of disembodied omniscience. This is not merely spiritual knowledge, as claimed for the Buddha, but all sorts of knowledge.

CHAPTER 13

Pure Awareness

> [T]here are no considerations of a logical or
> phenomenological nature that rule out the
> possibility of that experience [of pure consciousness].
>
> —MARK B. WOODHOUSE (Forman 1990, 267)

MODERN PSYCHOLOGY

The concept of consciousness is philosophically problematic in both the West and the East. The major difference is that in the East, it generally stands for transcendental Consciousness/Awareness (*cit, citi, cit-shakti, caitanya, drashtri, kshetrajna, parinishpanna, samvid,* and so on), whereas in the West, awareness is commonly understood as a property or function of the mind, if anything. "If anything" refers to behaviorism, which denies that consciousness is a meaningful concept at all and argues that we should concentrate on observable facts—a self-limiting position.

To begin with, behaviorism is the psychology without a "soul." Rejecting self-observation and espousing the idea that the inner life of another is not just difficult but impossible to understand, behaviorism relies on reflexes and measurable stimulus-response data elicited primarily from lower animals (such as rats and pigeons). It is thus applicable only to a certain range of noncognitive human behavior. Some would argue that this approach leaves out the most important part of the personality, but behaviorism has admittedly been helpful in modifying behavioral patterns involving only simple psychological mechanisms. Of late, it has—in an honest move—dropped the self-descriptive label *psychology.* After all, it is the psychology without a psyche.

In opposition to the early physiological psychologists who explored the body rather than the mind, the early mentalist psychologists followed the lead of scientists like Hermann Ebbinghaus (memory research), George Elias Müller (introspective investigation of the learning process), and

Oswald Külpe (founder of the Würzburg school for investigating the thinking process).

The great Wilhelm Wundt, who is often called the "father of psychology," still viewed consciousness as identical to the nervous system. For him, sensations and perceptions were the building blocks of the mind. During his long career, he revised his opinions on many points, and it is therefore difficult to get a clear sense of his views, though he held fast to his introspectionist track. Wundt's system lost its appeal by the 1920s and gave way to the mentalist approaches that had been in the offing for a few decades.

William James, a continent removed from Wundt, used introspection to establish the reality of the mind beyond the brain and nervous system. His approach of functionalism was contrary to Wundt's structuralist, biophysical orientation. James thought it would be premature for psychology to pronounce a definitive view about the connection between the mind and body. He did, however, feel that introspection reveals consciousness to be an ongoing process—a "stream"—of sensations, perceptions, emotions, intuitions, thoughts, and so forth. An integral part of this stream is the sense of self, which is uninterrupted by sleep or the passage of time. James refused to engage in metaphysical speculation about a transcendental Self but felt that, pragmatically, the empirical self that is accessible through introspective analysis of the "stream of consciousness" provided a sufficient unity to the psyche.

While James, who was aware of the newly formulated ideas about the unconscious, chose to focus on the stream of consciousness, European physicians and neurologists like Jean-Martin Charcot, Josef Breuer (an early supporter of Freud), and Sigmund Freud himself explored the hidden layers of the mind by closely studying the phenomenon of hysteria. Freud distinguished five structures, or layers, within the psyche: the unconscious, or id; consciousness; the preconscious; the ego; and the superego, or successor of the parents or educators, which has conscience as its main function. As this chapter is primarily interested in consciousness, we will ignore all layers but take the structures into account. Freud offered no special definition of consciousness but was content to say that he held this concept to be the same as the consciousness of the philosopher and everyday opinion and that whatever is not conscious is unconscious. Thus, Freud gave primacy to the unconscious; hence, the popular image of an iceberg, most of which is submerged. The visible part is consciousness and the ego, and the much larger, invisible part is the unconscious. The human personality acts reflexively by means of the unconscious, unless there is a significant stimulus from the outside world; only then is (the ego-driven) consciousness triggered.

An antistructuralist stance was also adopted by the pioneers of Gestalt psychology, for whom the whole was greater than the sum of its parts. This orientation eventually led to Gestalt therapy, which is one of the tributaries of the sweeping current of humanistic psychology. Gestalt theory contributed significantly to psychology by leading away from the unfruitful structuralist quest for the final components, or atoms, of the mind and by drawing attention to the integrity and contextuality of psychic activity. It was a major factor in the emergence of the cognitive perspective within psychology, which focused on thinking, intelligence, memory, and language. It did not, of course, solve the riddle of consciousness.

After Freud's establishment of psychoanalysis, the diverse lines of investigation issuing from his efforts broadened into what came to be called depth psychology. Freud's students and successors—Anna Freud, Carl Gustav Jung, Alfred Adler, Karl Abraham, Otto Rank, Sandor Ferenczi, Wilhelm Reich, Karen Horney, Melanie Klein, Henri Ey, Erik H. Erikson, Erich Fromm, and many others—spread and modified psychoanalysis in the postwar decades.

Of this group, the psychiatrist whose work was and continues to be the most influential is undoubtedly Carl Jung, the founder of the school of analytical psychology. He broke with Freud over major conceptual differences about the nature of the unconscious. While Freud understood the unconscious as the holding tank for repressed material (especially sexual impulses), Jung saw it as the creative matrix of consciousness. For him, it held both personal contents (composed of repressed, forgotten, or subliminal impressions in an individual's ontogenesis) and deeper collective contents (resulting from our species' phylogenesis). Jung was particularly interested in exploring the collective (prepersonal and transpersonal) unconsciousness, the seat of the universal archetypes as they appear in dreams, visions, reveries, art, and the world's mythological creations.

The central ("god") archetype, which regulates the psyche and is fundamental to the process of individuation (or becoming whole), is the Self; it stands in contrast to the conscious ego at the other end of an axis of complementarity. Supposedly, in the first half of life, the ego separates from the self, and if this does not occur, the psyche becomes dysfunctional, even "mad." At the same time, we must overcome the dualistic separation between the self and the ego, which Jung sees as the challenge of the second half of life, by means of the individuation process. In *The Integration of the Personality,* Jung writes,

> Consciousness and the unconscious do not make a whole when either is suppressed or damaged by the other. If they must contend, let it be a fair fight with equal rights on both sides. Both are aspects of life. (Jung 1939, 27)

Culturally and individually, of course, we have become alienated from the unconscious and place a premium on the ego, consciousness, and rationality. This alienation has led to widespread disorientation, despair, meaninglessness, aggression, and disconnectedness from others and from nature—far more widespread than the twenty-five hundred or so Jungian therapists in the world today could possibly handle.

Out of the creative and highly diversified group of psychiatrists of the so-called first force of psychology evolved humanistic psychology in the 1950s, largely thanks to the no-holds-barred work of Abraham Maslow. This proved a more complete approach than what went before. As Maslow explained in the opening chapter of his book *The Farther Reaches of Human Nature,*

> In the thirties I became interested in certain psychological problems, and found that they could not be answered or managed well by the classical scientific structure of the time (the behavioristic, positivistic, "scientific," value-free, mechanomorphic psychology). I was raising legitimate questions and had to invent another approach to psychological problems in order to deal with them. (Maslow 1971, 3)

Maslow's approach, by his own admission, became something of a weltanschauung, a worldview—the "third force" within modern psychology. "Psychology today is torn and riven," as Maslow (1971, 3) put it, consisting as it does of three "noncommunicating" groups—that of behavioristic-mechanistic psychologists, psychotherapists, and humanistic psychologists. Instead of looking only at the ground floor (behaviorism) or the cellar (psychoanalysis), Maslow was willing to boldly break with conventional psychology and, inspired by Jung, look at the higher human potential. He cast his conceptual net as wide as possible, using an evolutionary perspective and asking fundamental philosophical questions.

Thus, he invented his important theory of metamotivation—the superior values and attitudes cultivated by physically and mentally healthy self-actualizing, self-transcending people. Maslow explains,

> By definition, self-actualizing people are gratified in all their basic needs (of belongingness, affection, respect, and self-esteem)....
>
> In examining self-actualizing people directly, I find that in all cases, at least in our culture, they are dedicated people, devoted to some task "outside themselves," some vocation, or duty, or beloved job. (Maslow 1971, 299–301)

The attitudes of self-actualizers correspond with what Maslow identified as meta-needs, or B-values (Being-values): truth, goodness, beauty, unity, wholeness, aliveness, perfection, justice, order, simplicity, playfulness, meaningfulness, and so on. These values are at a premium in spiritual traditions like Yoga.

One of the key concepts Maslow formulated was that of "peak experience," which stands for moments of extraordinary happiness or meaningfulness, as they are present in experiences of ecstasy, rapture, bliss, or illumination. Again, such experiences are at home in the spiritual traditions, but apparently they are also reasonably common among certain kinds of people who may or may not have a religious-spiritual penchant. The British journalist, writer, and professed atheist Marghanita Laski (1961) administered a questionnaire to a small population sample and also applied content analysis to a good many literary texts to examine the varieties, triggers, and duration of "ecstatic" experiences, most of them being of the "intensity" (extravertive) rather than "withdrawal" (introvertive) variety. They last from a couple of minutes to up to one hour. Laski wisely abstained from passing judgment on these experiences but believed that it was legitimate to search for a rational explanation.

Abraham Maslow's theorizing benefited from the findings of drug experiments (LSD and mescaline) and the widespread use of hallucinogenic substances that shook up a whole generation, creating the counterculture of the 1960s. Significantly, he concluded that the meta-values associated with peak experiences and spiritual life in general are not only characteristic of morally and spiritually mature men and women—our "saints"—but are "the far goals of psychotherapy" (Maslow 1971, 109).

For those who have difficulty with the word *value* and ask what the term really means, Maslow has a sobering reminder that the term is simply a convenient label for wise motivation that leads to a healthy, sane way of life. He also reminds them that value is a well-considered "ought" and not a neurotic "should." As he put it, when we ask, "What ought I to do? How ought I to live?" we would do well to first ask, "Who am I?" Our answer to the last question inevitably implies an ought. All this is psychology merging into wisdom. If William James, two generations earlier, opened windows on the spiritual traditions, Maslow intrepidly opened doors for his scientific epigones of the transpersonal movement to step through confidently.

"The transpersonal model," writes the psychiatrist Roger Walsh and the psychotherapist Frances E. Vaughan (1996, 15), "clearly holds consciousness as a central dimension." They continue,

> A transpersonal model views "normal" consciousness as a defensively contracted state of reduced awareness. This normal state is filled to a remarkable and unrecognized extent with a continuous, mainly uncontrollable flow of fantasies which exert a powerful though largely unrecognized influence on perception, cognition, and behavior....
>
> Optimum consciousness is viewed as being considerably greater than normal consciousness and potentially available at any time, if the defensive contraction is relaxed. (Walsh and Vaughan 1996, 18)

This view of ordinary consciousness goes hand in hand with giving personality, which was previously an anchor point of psychological modeling, far less weight. This becomes possible through the kind of comprehensive spectrum theory, mutatis mutandis, developed by Ken Wilber (see, for example, Wilber 1977, 1980, 2000a), which endeavors to take into account the whole range of actual and possible human growth.

This was also Roberto Assagioli's purpose, though from a more practical perspective. Assagioli, born in Italy in 1888, first studied medicine in Florence and then turned to psychiatry under Freud's teacher, Eugen Bleuler, at the Burghölzli clinic in Zurich. His 1910 doctoral dissertation in medicine was a critique of psychoanalysis, which he felt was incomplete. Although he was the only Italian member of the Freud Society, he began formulating the principles of his own system of psychosynthesis (originally called bio-psychosynthesis), which represented a significant departure from Freudianism. Nevertheless, in the years before World War I, Assagioli, a polyglot, translated some of Freud's writings into Italian as authorized by Freud himself.

He was still in his early twenties when he hung up his shingle as a psychiatrist and, in 1926, established his Istituto di Cultura e Terapia Psichica (later Istituto di Psicosintesi) in Rome. Twelve years later, the institute was shut down by Benito Mussolini's fascist regime, and Assagioli was imprisoned and placed in solitary confinement for a month because of his Jewish descent and international humanistic activities. He used his time in prison well, practicing meditation for several hours a day, which gave him a taste of the peace that a *yogin* might enjoy. It also helped him formulate his ideas about the role of the human will (whose qualities and six stages are described in his book *The Act of Will* (1973). He was able to reestablish his institute only at the end of World War II, and in the late 1950s, students established the first foreign centers devoted to psychosynthesis in the United States, which was also when Assagioli collaborated with Maslow. Later, many other centers followed in more than thirty countries.

The unique feature of psychosynthesis is that it is spiritually based, and its sweep is as broad as that of transpersonal psychology, which Assagioli helped create. In *The Eye of Spirit,* Ken Wilber (1998, 267) appreciatively speaks of him as "an extraordinary pioneer in the transpersonal field, weaving the best of many important psychological and spiritual traditions together into a powerful approach to inner growth." Assagioli (1993, 193) declined to speculate about the metaphysical implications of "Spirit" and instead focused on the practical, psychological side of "spiritual," which he thought was as "basic as the material part of man." For him, *spiritual* meant "superconscious," that is, relating to that part of the unconscious that he labelled superconscious, as it becomes accessible through meditation, prayer, or some other form of inner discipline. This sounds like a contradiction, but it is not: The superconscious is unconscious as long as it is not realized as superconscious. This is not the same as the Self, which can only become immediately known through Self-realization. The superconscious can erupt into consciousness as intuitions and other extraordinary content, as in the case of geniuses. What Assagioli calls the superconscious, Wilber (2000a) refers to as the transpersonal bands of (psychic and subtle) consciousness.

This brings us back to peak experiences and psychotropic drugs (and nowadays biofeedback), the former opening the portal to the superconscious and the latter at least mimicking the superconscious.[1] The relevant research placed states rather than functions of consciousness in the limelight of psychological investigation. As Walsh and Vaughan (1996, 18) note, "The transpersonal perspective holds that a large spectrum of altered states of consciousness exist." The adjective *altered* is in relation to the normal or conventional state of mind that transpersonal psychology views "as a defensively contracted state of reduced awareness." Writing in the midst of the "psychedelic revolution," psychologist Charles T. Tart (1975) paid close attention to the concept of states of consciousness and formulated an elaborate model based on the systems approach.

He regarded the ordinary, everyday consciousness both as a complex system and a discrete state with specific characteristics. He argued that because all humans possess the same kind of body and nervous system, we all have available to us "a large number of human potentials" (Tart 1975a, 4). However, each culture selects or favors only some of these potentials, while rejecting others and remaining ignorant of a good many. These selected potentials make up the framework of our ordinary state of consciousness, which followers of "normal" science consider the best and the standard by which all other states are to be judged. From this narrow perspective, drug-induced or mystical states are deemed substandard and proximate to psychosis.

Careful study of the worldwide phenomenon of mysticism and unbiased research into artificially induced altered states belie this consensus view. Tart (1975a) reasonably proposes that awareness is fundamental and that consciousness is awareness modified by the nervous system. When these two terms refer to a psychological event, I will use all lowercase type. The question remains whether, in light of the spiritual traditions, *awareness* should be written with an initial capital letter.

Tart concludes that it should be possible, as claimed in the spiritual traditions, to magnify the awareness element within consciousness by systematically disciplining the mind. He explains the normal state of consciousness as a state of what the Indians called *samsāra,* or the round of conditioned existence. He is far less academic and more outspoken in his book *Wake Up.* Leaning strongly on the teachings of G. I. Gurdjieff, he characterizes our ordinary consciousness as "the sleep of everyday life," or the consensus trance:

> Consensus trance involves a loss of much of our essential vitality. It is (all too much) a state of partly suspended animation and inability to function, a daze, a stupor. It is also a state of profound abstraction, a great retreat from immediate sensory/instinctual reality to abstractions about reality. (Tart 1987, 85)

Tart argues that we are a "mass of potentials" when we are born, but our cultural environment, which is far from neutral, exerts all sorts of constraints to turn us into predictable, conforming individuals. Through enculturation and education, we are progressively turned into "normal," "sensible," "civilized" members of society, whatever that may mean in any given culture. When this fails to happen, we are dubbed "troublemakers," "deviants," or "crazy people"; worse, we may be evaluated psychiatrically, be emotionally and socially ostracized or physically punished, or be force-fed Ritalin or some other drug. Variations and degrees of these "trance-induction" methods exist in virtually every culture on earth.

We are considered normal when we can slip into the appropriate role for every occasion. Thus we have multiple identities, yet we assume that consciousness is a permanent unity that is also a notion to which we have been conditioned by our culture. That this presumed unitary "I" is something of an illusion becomes obvious when we are under the influence of a mind-altering substance, such as alcohol, or when we experience a mystical state of nonduality.

We ordinarily assume that we are genuinely self-aware. This is not the case, however. Most of our time is spent in a semiconscious state—the consensus trance. We do not tend to be *mindfully* present. We are not quite here. Our waters of consciousness are muddy and contain little of the oxygen of awareness.

AWARENESS

In his *States of Consciousness,* Tart (1975a, 27) argues that awareness is *not,* as is almost universally thought, inevitably a brain-dependent phenomenon; as he sees it, only consciousness is. He refers to altered states and parapsychological experiences that suggest that "awareness is at least partially outside brain functioning." This is the place to explain again that pure Awareness (capitalized) is utterly transcendental and hence transmental (*amanaska*), whereas pure awareness (lowercase) is a state of mind that is transconceptual (*nirvikalpa*). According to the spiritual traditions of Yoga, Sāmkhya, and Vedānta, the transcendental Subject (*purusha*) is pure, ultimate Consciousness/ Awareness. But Tart could not establish this on purely empirical evidence.

Assagioli (1993, 87), by contrast, unhesitatingly speaks of a "higher Self" or "spiritual Self," which we may equate with pure Awareness or, as he has it, "direct awareness." But he wisely does not introduce this notion in the treatment of patients unless they have spiritual problems or specifically seek out psychosynthesis for spiritual development. As he explains,

We consider that the spiritual is as basic as the material part of man. We are not attempting to force upon psychology a philosophical, theological or metaphysical position, but essentially we include within the study of psychological facts all those which make him grow toward greater realizations of his spiritual essence.... Psychosynthesis definitely affirms the *reality* of spiritual experience, the existence of the higher values and of the "noetic" or "noological" dimension (as Frankl aptly calls it). Its neutrality refers *only* to the second phase: that of the formulations and the institutions. (Assagioli 1993, 193–95)

Few transpersonal therapists, never mind psychiatrists, would risk going as far as Assagioli did, because the "consensus reality" is strong even in scientific circles. This is compacted by attachment to, or a bias toward, certain scientific models or the current paradigm.

Ken Wilber, who is the transpersonal movement's foremost theorist, does not shy away from speaking about the nondual Self or Spirit as the ultimate background of the entire spectrum of consciousness. In *The Atman Project* (1980), he explains that human development culminates in the transcendence of the ego, amounting to supreme enlightenment, which is the realization of the ultimate, unknowable, and unqualified Consciousness/ Awareness and which he apparently claims for himself.

Philosophically, the question of whether or not there is such a mental condition as pure awareness has been repeatedly considered since the 1960s. The standard view has been that of constructivism, as articulated by Steven T. Katz, a professor of religion at Dartmouth College in New Hampshire, in his edited volume *Mysticism and Philosophical Analysis*. According to this perspective, Katz (1978, 26) says, "*There are NO pure (i.e., unmediated) experiences*" (italics in original). In other words, the mystical experience is shaped by the concepts held in the mind of the mystic. Thus, a Hindu will have a Hindu mystical experience; a Christian, a Christian experience; and so on.

Needless to say, this contradicts the testimony of the mystical traditions themselves, which speak of an emptying of the mind, a release of attachment to the familiar conceptual categories. Not surprisingly, Katz's position has been reevaluated, and the most significant review is the one by Robert K. Forman, an assistant professor of religion at Vassar College in New York State. In *The Problem of Pure Consciousness* (1990), Forman and his contributors extensively critique Katz's position. Four of the contributors demonstrate in their essays that the spiritual traditions they represent (Christopher

K. Chapple, Sāmkhya; Paul J. Griffith, Yogācāra Buddhism; Robert K. C. Forman, Meister Eckhart; Daniel C. Matt, Jewish mysticism) clearly uphold the psychological reality of pure awareness. The other eight contributors debate the philosophical, hermeneutical, and methodological liabilities of constructivism. In other words, realizations of pure awareness are not only claimed to exist but cannot be explained (or dismissed) by constructivism.

I will not investigate this further here. Suffice it to say that in light of the arguments by Forman and his collaborators, there is no philosophical reason to question the Indian spiritual traditions to which we will turn next. They affirm that pure awareness realizations are possible and even highly desirable. The variability shown between systems is due entirely to the post-realization effort to present this direct realization in suitably communicative (and doctrinally "correct") terms. This is a major concession that leaves the conceptual mind out of the equation of what is considered the highest, or most advanced, "mystical" state. It is a concession that delimits the partiality toward constructivist explanations in the humanities and science, which is part of the general scientific paradigm.

YOGA AND OTHER INDIAN SPIRITUAL TRADITIONS

The transcendental Subject is called *purusha* in the traditions of Classical Sāmkhya and Classical Yoga, or *ātman* in Vedānta and the numerous Vedānta-dependent schools of post-Classical Yoga. This transcendental Subject in Yoga and Sāmkhya also bears the appellations "Consciousness/Awareness" (*cit, citi*), "Knower" (*jna*), and "Field Knower" (*kshetra-jna*). Vedānta insists that there is only one *ātman,* or transcendental Self. It is not the property of any one individual being but the backdrop or source of everything (whether sentient or insentient, material or immaterial). Important to note, this ultimate Self is pure Consciousness/Awareness, pure Being (*sat*), and pure Bliss (*ānanda*). Jainism's equivalent of the *purusha/ātman* Reality is called *jīva* ("life" or "sentient being"), which likewise has Consciousness/Awareness as its essence. This Awareness is at times equated with omniscience, which is a misleading concept in view of the fact that Awareness is transcognitive. While Buddhism rejects the concepts of *purusha, ātman,* and *jīva,* which it views as having serious philosophical/logical flaws, it at least acknowledges the mental state of pure or transconceptual awareness realizations.

Sāmkhya, Yoga, and Vedānta converge when they state that the ultimate principle of Awareness can be realized without mediating concepts. In both systems, the *purusha/ātman* in itself is unqualified, unconditional, and nonderivative. The major difference between these traditions concerns the relationship of the manifest universe to the transcendental Subject. In the case of Classical Yoga and Classical Sāmkhya, the phenomenal world is only in an apparent relationship or correlation (*samyoga*) to the transcendental Subject. In the case of the Vedānta tradition, the phenomenal world is either a real emergent out of the singular *ātman* or a completely illusory appearance in the state of unenlightenment. Either option involves a heavy conditioning, or bondage (*bandha*), on the part of the unenlightened individual whereby the transcendental Subject is occluded, which is also the position of Jainism and the various forms of Yoga and Sāmkhya.

More than as an ontological statement, this can be understood epistemologically and psychologically: We are deluded in our perception of the world. The mind structures what we see, and our structuring is not always readily recognizable except perhaps in broad outlines. This is a major handicap on the spiritual path, as it is in our relationship to the world and other people.

In the *Yoga-Sūtra* (1.3), Patanjali states that when the activities (*vritti*) of the mind are brought under control, the Seer (*drashtri*) stands revealed in its true nature. The Seer, as I will explain in the next chapter, is the transcendental Subject or Witness. This description must be understood metaphorically. Nothing happens to or within the transcendental Subject itself, which is eternally the same. The event is an intrapsychic one. It is only the mind that becomes illuminated, not the ultimate Reality. In the next aphorism (1.4), Patanjali tells us that "At other times, [the transcendental Subject] is in conformity (*sārūpya*) with the activities [of the mind]." In other words, outside enlightenment, our possible view of the Self gets lost in mental activity. Again, this is entirely an intrapsychic event and not something that happens to the *purusha*.

The *purusha* stands revealed only in the highest ecstatic state, which is *asamprajnāta-samādhi*. As the word *asamprajnāta* indicates, this realization is beyond all cognition (*prajnā*). Here, we must interpret the initial *a* as an alpha privative and not as a mere alpha negative. Negation alone is insufficient to describe the essential event of this state, which suggests transcendence ("beyond"). This form of ecstasy is touched on in aphorism 1.18 of the *Yoga-Sutra*. From the perspective of its fruition, this also bears the technical designation of "seedless ecstasy" (*nirbīja-samādhi*), which is the transition phase to the spiritual. This lofty state of pure awareness is again referred to in aphorism 3.50.

Since Classical Sāmkhya has a very similar ontology to Classical Yoga, the higher stages of the process of transformation also allow for pure Awareness. As Chapple notes, "A pure state of awareness emerges, not in the sense that a self is aware of something pure, but in the sense that one is purely aware" (Forman 1990, 59). The state of liberation is known as *kaivalya* ("aloneness/isolation") as in Patanjali's work, which suggests the purity of Consciousness/Awareness. In his *Sāmkhya-Kārikā* (59), Īshvara Krishna states, "As a dancer ceases from the dance after having been seen by the audience, so also the *prakriti* ceases after having revealed herself to [or been "seen" by] the *purusha.*" The Cosmos (*prakriti*) ceases in the sense that the mind is transcended, which is tantamount to the realization of the impartite *purusha*.

A similar situation prevails in the Vedānta tradition. In one of its earliest layers, the many-branched philosophical tradition of Vedānta acknowledges in a classical passage that the Hearer cannot be heard, the Seer cannot be seen, and so forth (see the pre-Buddhist *Brihadāranyaka-Upanishad* 3.7.23). The speaker of this esoteric knowledge was the great sage Yājnavalkya in response to his teacher Uddālaka's questions.[2]

In the *Upadesha-Sāhasrī* (14.39), an authentic tract of Shankara's (c. 700–750 C.E.),[3] we read that the Self (*ātman*) is beyond time, space, and causation. All characteristics that we bestow on the transcendental Subject are superimposed on it because of spiritual ignorance (*avidyā*). When we eliminate those imputed characteristics through the apophatic process of *neti neti* ("not this, not that"), Shankara tells us in verse 14.48 that the transcendental Self alone remains. The sun shines regardless of the clouds that seem to cover it. When the clouds drift off, we can see the self-same sun as radiant as ever.

Countless metaphors of this kind make it clear that the transcendental Subject is, by definition, imperceptible. Thus, it can be "realized" only when we become identical with it or rather when we eliminate all our false identities and have the Self as our only and true Identity. Paradoxically, the Self can be "known" in the transconceptual ecstasy (*nirvikalpa-samādhi*). This is a mental condition often called the Fourth state (*caturtha-avasthā*). How is this extraordinary "knowledge" even possible? I believe that it is an ex post facto reconstruction of what happened in the nonconceptual state of ecstasy: As we emerge from this sublime "oblivion," the mind seeks to grasp what just happened and constructs its answers based on extrapolations from its present experience. This is not likely to involve much analytical thought but probably is a matter of instant intuitive understanding. The difficulty of describing this paradoxical circumstance, where the contemplator becomes the contemplated, is insurmountable. As the *Upadesha-Sāhasrī* (15.31) says,

> Words turn back along with the mind without reaching [that ultimate Reality] on account of [Its] having no qualities (*guna*), having no activity, and having no characteristics.

That is to say, as we approach ultimate Reality, words fail us and the mind itself is neutralized. The difference between conceptual ecstasy (*savikalpa-samādhi*) and transconceptual ecstasy (*nirvikalpa-samādhi*) is the absence of mental "whirls" (*vritti*) in the latter state.[4]

Jainism has comparable utterances. Thus, the twelfth-century adept Hemacandra makes it clear in his *Yoga-Shāstra* (12.35–36) that Self-realization involves the "annihilation" (*vināsha*) of the mind, which entails the forfeiture of thinking (*cintā*) and memory (*smṛti*). There could be no clearer statement about the transconceptual nature of realization.

Similarly, there are numerous statements in the Buddhist scriptures confirming that the highest ecstatic realization is transconceptual. Buddhism recognizes eight levels of ecstatic absorption, called *jhāna* in Pāli (*dhyāna* and *samādhi* in Sanskrit). The eighth level is termed *naivasamjnānaivāsam-jnā*[5] ("neither perception nor nonperception"). As with Patanjali's *asam-prajnāta-samādhi*, this state of consciousness has only a minor residue of unconscious content, but no conceptual knowledge is present. The terminus of the Buddhist path is "extinction" (*nirvāna*), which lies beyond even this rarefied state of mind. As the *Hevajra-Tantra* (2.43a) restates a Pāli testimony by the Buddha himself,

> Neither existence (*bhāva*) nor the condition of nonexistence (*abhāva-rūpa*) [applies to] the Buddha.

There can be no question, then, that the Hindu/Jaina and Buddhist traditions have a clear sense of the role and importance of pure awareness in the liberative process. This is an important finding that places the Indian spiritual traditions ahead of the Western depth (or height) psychologies, confirming Jung's appraisal as well as that of other psychotherapists.

CHAPTER 14

The Invariable Witness and the Variable Self

> In my days at Oxford and since then, I have been
> impressed by some of the genuine strengths of western
> psychology. It is open to new viewpoints and discoveries.
> It maintains a critical attitude toward itself. And it is the
> most experiential of western intellectual disciplines.
>
> —CHÖGYAM TRUNGPA (Katz 1983, 1–7)

THE TRANSCENDENTAL WITNESS

Pure Awareness is not an empirical experience. It is equivalent to the transcendental Reality; however, it may be conceived as Self (*ātman*), Absolute (*brahman*), Omniscience (*sarvajnātā*), Emptiness (*shūnyatā*), Thusness (*tathātā*), and so on.

As Christopher Chapple (1990) shows in his essay "The Unseen Seer and the Field: Consciousness in Samkhya and Yoga," the concept of the Witness has its mythological origin in the *Rig-Veda* (1.164.20ff.), where the evocative symbolic image of two birds in the same tree is given—one bird is eating the tree's fruit, while the other is simply watching. This powerful image is reiterated in many texts of the subsequent Upanishadic literature. What could the metaphoric image of the two birds stand for if not the individuated self (*jīva*) and the transcendental Self (*ātman/purusha*), respectively—ideas instrumental in Vedānta, Sāmkhya, and Yoga? This decipherment of the Vedic image is confirmed in the *Shvetāshvatara-Upanishad* (4.6–4.7), which, following Nakamura (1990), was probably composed circa 300 B.C.E.

The metaphor of the witness is not entirely convincing, because when we think of human witnesses, we know they are unreliable. They bring to their observations all sorts of cognitive disadvantages: the mind interprets perceptual information and makes up incomplete evidence, and there are inevitable mental biases and emotional reactions. At any rate, the transcendental Witness is, by definition, impartial and inactive. It is pure Consciousness/

Awareness and is called pure because it has no content and therefore can be regarded as inactive. We must understand this notion as being rooted in an actual "ecstatic" realization rather than as a mere conceptual invention.

The American psychotherapist Arthur J. Deikman deserves credit for recognizing the important role of the witnessing self in Western psychotherapy. In his book *The Observing Self: Mysticism and Psychotherapy*, he admits that thus far, the witnessing Self "has been ignored by Western psychology because it is not an object and cannot fit the assumptions and framework of current theory" (Deikman 1983, 11). We can appreciate the oddity of this when we realize that the observing Self "is located in awareness itself, not in its content" (10) and that the ego/self is to be found in that awareness. As Deikman also states, Western psychological theory describes "the self in terms of everything but the observer." He retrieved the idea of the witnessing Self—"the transparent center, that which is aware" (94)—from the mystical tradition.

In the process, Deikman had to restore the legitimacy and respectability of mysticism, which really helped establish a new paradigm for the psychological disciplines. Instead of seeing mysticism as a nebulous, unscientific affair, he showed how mystical routines like concentration and meditation can have a valid place in psychotherapeutic practice.

With Mark Epstein (2007), I here distinguish concentrative meditation from mindfulness meditation. The former is the typically yogic meditation that involves the narrowing of attention; the latter allows the splitting of the ego so that it can scrutinize itself in order to penetrate thoughts, feelings, and identifications until they are seen to be transitory. In other words, mindfulness helps us to become transparent. Although mindfulness meditation is mainly a practice from Theravāda Buddhism, it is beautifully consonant with the Madhyamika philosophy of "form is emptiness, emptiness is form."

In equating the observing self with the transcendental dimension, Deikman (1983) did, however, take a step beyond Immanuel Kant, who denied that we could ever know a transcendental principle. Despite the unresolved problem of how the transcendental Witness can be effective at the empirical level, I agree with Mircea Eliade when he says,

It is impossible...to disregard one of India's greatest discoveries: that of consciousness as witness, of consciousness freed from its psychophysiological structures and their temporal conditioning, the consciousness of the "liberated" man. (Eliade 1973, xx)

Interestingly, what we must regard as the same realization has given rise to both the nondualistic teachings of Vedānta on the one side and the contrasting dualistic teachings of Classical Sāmkhya and Classical Yoga on the other. Jainism and Buddhism developed their concepts about ultimate Reality independent of the Vedas, which is why they are considered heterodox by the brahmins. While Jainism attributes Consciousness (and hence Seership) to the *jīva,* Buddhism originally took an altogether different tack in that it refused to speculate about an eternal transcendental Reality. The Buddha was more interested in demonstrating that the phenomenal world and psyche hold nothing permanent in them but that everything is constantly shifting. The process approach of early Buddhism made room for the idealistic position of the Mahāyāna branch around the turn of the first millennium, notably the Vijnānavāda and Yogācāra traditions, which treat the absolutized Buddha as a perennial Reality that consists of pure Consciousness/ Awareness.

THE VEILING OF THE WITNESSING SELF

For the Hindu traditions, the ultimate Reality is not only the transcendental core, or (according to some schools) the source, of the objective world but also the nucleus, or Self, of the human psyche. In early Upanishadic teachings, this center is envisioned as being surrounded by several successive sheaths, which we can conceive as "fields" (*kshetra*). Five such casings, envelopes, or layers are distinguished (from the inside out) as follows:

- *ānanda-maya-kosha,* or "casing made of (*maya*) bliss"
- *vijnāna-maya-kosha,* or "casing made of awareness"
- *mano-maya-kosha,* or "casing made of mind"
- *prāna-maya-kosha,* or "casing made of psychosomatic energy"
- *anna-maya-kosha,* or "casing made of the food [that is, the physical body]"

This model of the five casings (called *panca-maya-kosha*) is found in the pre-Buddhist *Taittirīya-Upanishad* (2.2ff.). In this Sanskrit text, the first sheath is equated with the transcendental Reality itself, which is conceptualized as Existence-Consciousness-Bliss (*sac-cid-ānanda = sat + cit + ānanda*). Strictly speaking, it is not a sheath at all. Some later Vedānta schools, however, prefer to think of it more sensibly as one of the veils around the Self.

Each of the five layers corresponds to a state of mind, and the terminology hints at the predominant contents of the diverse layers, with bliss being most proximate to Self-realization and so forth.

Western anatomy and physiology have amassed a huge amount of data about the "food body." Some research has been done about the *prānic* body (or aura), but this is considered more the domain of parapsychology (see chapter 11) than of medicine or psychology. The mental sheath is the forte of psychology, while the phenomenon of awareness (*vijñāna*) is only a recent concern of psychology, and the phenomenon of bliss is altogether disregarded or cursorily relegated to mysticism. The term *vijñāna* in this context has been variously translated as "consciousness" or less convincingly as "intelligence" or "knowledge." Bliss, or *ānanda,* is not the pleasure that is derived by triggering the so-called pleasure center of the brain, even if Silvan S. Tomkins (1962) calls it "joy" in his three-volume work *Affect, Imagery, Consciousness.* Bliss is not a mental quality but is uncaused and intrinsic to the Self.

Graphically, we can imagine the five sheaths as concentric circles around the innermost center, which is the Self, except that the Self is infinitely larger than the conglomeration of veils that block it from our view. In fact, the veils are illusory and temporary obstructions of the timeless omnipresence that the Self represents. The Self is never occluded to itself. Rather, it is always self-illuminating. Only the finite mind undergoes the experience of lacking Self-realization. From the mind's point of view, Self-realization calls for a quantum leap, as suggested by quantum physicist Amit Goswami (pers. comm.).

"Veiling" (*āvarana*) is also acknowledged in the Buddhist tradition, but the notion of sheaths is not used. The veiling agents are considered to be obstacles, and the Cittamātra (Mind Only) school of Mahāyāna distinguishes ten of them (see Ganguly 1992, 59–60). In Jainism, the material karma is regarded as the veil, which prevents the manifestation of wisdom.

From the perspective of the nondualist tradition of Vedānta, the Self is the singular Identity comprising all empirical selves and worlds. In other words, there is one and the same Self for every single being. By contrast, the classical systems of Yoga and Sāmkhya teach that there are innumerable transcendental Selves, but we might think of them as mutually intersecting each other in eternity and then arriving at a semblance of unity. Whatever metaphysics is adopted, the transcendental Reality is invariably given the quality of the Witness, because the Awareness associated with it is omnipresent and omnitemporal.

EGO AND SELF

Western philosophy and psychology are riddled with a central problem: What is our true identity, ego, or self? The ego is a problematic concept with numerous definitions attached to it.[1] Is the self a psychological or an existential concept? Or are ego and self the same? Here, we understand the ego to be our assumed identity with the body and mind rather than the functional self.

In the context of Hinduism, the ultimate Reality is the transcendental Self, our final identity, which is the identity of everything. Whatever its philosophical explanation may be, the Self—whether singular or multiple—is beyond the ken of the mind and senses. It is pure, transcendental Awareness. What we know as the selfhood of our personality is a finite, empirical structure or function, which is often equated with the ego. In Jungian analytical psychology, the self—generally capitalized—is the central archetype of the unconscious standing for wholeness and transcendence. It is the psychological god.

To distinguish the transcendental Self from the empirical self, the latter is often referred to as *jīvātman* in the Hindu literature—from *jīva* ("individual") and *ātman* ("self"). The ego, as Jung (1933, 4) states, is the "center of consciousness." The problem with the ego is that while it appears to be constant, it is not. As research on altered states of consciousness has amply demonstrated, the ego is capricious and not even present in some states. Thus, it is a construct of the consensus reality explained earlier. As we grow up, we learn to have an ego identity. Tart captures the situation well when he states,

> In terms of the systems approach, we can characterize ego as a continuity and consistency of functioning to which we attach special importance, but which does not have the reality of a solid *thing* somewhere, which is only a *pattern* of operation that disappears under close scrutiny. (Tart 1975a, 133)

India's spiritual traditions have demonstrated great ingenuity in devising many ways of understanding the relationship between the ultimate Reality and the finite world. The principal solutions to this metaphysical problem include various forms of nondualism and dualism, as well as the agnosticism of early Buddhism. Here we are primarily interested in the practicalities of the relationship between the Absolute and the relative.

Classical Sāmkhya envisions this relationship as one of proximity (*samni-dhi*) between the *purusha* and *prakriti*. This spatial metaphor is as unhelpful as the term used in Patanjali's *Yoga-Sūtra* (2.17, 2.23, 2.25), which is *sam-yoga*—"connection" or, as some translators would have it, "correlation." No further explanation is given other than that this relatedness is entirely due to spiritual ignorance (*avidyā*), which is defined in aphorism 2.5 as follows: "Ignorance is seeing [that which is] eternal, pure, joyful, and the Self in [that which is] ephemeral, impure, sorrowful, and the nonself." In other words, *samyoga* consists of mistaking the ego-personality for the transcendental Self, which then colors the way we see the rest of the world.

The fact is that two ultimate reals that, by definition, are separate cannot have a connection. But this leaves the question of how Self-realization is ever possible in a dualistic system. Īshvara Krishna and Patanjali believed that when the unenlightened mind is duly (perfectly) purified or refined, the *purusha* wakes up to itself. Unfortunately, this is loose language, because we already know that the *purusha* is pure Awareness and unchangeable. Therefore it must always be awake. The change, then, is in the mind alone. Through ignorance, we are unable to be the ever-present, ever-aware Self, our true Identity. All of a sudden (upon enlightenment), we *are* the Self. How can this leap be accomplished if the *purusha* is utterly separate from the mind? Both Classical Sāmkhya and Classical Yoga are saddled with philosophical confusion arising from the intermittent use of ordinary language, which is most strikingly witnessed in their insistence that there are multiple *purushas*, one for each individual. The Sāmkhya philosophers argue that if there were only a single *purusha*, everyone would be liberated at the moment the first person is, which is evidently not the case.

The diverse branches of the nondualist tradition, although perhaps less awkward in their arguments, are still philosophically unsatisfactory. When we examine the nondualist metaphysics of the early Upanishads, we find that they are neither sufficiently explicit and uniform nor systematized. Their arguments proceed almost exclusively along mythological or, more sparingly, metaphysical lines and are not entirely clear; consequently, they have given rise to divergent scholastic opinions.[2] From the various passages in the Upanishads, we can distill the following common features:

· The transcendental Self (*ātman*) and the transcendental Reality, or Absolute (*brahman*) are one and the same.

- The Self is pure, formless Awareness as well as pure Being and pure Bliss.
- It cannot be grasped with the mind or the senses.
- It can be realized through direct apprehension simply by waking up as the Self; this involves the renunciation of all desires.
- The Self is somehow connected with the heart as its empirical point of contact, but this is left unexplained.
- Its symbolic expression is the syllable AUM (or OM).
- Realization of the Self makes a person effulgent ("the face shines").

The question of the relationship between the transcendental Reality and the empirical world is not specifically addressed until the time of the Advaita Vedānta philosophers, starting with Gaudapāda and Shankara.

Occasionally (see, for example, *Brihadāranyaka-Upanishad* 3.7.1), the Self is described as the "inner ruler" (*antaryāmin*), which suggests that it was thought to have governing control over the empirical dimension, comprising both the human personality and the macrocosmic world. Thus, much later, the *Katha-Upanishad* (2.3.3) states, "Through fear [of that Self], fire burns; through fear [of that Self], the sun [gives off] heat...." Here, *fear* refers to the basic state of fear that is inherent in all beings who experience duality. Sun and fire are deemed beings rather than things. The idea of the *antaryāmin* was taken up as a major theme by the medieval Vedānta master Rāmānuja (1017–1127 C.E.), who formulated the school of Vishisthādvaita, or nondualism with differentiation. The concept of the *antaryāmin* suggests that the transcendental Self is somehow related to the empirical personality, though the implied relationship is not explained. Strictly speaking, no such relationship can exist as long as the Self is defined as the transcendental Subject.

The surviving literature of the period between the early Upanishads and Shankara, who has tentatively been assigned (Nakamura 1990, 88) to 700–750 C.E., is surprisingly scant.[3] The post-Buddhist *Katha-Upanishad,* which is a composite text consisting of an older and a newer part, for the first time contrasts the "light" (*tapas*) of the transcendental Self with the "shadow" (*chāyā*) of the ego-personality. In this scripture (1.3.3–4), we also find the well-known metaphor of the body as a chariot (*ratha*) and the Self as the chariot's lord (*rathin*), while the senses are compared to horses, the higher mind (*buddhi*) to the charioteer, the lower mind (*manas*) to the reins, and the sense objects (*vishaya*) to the pathways. We have a simplistic version of Sāmkhya ontology relative to the embodied being. Several verses later (1.3.10), we learn that beyond the higher mind is the "great self" (*ātmā mahān = mahātman*), which is a transpersonal or cosmic principle. Beyond this undefined principle is said to be the unmanifest (*avyakta*), which we may equate with *prakriti-pradhāna*. Transcending all this is the *purusha*, or Spirit, who resides thumb-sized in the heart (2.1.12–13). When the embodied self (*dehin*) disintegrates completely, only the transcendental Self remains. But at the time of death, the embodied self that is not liberated by "knowing" the Self enters another womb, depending on its karmic stock (2.2.6). The condition of inner stability or equilibrium is attained by the control of the distracting senses (2.3.11), which is considered Yoga.

The *Bhagavad-Gītā* teaches a form of panentheism, with Krishna both as the God-realized teacher and the ultimate Reality, who speaks personally in this work. Following Sāmkhya contours of thought, the world composed of the three primary qualities (*gunas*) is said to be inherent in the transcendental supreme Person (*purushottama*), who is beyond the *gunas*. This text maintains a syncretism of three paths—Jnāna-Yoga, Karma-Yoga, and Bhakti-Yoga, with the last being the most sublime method. Krishna speaks of himself as having come into the world repeatedly as an illumined master (the *tulku* ideal of Tibetan Buddhism).

The *Shvetāshvatara-Upanishad*, which is from a somewhat later time than the *Bhagavad-Gītā*, has similar metaphysics but glorifies Shiva (also named Hara) as the supreme Lord. Shiva is said to preside over both the immortal Self and the perishable *pradhāna* (1.10). The Self is considered to be one with the divine Lord in whom all the worlds abide and who is the maker of all the worlds (*vishva-krit*, 6.16). This teaching is called "the highest mystery in Vedānta" (*vedānte pramam guhyam*).

The *Brahma-Sūtra*, ascribed to Bādarāyana, is one of three mainstays of Vedānta; the other two are the (old) Upanishads and the *Bhagavad-Gītā*. This scripture summarizes earlier Vedānta teachings and refers to previous preceptors, and it is clear from the references and the surviving fragments of their teachings that a variety of interpretations of the Upanishads were in circulation. Bādarāyana's was the most successful aphoristic composition and hence survived to our time, even though most of its aphorisms are so succinct that they are obscure. This very obscurity, however, allowed for many pathways of interpretation, some of which are mutually contradictory.

However we may wish to characterize the Upanishadic teachings, they were not of the order of Shankara's authoritative system of Advaita

Vedānta, or radical nondualism. The first work of this particular school was the *Māndūkya-Kārikā* by Gaudapāda, who was the teacher of Shankara's teacher, Govinda. According to Gaudapāda, all phenomena are as vacant as the sky; they are superimposed on the nondual Reality by the mind under the spell of illusion (*māyā*). Nothing whatsoever is born, and therefore nothing is ever destroyed. The world of duality is a mere "quivering of the mind" (*citta-spandita*). This innovative position and its vocabulary is so similar to certain schools of Buddhism that Gaudapāda, who seems to have saluted the Buddha as a great teacher (4.1), has often been styled as crypto-Buddhist. In his commentary on the *Māndūkya-Kārikā* (for example, 4.28), Shankara, who has been subjected to the same criticism, vigorously defends Gaudapāda against this charge. In particular, he criticizes the Vijñānavāda and Shūnyavāda Buddhists for their metaphysical idealism and nihilism, respectively. The former makes the existence of the world dependent on consciousness; the latter upholds the idea of emptiness (*shūnya*), which Shankara misunderstood.

Shankara, who fiercely attacked the Buddhists, laid down his own philosophical path. He interpreted the *Brahma-Sūtra* as offering a coherent view, and to demonstrate that this was so, he was not above bending the meaning of aphorisms in his favor. *Brahman,* or *ātman,* is pure Awareness without any attributes. In regard to the individual being (*jīva*), this Awareness is the Witness (*sākshin*). Upon the dawn of true knowledge ("I am the Absolute"), the wrong knowledge generated by *māyā,* which is really indeterminable (*anirvacanīya*), is removed, and the individual being appears as *brahman.* Phenomenologically speaking, the individual being is as real as the world it confronts. In other words, neither is merely illusory as in the schools of radical philosophical idealism. *Māyā* is understood as spiritual ignorance (*avidyā*), or mistaking the Absolute for the finite endowed with certain false characteristics.

Some three centuries after Shankara, the long-lived South Indian teacher Rāmānuja developed his Vishishtādvaita by interpreting the *Brahma-Sūtra* along lines that were markedly different from those of his predecessor and more in keeping with the spirit of the *Bhagavad-Gītā.* While Shankara's radical nondualism has won much interest and appreciation in the West and is also the preferred philosophy of many of India's traditionalist intellectual elite, Rāmānuja's philosophy of qualified nondualism has long appealed to the majority of Indian religionists, especially those of the Bhāgavata camp. The latter puts forward a theistic interpretation "with great feeling, vast learning and brilliant logic" (Radhakrishnan 1960, 51). For Rāmānuja, the world and the individual beings inhabiting it are the body of the all-comprising Divine (*brahman* = *īshvara* = Nārāyana). He does not regard embodiment itself as a problem—only ignorance and karma. Upon liberation, the individual retains its individuality, and the yogic ideal of *kaivalya* ("aloneness") is deemed lower than that of *mukti* ("release"). The relationship between God and the individual is one of similarity rather than identity. Unlike Shankara and most other teachers of Vedānta, Rāmānuja insists that both knowledge (*jnāna*) and action (*karman*) purify the mind but that only devotion (*bhakti*), or surrender to the Divine, is ultimately salvific. He understands *bhakti* as a special form of knowledge—*jnāna-vishesha*.

Still further removed from Shankara's system is the dualistic (*dvaita*) Vedānta school of Madhva (thirteenth century). He was openly antagonistic toward radical nondualism and its "demon" teachers and has the questionable distinction of being the only Hindu preceptor on record who taught the doctrine of eternal damnation (for demons). Like Rāmānuja, he believed that only devotion is capable of stilling the mind; *bhakti* can absolve a person from the worst sin and bring him or her closer to God, but the kind of complete merging or identification envisioned by Shankara is impossible. Since upon enlightenment both the individuality and distinctive characteristics remain intact, it can be said to vary from one individual to the next. It is really salvation, because it requires the grace of God. The world and its individual beings are not the body of God but his creations. Enlightenment is thought to have four degrees: (1) *sālokya,* or dwelling in the "vicinity" of God; (2) *sāmīpya,* or being close to God; (3) *sārūpya,* or having a spiritual "form" similar to but not the same as God; and (4) *sāyujya,* or having a direct connection with God, which still only qualifies the individual for a partial partaking in the bliss of God.

Madhva explains the Witness as an "I-notion" (*aham-dhī*), which he strictly differentiates from the "I-maker" (*ahamkāra*), or *principium individuationis* ("individuation") of the empirical personality evolving out of *prakriti.* The Witness is identical to the *ātman,* which is absolutely dependent on God but, through ignorance, experiences itself as being enmeshed in cosmic existence and apart from God. While the Witness only perceives time and space, which evolve out of *prakriti,* the ego-personality does not. Madhva apparently also recognized various degrees of Witnessing, the *ātman* being only the first degree; at a higher level, there is the Witnessing of the Golden Germ (Hiranyagarbha), or Cosmic Person, and last is the omniscient Witnessing of God. This is one of the less lucid aspects of Madhva's metaphysics.

Other teachers have elaborated their own distinct philosophical edifices, either modifying Shankara's system or opposing it. Like any philosophical framework, none of these creations are entirely satisfactory from a logical perspective. The critical issue of how a transcendental Reality can be functionally related to a finite mind and body remains problematic.

AWARENESS, SELF-CONSCIOUSNESS, AND SELF-OBSERVATION

We have already dealt with *pure* awareness, so here we will focus on awareness as a property of the mind and also address related questions of self-consciousness and self-observation, which fall under the category of the lower mind (*manas*). The lower mind is defined vis-à-vis *vijñāna*, which is deemed higher because it is more proximate to the Self in the model of successive layers and because it becomes accessible higher up on the *scala mystica* (mystical ladder).

Interestingly, the Witness is regarded as purely transcendental, being identical to the Self. Yet witnessing is obviously a function in which the mind can engage. The practice of mindfulness, as promoted especially in Buddhism, is essentially a form of witnessing. At a lower level, self-observation also has an element of witnessing in it. So it is curious that the Indian traditions banish the Witness to the transcendental level, especially since the transpersonal aspect of the mind—called *buddhi* in the Sāmkhya and Yoga traditions—has all the qualities necessary for witnessing. It is almost pure *sattva,* or lucidity, and therefore reflects the Witness-Self as faithfully as can be expected of any structure within the Cosmos (*prakriti*). Certainly, ordinary awareness, self-consciousness, and the capacity for self-observation must be credited to *buddhi*. Patanjali, in his *Yoga-Sūtra* (3.55), even defines the seeming equality in the purity between *sattva* and the Self. Here *sattva* stands for the *buddhi*.

Although India's spiritual traditions do not discuss the involvement of the *buddhi* in more conventional witnessing, this is always implied. As the higher mind becomes dominant in the spiritual process through increasing "sattvification," the witnessing function gets more and more prominent. Practically speaking, the transcendental Witness (*sākshin* = *ātman/purusha*) could be said to be present, via the reflective "mirror" of the higher mind, in the transformative life of the *yogin*; hence, the importance of the concept of purification in Yoga and similar spiritual disciplines.

The mental function of consciousness entails self-consciousness: We can be conscious of an object and at the same time know that we are thus conscious. This is a matter of a rudimentary kind of self-awareness. It is involved in self-observation, which is the next level of the mind looking at itself in a purposive manner. Self-observation is notoriously difficult, imprecise, and unreliable, which is why it has often been rejected as a method of gathering information in psychology.

Self-observation is, however, an important aspect of the meditative disciplines, notably *vipassanā* meditation in Theravāda Buddhism. Since self-observation is an event within the conscious mind, it is embedded in the nervous system. Self-observation is replaced by Self-Awareness only in the transconceptual ecstatic state (*asamprajnāta-samādhi*), which is beyond the functioning of the brain and nervous system.

The observing self cannot become the object of observation. Thus, it functions at least somewhat like the transcendental Self, which is why Arthur J. Deikman equated the two.[4] My own idea is that it is a function of the *buddhi*, since a transcendental principle is, by definition, above the mind.

PART THREE

Mind in Transition

CHAPTER 15

The Transformative Path

> Yoga is nothing but practical psychology.
>
> —SRI AUROBINDO (1955, 39)

Both Yoga and Western therapeutic approaches in psychology are best viewed as occupying different bands of the same developmental spectrum. The Western approaches (from Freud on) can be regarded as primarily dealing with maladaptations and the goal of restoring the person to normalcy (however this is understood). With Jung, this range widened to include those groping for existential meaning at a time when our culture was (and still is) riddled with uncertainty. Thus, in a lecture given at the Alsatian Pastoral Conference held in Strasbourg in May 1932, Jung talked about Protestants and Catholics who sought out a psychiatrist rather than a pastor or priest for help with their existential worries, because they didn't want to hear doctrinal answers (see Jung 1958b). He reasonably suggested a collaboration between psychiatrists on one hand and parsons or priests on the other.

After Jung, others—notably Sandor Ferenczi, Melanie Klein, Erich Fromm, Victor E. Frankl (1985; see also 1959, 1965, 1967, and 1969), Karl Abraham, Anna Freud (Freud's daughter), Abraham Maslow (1971), and Rollo May (May 1953)—claimed the limelight. At the extreme outer edge of the psychotherapeutic band of the developmental spectrum stood Roberto Assagioli (1965), whose orientation conveniently leads to the yogic band. Ideally, Yoga starts with the reasonably well-adjusted individual who is not suffering from psychoses or major neuroses, and it seeks to conduct him or her to the farther reaches of the developmental spectrum, particularly to the realization of the very essence of the human being (however this essence may be conceived). In Hindu yogic terms, this is the goal of liberation through Self-realization.

In *Psychosynthesis*, Assagioli wrote,

Man's spiritual development is a long and arduous journey, an adventure through strange lands full of surprises, difficulties and even dangers. It involves a drastic transmutation of the "normal" elements of the personality, an awakening of potentialities hitherto dormant, a raising of consciousness to new realms, and a functioning along a new inner dimension. (Assagioli 1965, 39)

This is as far as psychotherapy can probably go, and Assagioli's method is based partly in psychotherapy and partly in spirituality. Some critics feel that he stepped over the boundaries of psychotherapy and was dabbling with the spiritual. While we must admire Assagioli's vision and daring, we cannot help but wonder about the legitimacy of his approach. Unless we assume that he was a Yoga master, which he does not seem to have been, we are right to wonder to what degree he could safely guide a person to actual Self-realization.

THE STEPS OF HINDU YOGA

Early on, traditional Yoga authorities sought to systematize the yogic path. In the post-Buddhist *Shvetāshvatara-Upanishad* (2.8ff.), we find an archaic *scala spiritualis* (spiritual ladder) of four steps that later acquired the technical term of "limbs" (*anga*): sitting straight and steady (*āsana*); causing the senses to enter the heart (*pratyāhāra*); restraining the mind in the heart (*dhārana*); and controlling the breath (*prānāyāma*). The *Katha-Upanishad* (1.3.13) taught the following sequence: restraint of the speech in the mind; restraint of the mind (*manas*) in understanding (*jnāna* = *buddhi*); restraint of understanding in the great self; and restraint of the great self in the tranquil.

Clearly, disciplining the mind—which involves sensory restraint—has been crucial from the outset. Without a doubt, the mind was recognized as the crux of the matter: if the mind could be transformed, a person's entire life could be transformed, and transformation was seen as instrumental to enlightenment.

The path of Hindu Yoga attained its classical form in Patanjali's eight-limbed path (*ashta-anga-mārga*):

1. Moral discipline (*yama*): This branch comprises nonharming (*ahimsā*), truthfulness (*satya*), nonstealing (*asteya*), chastity (*brahmacarya*), and nongrasping (*aparigraha*).

2. Self-restraint (*niyama*): This branch is composed of purity (*shauca*), contentment (*samtosha*), asceticism (*tapas*), study (*svādhyāya*), and dedication to the lord (*īshvara-pranidhāna*).

3. Posture (*āsana*): Contrary to contemporary popular opinion, Patanjali did not teach any postures specifically but sought to capture the essence of meditational posture.

4. Breath control (*prānāyāma*): This involves the control of the in- and out-breath; again, Patanjali offers no specifics.

5. Sensory inhibition, or "sense withdrawal" (*pratyāhāra*): This branch comprises control of the senses that normally hurl attention into the outside world.

6. Concentration (*dhāranā*): This branch consists of fixing attention on whatever inner object has been selected for the contemplative process.

7. Meditation (*dhyāna*): This is the process of sustained mental concentration.

8. Ecstasy (*samādhi*): This branch consists of the temporary merging of subject and object (that is, meditator and meditative focal point in the mind) in a state of supernormal lucidity.

The practices of the first limb are to be performed without fail under all circumstances. If we subscribe to a deep ethical/philosophical teaching, we will likely seek to be benevolent. I discuss these practices in more detail in my book *Yoga Morality* (2007).

I also deal with the second limb at length in *Yoga Morality* and therefore will not go into it further here. Let me just say that in *īshvara-pranidhāna*, or "dedication to the lord," *īshvara* does not stand for "god." Here, the lord is simply a special *purusha,* or transcendental Self, without any creative function. As is evident from aphorism 2.45, the lord has the ability to grace the *yogin* with the perfection of ecstasy.

Psychologically, the aforementioned ethical restraints can be understood as mental preparations for the higher stages of Yoga. The mind *cannot* be stilled in the absence of ethical integrity. Physiologically, this means that we must be able to exercise control over the animal part of our brain.

The yogic path can be interpreted as a course of progressive inner control, mental simplification, or inner purification. At its purest, the person stands revealed as the Self, which is utterly simple (*kevalin*).

In later times, Patanjali's eight-limbed path was expanded into a fifteen-limbed approach (see, for example, the *Tejobindu-Upanishad* 1.15–16) and more complex arrangements (see, for example, the sixteen limbs of Mantra-Yoga according to the *Mantra-Yoga-Samhitā* [31ff.] of the seventeenth or eighteenth century). Thus, the fifteen steps given in the *Tejobindu-Upanishad* comprise the following:

1. Moral disciplines
2. Self-restraint
3. Renunciation (*tyāga*)
4. Silence (*mauna*)
5. Place (*desha*)
6. Time (*kāla*)
7. Posture
8. "Root lock" (*mūla-bandha*)
9. Bodily balance (*deha-sāmya*)
10. Steadiness of vision (*dhrik-sthiti*)
11. Breath control (*prāna-samyama*)
12. Sense withdrawal (*pratyāhāra*)
13. Concentration (*dhāranā*)
14. Meditation (*dhyāna*)
15. Ecstasy (*samādhi*)

This path is a combination of the eight practice categories of Patanjali's Yoga and select physical techniques of Hatha-Yoga from the medieval period.

According to the *Goraksha-Samhitā* (1.7), an early text of this branch of Yoga, Hatha-Yoga has six limbs that correspond to the limbs of Pātanjala-Yoga, without the first two (*yama* and *niyama*). These six limbs comprise Classical Yoga's ethical rules, which are to be universally observed. Their absence in Hatha-Yoga often leads to the incorrect assumption that this branch of Yoga is ethically neutral, but they are assumed by all practitioners.

Bhakti-Yoga, which first emerged in the *Bhagavad-Gītā* (for example, 18.54), has nine limbs, such as listening, praising (through songs), and prostration, in its medieval form.[1] According to the *Kulārnava-Tantra* (9.34ff.), tantra, which formed itself around the middle of the first millennium C.E., consists of spontaneity (*sahaja*) at the highest level, concentration and meditation at the middle level, laudation and recitation at the penultimate level, and sacrifice and worship at the lowest level.

THE PRACTICE (JNĀNA-YOGA) OF VEDĀNTA
AND OTHER HINDU TRADITIONS

All liberation systems of Hinduism have the same goal—*moksha*—and a path that is thought to lead to that goal. In the case of early Vedānta, as we encounter it in the Upanishads, there are the three practices of hearing (*shravana*), reflecting (*manana*), and contemplating (*nididhyāsana*), which make up Jnāna-Yoga, the path of wisdom.[2] In later Vedānta, we generally find the path of Patanjali, suitably reinterpreted along nondualistic lines. "Hearing" refers to the practice of imbibing the wisdom of Vedānta, either by listening carefully to one's teacher or by studying the scriptures. It is not simply tacit assent but calls for study of the Vedānta tradition.

The discipline of reflecting stands for the constant consideration of the truth of nonduality, as taught by Vedānta. There are two kinds of contemplating: (1) *savikalpaka,* or with form (*kalpa*), and (2) *nirvikalpaka,* or without form. In the first variety, the contemplative experience is based on the distinction between subject and object (even though this distinction is experientially not in place in the state of ecstasy). The form is the object of contemplation with which the practitioner achieves a sense of identity. The second variety is formless, that is, the practitioner has transcended the ecstatic identification with the contemplated object and attained the realization of the singular Reality (or *ātman/brahman*). Interestingly, the *Vedānta-Sāra* by Sadānanda Yogendra, which belongs to the medieval period, mentions both varieties (sections 12–13) as authoritative and valid. The apex of either approach is the transconceptual ecstasy (*samādhi*) about which Swami Satprakashananda has written the following:

> In nirvikalpa samādhi, contrary to deep sleep, all the features and functions of the mind, including even the ego-idea, are absorbed in unspecified, undifferentiated awareness, or Pure Consciousness beyond the distinction of the knower and the known. Whereas in deep sleep the mind is completely engulfed in ignorance or darkness, in nirvikalpa samādhi it is thoroughly suffused with the light of Pure Consciousness.... From sleep a person returns with all his ignorance. His doubts, fears, wrong notions, and tendencies root in ajñāna remains just the same. But from nirvikalpa samādhi one returns as an illumined person freed from ajñāna [spiritual ignorance]. (Satprakashananda 1965, 280)

Nirvikalpa-samādhi fulfills itself in liberation (*moksha*). If little can be said about this ultimate level of ecstasy, liberation is even less amenable to the conceptual contrivances of language. It is the undoing of everything we may call human, and the only appropriate response to the question of what liberation is, is silence or paradoxical language. Liberation, which is the termination of the spiritual path, makes the adept transhuman. As the Buddha responded, the liberated being neither exists nor does not exist. This nonexplanation leaves the ordinary individual delightfully perplexed.

According to the *Yoga-Vāsishtha*,[3] which we may assign to about 800 C.E., the spiritual path comprises the following seven steps:

1. *shubha-icchā,* or "the urge toward the auspicious": This involves the desire for liberation, which corresponds to right view.
2. *vicāranā,* or "consideration": By contemplating the philosophical matters of Vedānta (such as by asking "Who am I?"), a practitioner stimulates his or her commitment to the spiritual path; this second element corresponds to the practice of *manana.*
3. *tanu-mānasā,* or "refined thinking": Here thinking assumes a new quality that makes a practitioner weary of the world and he or she is moved toward dispassion (*vairāgya*); this corresponds to a higher phase of *manana.*
4. *sattva-āpatti,* or "attainment of lucidity": This is a virtue similar to Classical Yoga's ecstatic "vision of discernment" (*viveka-khyāti*) in which the Self comes into view.
5. *asamsakti,* or "nonattachment": This element is analogous to the act of supreme dispassion (*para-vairāgya*) in Pātanjala-Yoga.
6. *padārtha-abhāvanā,* or "the nonimagining of reality": All mental projections are withdrawn and reality is seen for what it is in itself, which is like a dream; possibly, this level corresponds to *nirbīja-samādhi* in Pātanjala-Yoga.
7. *turya-gā,* or "abiding in the Fourth": This element corresponds to the attainment of living liberation.

The *Yoga-Vāsishtha,* which consists of nearly thirty-two thousand stanzas, subscribes to a radical form of nondualism that, in keeping with philosophical idealism, regards the world as a mere mental phantom (hence step 6). In reality, the world is the ultimate Reality, though a person may only believe this until there is direct realization (*sākshātkāra*) in the highest ecstasy.

Most Vedānta schools do not subscribe to this kind of philosophical idealism. Even the radical nondualist school (Kevalādvaita) of Shankara does not deny the existence of the world and only claims that we interpret it incorrectly. Thus, only a limited illusion (*māyā*) is involved. This is explained by invoking the visual illusion of seeing a snake instead of the rope it really is or mistaking a person for a tree trunk. *Māyā*, then, is distortion, or erroneous knowledge. The moon reflected in the water is not the moon itself. Similarly, the mind riddled with unconscious activators and their products (*vrittis*) does not reveal its true nature to us. When it is completely pacified, it acts like a mirror in which the ultimate Reality stands faithfully revealed.

Most Vedānta schools belong to what is known as qualified nondualism (Vishishtādvaita), as taught by Rāmānuja in the tenth to eleventh century C.E.; the Dvaitādvaita school of Nimbārka; the Shuddhādvaita school of Vallabha; or other similar metaphysical systems. The school of Shankara's Kevalādvaita, which is best known in the West, is mostly confined to the brahmanical intelligentsia in India.

Shankara's form of Vedānta was close to Mahāyāna Buddhism, and Kevalādvaita—which has its roots in the teachings of Gaudapāda, Shankara's grand teacher—has often been branded as crypto-Buddhism. It was perhaps this misperception that was reponsible for the ousting of Buddhism from India. More importantly, however, the Muslim invaders found Buddhism's atheistic stance more offensive than the putative "pantheistic paganism" of the Hindus.

THE BUDDHIST FLOW TO *NIRVĀNA*

The Buddha can be said to have revolutionized philosophical thinking in India by favoring a process method that broke away from structuralist models like Sāmkhya and Vedānta. For him, everything was interlinked in an unbroken nexus. This teaching is captured in the idea of "dependent origination," or as some call it, "conditioned coproduction" (*pratītya-samutpāda*), which states that everything is dependent on everything else and nothing exists in isolation.

The Buddha thought that liberation (*nirvāna*, or "extinction") is not the attainment of a static state of existence beyond all other states but is also subject to the inevitable processual march of things. Admittedly, this teaching is hard to grasp, and we may perhaps derive more meaning from his mystical/paradoxical confession that an enlightened being cannot be said to exist or not exist.[4]

Like all liberation teachings, however, the Buddha understood the path as a movement from ignorance (or false view) to true knowledge (*jnāna*). His formulation of the path has the following eight steps (see Goddard 1981):

1. Right view (Pāli: *sammā-ditthi;* Skt.: *samyag-drishti*): the view that sees things as they are and is not marred by the usual delusions
2. Right resolve (Pāli: *sammā-sankappa;* Skt.: *samyak-samkalpa*): the resolution to proceed without causing harm to others and to further their welfare
3. Right speech (Pāli: *sammā-vāca;* Skt.: *samyag-vākya*): speech that is spiritually sound
4. Right conduct (Pāli: *sammā-kammanta;* Skt.: *samyak-karmantā*): conduct that follows and promotes the basic ethical norms of Buddhism
5. Right livelihood (Pāli: *sammā-ājīva;* Skt.: *samyag-ājīva*): livelihood that does not infringe on the major ethical norms of nonharming and nonstealing
6. Right effort (Pali: *sammā-vāyāmā;* Skt.: *samyag-vyāyāma*): effort that furthers the spiritual values of Buddhism
7. Right mindfulness (Pāli: *sammā-sati;* Skt.: *samyak-smṛti*): the ongoing wholesome exercise of attention
8. Right concentration (Pāli: *sammā-samādhi;* Skt.: *samyak-samādhi*): the higher meditation practices that simplify the mind and tap into its subtle potential

These eight steps are usually grouped into three sets as follows: Steps 1 and 2 make up wisdom (*prajnā*); steps 3 through 5 make up morality (*shīla*), and steps 6 through 8 constitute concentration (*samādhi*).

The first step recalibrates the mind by getting us to abandon our wrong views of the world. The *Brahma-Jala-Sutta* of the *Dīgha-Nikāya* (1.1) lists as many as sixty-two wrong views. These are views or opinions about the world that, if followed, would lead us into suffering. As part of the teaching about right view, we mainly ought to understand that *duhkha,* or "suffering," is woven into the very fabric of life and that there can be no lasting happiness through any worldly experience. Likewise we ought to grasp that it is perfectly possible to remove suffering by means of the noble eightfold path. We should not look for permanence in this impermanent world, for a Self in the nonself, or for beauty in what is really ugliness. Once we understand things correctly, we should also embark on the spiritual path correctly. Right view must be followed by right action, or nothing is accomplished. The Buddha was not merely a teacher of ethics, as is often thought in Western circles; at the same time, he was not a teacher of mere abstract philosophical principles. He duly integrated body and mind.

Right resolve precedes right action. It includes the desire to not harm any living being but to seek their welfare and practice renunciation (or what we would perhaps call voluntary simplicity today).

Right speech is vitally important, especially today when we generally do so much harm verbally through harsh speech, idle talk, gossip, abusive talk, or slander. All these forms of wrong speech merely do harm and increase our store of inauspicious mental phenomena, which inevitably ripen into undesirable karma.

Right conduct is concerned with how we behave in the world. The idea behind this step on the path is to minimize the production of negative, or inauspicious, karma. Wrong behavior includes grave offences like killing, stealing, and debauchery (which earns expulsion from the order in the case of a monastic).

Right livelihood relates to how we earn a living, and here the Buddha had all kinds of commonsensical recommendations, notably those relating to the virtue of abstention from harming in the course of procuring one's livelihood. Thus, he thought it ignoble for a follower of his teaching to kill other beings, which made it impossible to pursue professions such as those of a butcher or a soldier. Reasonably, he even forbade his lay followers to trade in arms, human beings, meat, intoxicating drinks, and poisons.

Right effort means lawful exertion. The Buddha indulged in extreme asceticism for six years before finding the middle path. He thought it wrong to pursue liberation by such destructive means, which merely weaken the body and the mind.

Right mindfulness primarily applies to the lifestyle of a monastic. This consists in moment-to-moment attentiveness to all arising physical, mental, and emotional experiences. In this way, a monk or nun can move toward auspicious states of mind and away from inauspicious, or karmically detrimental, states.

Right concentration refers to the advanced ecstatic practices a Buddhist monastic is encouraged to cultivate. They are deemed important in reaching *nirvāna,* though it is held by some authorities that one can also attain the supreme state of enlightenment without them. The most important concentrations are the four formative and the four formless *jhānas*.

Mahāyāna Buddhism recognizes ten levels in the development of a bodhisattva, a being who has dedicated him- or herself to the welfare of all beings, both before and after enlightenment. The ten stages are as follows:

1. Joyous stage (*pramuditā bhūmi*), which is associated with the perfection of generosity (*dāna*), allowing the bodhisattva to implement his or her vow unencumbered by egoic motivations
2. Immaculate stage (*vimalā bhūmi*), which correlates with the perfection of moral conduct (*shīla*) whereby the bodhisattva's spiritual discipline becomes unshakeable
3. Radiating stage (*prabhākārī bhūmi*), which is connected with the perfection of patience (*kshānti*), permitting the bodhisattva to endure any kind of adversity
4. Blazing stage (*arcishmatī bhūmi*), which is associated with the perfection of vitality or irresistible willpower (*vīrya*)
5. Very-difficult-to-conquer stage (*sudurjayā bhūmi*), which is connected with the perfection of meditation (*dhyāna*) in which the bodhisattva masters the keyboard of mental states
6. Facing-toward-[wisdom] stage (*abhimukhī bhūmi*), which is associated with the perfection of wisdom (*prajnā*) and in which the bodhisattva, understanding him- or herself as an illusory being, is committed to freeing all other illusory beings from an illusory world
7. Far-going stage (*dūrangamā bhūmi*), which is correlated with the perfection of skillful means (*upāya*), when the now-disembodied transcendental bodhisattva can appear in any form whatsoever and skillfully guide others
8. Immovable stage (*acalā bhūmi*), which is connected with the perfection of [right] resolution (*pranidhāna*), enabling the bodhisattva to transfer his or her own karmic merit to others
9. Good stage (*sādhumatī bhūmi*), which is associated with the perfection of strength (*bala*), allowing the bodhisattva to begin to make good on his or her initial vow to liberate all beings
10. Cloud-of-teaching stage (*dharma-megha-bhūmi*), which correlates with the perfection of knowledge (*jnāna*)—that is, omniscience

The progression through these ten levels is slow and arduous.

THE JAINA LADDER TO PERFECTION

In Jainism, the ladder to enlightenment, or omniscience (*kevala-jnāna*), comprises the following fourteen steps:

1. False view (*mithyā-drishti*): Our starting point in regular life is marked by many mistaken opinions and views; we grow by giving them up. The inclusion of this step suggests that even wrong view entails the possibility of correct view. Otherwise, none of us would ever wake up.
2. Mixed taste (*sāsvādana*): This step can only be reached when the practitioner has fallen from a higher level of spiritual attainment.
3. From false toward correct view (*samyag-mithyātva*): This is a transitional stage during which the practitioner proceeds from the first to the fourth step.
4. Correct view (*samyag-drishti*): This is where most traditions start the path.
5. Restraint of place (*desha-virata*): At this level, a layperson receives the vows (*vrata*) appropriate for him or her, which are watered-down (partial) versions of the vows for an ascetic. The idea behind all vows—nonharming, truthfulness, nonstealing, chastity, and the renunciation of possessions—is to reduce or stop the "influx" of karma.
6. Restraint of all (*sarva-virata*): At this stage, the "great vow" (*mahā-vrata*) of an ascetic is received.
7. Attentive restraint (*apramatta-virata*): Here virtuous contemplation (*dharma-dhyāna*) is the means of combating carelessness (*pramāda*).
8. Gross struggle with cessation (*apūrva-karana*): Here there is the capacity for deep meditation leading to great joy; moreover, the ascetic gains even greater power over himself or herself.
9. Cessation of cause (*anivritti-karana*): Here the vision of truth becomes manifest, and things are seen as they really are. The passions (*kashāya*)—anger, pride, deceit, and greed—are overcome.
10. Subtle struggle (*sūkshma-sāmparāya*): Only subtle greed—such as the subconscious attachment to the body—is able to disturb a practitioner occasionally.
11. Tranquil delusion (*upashānta-moha*): This is equivalent to the conquest of all the passions called *vita-rāga*. Here a twofold ladder (*shreni*)—of control (*upashama-shreni*) or of annihilation (*kshapa-shreni*)—presents itself.

12. Dwindled delusion (*kshīna-moha*): This is the summit of the ladder of annihilation, and it destroys the karmas that conceal knowledge and intuition.
13. Active omniscience (*sayoga-kevalin*): This is the level of a *jīvanmukta*. The karmas that are produced at this level are no longer obscuring.
14. Inactive omniscience (*ayoga-kevalin*): This is the last stage before full disembodied liberation (*moksha*) is attained. The mind and body become completely tranquil. The means to this stage is the highest level of *shukla-dhyāna*—based on forbearance, humility, straightforwardness, and freedom from greed—that lacks all vibration (*samducchinna-kriyā*) and has neither coarse thought (*vitarka*) nor subtle thought (*vicāra*).

Liberation, which is understood as omniscience, is the state of a *siddha* (adept) who, without a physical body, lives permanently in the realm of adepts (*siddha-loka*). This realm is curiously pictured as cresent-shaped and constituting the apex of the world (*loka-ākāsha*) beyond the divine realms.

CHAPTER 16

The Yoga of Sound and Dance

> Rhythmic sound, in cosmogonic myths,
> is at the root of all creation.
>
> —MARIA-GABRIELE WOSIEN (1974, 8)

Rhythmic sound (voice, drums, rattles) and dance belong to the earliest techniques of altering consciousness. As Mircea Eliade (1972, 416) notes, the commonalities between Yoga and shamanism are numerous. In his monograph on Yoga (1973, 106ff.), Eliade singles out *tapas* ("ardor/heat"), which has a clear shamanic precursor. To master inner heat is a prominent feature of Yoga. According to the *Rig-Veda* (10.167.1), Indra stormed heaven by means of *tapas,* and all the deities (*deva*) gained their celestial status by the same means (see *Taittirīya-Brāhmana* 3.12.3.1). We may associate the deities' luminosity with the same source (*deva* stems from the grammatical root *div,* meaning "to shine").

One entire Vedic Samhitā—the *Sāma-Veda*—is dedicated to the chanting of certain hymns from the *Rig-Veda* during the sacrificial rituals. A mantra is best defined as a "conduit of power." Power (*shakti*) and empowerment are essential qualities of the mantra, and this also connects it to the shamanic era, which is concerned with power. The hymns are measured out in meters (such as the *gāyatrī,* the *anushtubh,* and the *chandāmsi*) and are therefore rhythmic. As rhythmic creations, they are psychologically potent. The entire sacrificial ritual is first and foremost concerned with the strategy of power. As the Upanishads express it, "Speech verily is the Absolute" (*vāg vai brahman*). We must visualize the Absolute as a network of power, of potent forces. Speech is just one node in this network and, according to Mantra-Yoga, the most important one.

Another aspect of Yoga that correlates well with shamanism is the paranormal (or magical) powers, which are given great prominence in the *Yoga-Sūtra* of Patanjali (chapter 3), the textbook of Classical Yoga.

MODERN RESEARCH

Mantras vary from tradition to tradition, and to strip them of their religious or sacred background, some authors have made up their own. The best-known book of this kind is *Freedom in Meditation* by the American psychologist Patricia Carrington (1978). She went so far as to suggest that any word can function as a mantra and focus the mind. This counsel ignores the fact that a mantra is traditionally rendered effective by being "seen" by a seer (*rishi*)—that is, a qualified *guru*—and is transmitted by way of initiation (*dīkshā*). In her later years, Carrington turned to Emotional Freedom Technique (EMT), which is also known as "tapping."

For a mantra to be effective means that it can generate the *mantra-caitanya,* or mantric consciousness. It is through this consciousness that the mantra's recitation becomes automatic (or an unconscious process) and, in due course, will bear fruit. To jump-start a mantra, it is generally repeated at least one hundred thousand times. Since some mantras are not just phonemes but entire phrases, this process can take several weeks or even several months to complete.

Research on mantras started in the 1960s with Transcendental Meditation (TM), which is a supposedly "easy" mantric practice invented by Maharishi Mahesh Yogi. Research on TM is voluminous but apparently unreliable. The technique is supposed to calm the nervous system and enhance intuition, creativity, and social coherence. Unfortunately, in the mid-1970s, TM became associated with the Maharishi's Sidhi Program, which promoted the paranormal power of "flying" (or levitation). The available evidence does not bear out this ambitious claim, which came at a time when the number of TM students was dwindling. Founded in 1957, TM probably reached its peak by 1975 when Merv Griffin endorsed it on his TV show.

The sweeping theory behind TM is known as Science of Creative Intelligence (SCI), which seems to be a reformulation of the Advaita Vedāntic teachings of Shankara for Western students. Among other things, SCI predicted that social transformation kicks in when 1 percent of people in a given area practice TM. Thus, in 1982, Maharishi Mahesh Yogi confidently announced that he would transform the entire world and prevent war and social disharmony by establishing thirty-six hundred centers around the world. Each center would have one TM teacher who would attract one thousand trainees. The world would change when the magical figure of 1 percent was reached.

But the immediate goal of TM is "cosmic consciousness," or enlightenment, as Maharishi Mahesh Yogi explains about the enlightened being:

> He is engaged in fulfilling the cosmic purpose and therefore his actions are guided by nature. (Maharishi 1969, 287)

Beyond cosmic consciousness is the stage of "God consciousness," which adds devotion to the qualities of the former condition. The inner space is filled with God—a notion that brings us close to the teachings of Krishna in the *Bhagavad-Gītā*.

Of course, not all research is about TM, and the field has become replete over the years with all kinds of electroencephalographic and other data. We have become clearer about the benefits of meditation and its limitations, as well as its types.[1]

POST-VEDIC MANTRA-YOGA IN HINDUISM

Mantra-Yoga is intimately connected with the rise of theistic Yoga. Apart from Vedic Yoga, which has a distinguished mantra practice, we see Mantra-Yoga closely associated with the emergence of the god Vishnu in the *Bhagavad-Gītā* (c. 400 B.C.E.), the god Shiva in the *Shvetāshvatara-Upanishad* (c. 300 B.C.E.), and the goddess Devī in the *Devī-Gītā* of the *Devī-Bhāgavata-Purāna* (7.31–40; c. 1300 C.E.).

Vishnu (as Krishna) claims OM is a superior manifestation of himself (*Bhagavad-Gītā* 9.17). In stanzas 17.23–27, he expounds on the Upanishadic mantra OM TAT SAT ("Oм. That is real/true."). The *Shvetāshvatara-Upanishad* (1.14) offers this simile: By making one's body the lower friction stick (*arani*) and the *pranava* the upper one, it is possible to see the hidden God by the practice of meditation. It seems that mantra recitation was essential to Yoga. The *Maitrāyanīya-Upanishad* (c. 200 B.C.E.) mentions that AUM (= OM) is the formative, solar aspect of *brahman*. The formless *brahman*, however, is reality that can be reached via the sacred syllable AUM. This syllable is also known as the *shabda-brahman*, or sonic Absolute. It is the same as the ether-space in the middle of the heart (see *Maitrāyanīya-Upanishad* 7.11.3).

In post-Vedic Yoga, the recitation or "muttering" (*japa*) of *mantras* is given preeminence. The "seed syllables" (*bīja-mantra*) are credited with heightened power, and the syllable OM—or *pranava* (humming sound)—is thought to be charged with particular power. It is the *mantra* par excellence that symbolizes the Absolute, or God (see *Yoga-Sūtra* 1.27), the holder of all power. The syllable OM, which is not mentioned but was undoubtedly known in Vedic times (see, for example, *Rig-Veda* 1.164.39), is first mentioned in the "white" (unmixed) recension of the *Yajur-Veda* (1.1). By the time of the Upanishads—the oldest of which are conventionally assigned to about 1000 B.C.E.—a rich speculation had become associated with OM.

In the *Mundaka-Upanishad* (2.4), composed by about 300 B.C.E., we can read,

> The humming-sound [that is, OM] is the bow; one's self indeed is the arrow.
> *Brahman* is said to be the target of that. It is to be pierced with care. Thus [the *yogin*] becomes one with it, as the arrow [becomes one with the target].
> (Nakamura 1990, 40)

According to the *Bhagavad-Gītā* (8.13), which was created earlier than the *Mundaka*, the *yogin* is supposed to pronounce this mantra at the time of death. Death requires the utmost concentration, the kind of attentiveness that one must also muster in everyday life. The *Katha-Upanishad* (1.2.17) explains that by reciting OM, we can win the higher or the lower *brahman*. The lower *brahman* is not the Absolute but *prakriti,* which is also a teaching found in the *Bhagavad-Gītā*.

Mantras became the center of Mantra-Yoga with the rise of Tantra. About 1000 C.E., Abhinavagupta—a great Kashmiri master—developed the Trika system, which was built around the practice of *mantras.* The degree to which Trika is mantrically based is obvious from Abhinavagupta's *Parātrīshikā-Vivarana,* which is available in a fine English rendering. As Abhinavagupta (1989, 180) says in this text, "Here (i.e., in Trika)... every object rests on the superb splendour of the *mantra*." Mantric theory was greatly embellished in the Tantric schools. Mantra-Yoga acquired sixteen limbs in the early modern era, including devotion (*bhakti*), serving the sacred (consecrated) space, offering water libations to the deities, invoking, and making food offerings (see *Mantra-Yoga-Samhitā* 31, which was probably authored in the seventeenth century). A century earlier, the well-known *tāntrika* Pūrnānanda wrote several works on *mantras,* not least of which were the *Mantra-Mahārnava* (Great Odean of Mantras), the *Mantra-Muktavalī* (Independent Tract on Mantras), and *Mantra-Kaumudī* (Moonlight on Mantras).

MANTRAS IN BUDDHIST AND JAINA YOGA

Buddhism has known many *mantras* from its beginnings. They achieved great prominence in Tantric Buddhism (or Vajrayāna). The sacred syllable OM is steadily present in all branches of Buddhism. *Mantras* are particularly important in Vajrayāna, as it is still practiced in Tibet. They play a major role in the cultivation of the development, or first, stage of Deity Yoga, which is most widely practiced and also very challenging. The purpose of the development stage (Tib.: *bskyed rim*, pron. *kye rim*) is not only to gain identity with the visualized deity but to recognize that the deity and every other being has absolutely no essence—that is, they are all illusory. The development stage is accompanied by the recitation of *mantras*, which are employed to protect the practitioner and to invoke the deity and his or her retinue (Jigme et al. 2006).

MEDITATION IN JAINISM

Mantras play a role in Jainism mainly in conjunction with doctrinal formulas such as the *namaskāra-mantra*. Mantric recitation was boosted in Jainism's brush with Tantra. *Mantras* are often written in an elaborate, ornamental style. In Jainism, the word *yoga* does not have the usual meaning. It generally stands for "vibration," by which karma is attracted. In 800 C.E., the scholar Haribhadra Sūri wrote several Sanskrit works that sought to integrate Yoga with Jainism.

In his *Yoga-Bindu* (31), Haribhadra distinguishes various kinds of Yoga: *adhyātma-yoga*, or Yoga of the inner self; *bhāvanā-yoga*, or Yoga of meditative cultivation; *dhyāna-yoga*, or Yoga of meditation; *samatā-yoga*, or Yoga of equanimity; and *vritti-samkshaya-yoga*, or Yoga of the destruction of the fluctuations (of the mind). Elsewhere in the same text (369ff.), he has *tāttvika-yoga*, Reality-based Yoga; *atātvika-yoga*, or Unreal Yoga; *sānubandha-yoga*, or Yoga with Continuity; *niranubandha-yoga*, or Yoga That Is Discontinuous; *sāsrava-yoga*, or Yoga with (Karmic) Influx; and *anasāsrava-yoga*, or Yoga Free from Influx.

Hedistinguishes four kinds of Yoga for the mind: *satya-mano-yoga*, or Yoga of Truthful Mind; *asatya-mano-yoga*, or Yoga of Untrue Mind; *mishra-mano-yoga*, or Yoga of Mixed Mind; and *vyavahāra-mano-yoga*, or Yoga of the Ordinary Mind. There are also four kinds of Yoga for speech: *satya-vacana-yoga*, or Yoga of True Speech; *asatya-vacana-yoga*, or Yoga of Untrue

Speech; *mishra-vacana-yoga,* or Yoga of Mixed Speech; and *vyavahāra-vacana-yoga,* or Yoga of Ordinary Speech. Then there are seven kinds of Yoga for the body: *audarika-kāya-yoga,* or Yoga of the Gluttonous Body; *audarika-mishra-kāya-yoga,* or Yoga of the Mixed Gluttonous Body; *vankrya-kāya-yoga,* or Yoga of the Crooked Body; *vankrya-mishra-kāya-yoga,* or Yoga of the Mixed Crooked Body; *āhāraka-kāya-yoga,* or Yoga of the Food Body; *āhāraka-mishra-kāya-yoga,* or Yoga of the Mixed Food Body; and *kamana-kāya-yoga,* or Yoga of the Enamored Body.

Haribhadra Sūri (381) goes on to say that a novice practices the Yoga of the inner self in the form of mantric recitation (*japa*), which is connected with a deity whose favor he or she seeks.

Meditation is central to all Indian spiritual traditions. The Jaina Sutras categorize meditation into *ārta-dhyāna, raudra-dhyāna, dharma-dhyāna,* and *shukla-dhyāna.*

ECSTATIC DANCE

Dance movement therapy (DMT) has been around since the 1940s. One of the founders was Marian Chace, who was influenced by Carl Jung. In the 1970s and 1980s, DMT experienced a florescence that led to today's dance therapeutic efforts (see Lewis 1984, Siegel 1984, Stanton-Jones 1992, Meekums 2002, and Payne 2006). Modern Western Yoga has likewise shown an interest in dance.

This is not as extraordinary as it sounds, because the god Shiva—a rascal ascetic—is known both as a prototypical *yogin* and as a master of dance.[2] Iconographically, Shiva as the King of Dance (*nata-rāja*) is depicted standing in a dance posture surrounded by an aureole of flames, with his right foot planted on a dwarflike figure. This figure is known as the *apasmara-purusha,* or amnesiac man, symbolizing the human being who fails to remember his or her divine nature at birth. Shiva's dance disturbs the ordinary human. Shiva's right hand is in *abhaya-mudrā,* suggesting that the individual need not fear his dancing action.

With an ash-besmeared naked body and matted hair, Shiva performed his cosmic dance before sages and *yogins* in the forest. He also danced in a gorgeous form when he was wooing Pārvatī, the daughter of Himālaya, and his future mother-in-law, Menā, was suitably impressed. Despite all of Shiva's sexual overtures, he was fully renounced. This became obvious when a blade of grass cut his hand, and instead of blood, vegetable juice issued forth.

The seer Mankanaka was overly elated, and the gods asked Shiva to curb his pride. Shiva appeared before him and pierced his thumb. The wound produced ashes, and the seer stopped his euphoric dance in shame.

Shiva is associated with the *damaru,* the small hand drum that produces a staccato rhythm (*tala*). The *tala* is equated with the male gender, while the melody (*rāga)* represents the female gender. The *damaru* is fashioned from two joined cranial sections of the skulls of a fifteen- or sixteen-year-old boy and girl. The skulls are tightly covered with animal skin and equipped with beaters made of string and ending in balls. It was Shiva who taught not only Yoga but music and all the arts and sciences to the sages.

Swami Sivananda Radha, a German-born woman whose former name was Sylvia Hellman (née Demitz) and who was initiated into Yoga by Swami Sivananda of Rishikesh, learned Indian dance at her teacher's behest. In 1951, she emigrated to Canada where she founded a prominent ashram at Kootenay Bay. She once remarked,

Yoga is dance.
Dance is Yoga.
Life is dance.
Dance together in
Divine Light.

CHAPTER 17

Authority and Discipleship

The teachings of the masters have left
an eternal influence on humanity.

—MENOS KAFATOS and
THALIA KAFATOU
(1991, 259)

Wherever a course of initiatory disciplines is involved, the question of authority rears its head and often becomes a knotty problem. Who is authorized to initiate, and what does this entail? Especially in modern times, under the influence of widespread democratization, authority is a tricky subject and is often couched in terms of power symmetry and asymmetry. The *guru*-disciple relationship is typically seen as being asymmetric: the *guru* is invested with power that the disciple does not have. This may be so in the context of Eastern social arrangements, but even the psychotherapist-analysand relationship of the West is asymmetric: the psychotherapist knows, while the analysand is enmeshed in ignorance. Those who see relationships in symmetric/asymmetric terms are bound to perceive and critique either type of relationship as one of unwholesome power inequality. Thus, Anthony Storr, who assures his readers that by no means are all *gurus* bad, writes in *Feet of Clay,*

> Gurus tend to be intolerant of any kind of criticism, believing that anything less than total agreement is equivalent to hostility. This may be because they have been so isolated that they have never experienced the interchange of ideas and positive criticism which only friends can provide. (Storr 1996, xii)

While this may be true of some religious *gurus* and many authoritarian figures, as Storr believes—he lumps together Bhagawan Rajneesh, Jim Jones, and David Koresh with Sigmund Freud, Carl Jung, Rudolf Steiner,

Paul Brunton, and G. I. Gurdjieff—it is probably truer of disciples in the grip of irrational idealization or adoration of their teacher or those who have an irrational fear of him or her.

Storr, an Oxfordian psychiatrist, is convincing only to those who are a priori against *gurus* or who blindly subscribe to the doctrines of conventional psychiatry. His book is written in a style that is bound to attract readers who are fond of sensationalism, and some of his accounts—such as the one on Paul Brunton—are little more than ill-researched character assassinations. If Brunton suffered from "compensatory phantasies" and was subject to "wildly improbable premises," one would have to write off every spiritual teacher of his caliber, which is unreasonable.

THE PSYCHOTHERAPIST

The relationship of the therapist/analyst and the analysand has often been compared to that of the *guru* and the disciple, especially when the analysand does not desire help with a life problem but seeks to further his or her individuation.[1] Both relationships require intimate trust—in psychological terms, transference and countertransference. The *guru*, at his best, is traditionally expected to live out of the mode of Self-realization (or enlightenment) and to be able to initiate the disciple into Self-realization (even if it is only a glimpse). If a *guru* is not Self-realized, he (or more rarely, she) is expected to firmly aspire to Self-realization or at least to be able to guide the disciple toward this highest goal of Yoga.

The psychotherapist also endeavors to lead the analysand's psyche, to be a psychopompos, though for the most part his or her goal is to conduct that psyche from neuroses to ordinary health and, more seldom, from average functioning to wholeness (or individuation). He or she is inspired by science (or scientism). Even Carl Jung, whose father was a Lutheran pastor and who saw his role as a therapist as having religious (spiritual) objectives, ventured to be true to the canons of science. Like the *guru*, the therapist is concerned with wisdom, which should grow especially in the latter part of life. But whereas the *guru*'s wisdom, at least in theory, sets the disciple free existentially, the therapist's wisdom only increases the analysand's understanding. In comparison with the Eastern teachings, it is not truly liberative.

Although Carl Jung assured us that "I am a researcher and not a prophet,"[2] he also admitted that unless psychotherapy digs down into religious humus, it cannot effect a real change. In *Modern Man in Search of a Soul*, he wrote,

Among all my patients in the second half of life—that is to say, over thirty-five—there has not been one whose problem in the last resort was not that of finding a religious outlook on life. (Jung 1933, 229)

Joel Kramer, a well-known Yoga teacher, and his partner, Diana Alstad, take a highly critical stance about authoritarianism, which they perceive everywhere in our civilization (Kramer and Altstad 1993, xi, 32, 33). They understand that authoritarianism "has been part of the structural weave holding social orders together" and, popular opinion to the contrary, "has been and largely still is a primary mode of social cohesion." For Kramer and Alstad, the *guru* role or function is problematic. They tell us that the "guru/disciple relationship is a formal structure of extreme authoritarianism" that elucidates "in bas-relief the workings of what may be called the cult mentality." This is inherently dangerous, because "[s]hould the *guru* become paranoid, greedy, or merely bored, as many do, they can get their disciples to do most anything." This is, of course, the popular Western stance—the *guru* as rascal. When we examine a genuine teacher, we find that the scriptural demands made on him or her are contrary to what we assume or what has been played out in recent history by immature or deluded *gurus*. The moral demands are actually so high that no one in his right mind would want to don the mantle of a *guru*.

What is especially interesting about Kramer and Alstad's book is that their commanding tone suggests, if we rigorously apply the standards of their book, a hidden and therefore more virulent authoritarianism that undoubtedly seeks to manipulate us away from traditional values and expectations. It would undoubtedly have been more honest to highlight recent fiascos as moral failures amd as spiritual/yogic bankruptcies. They are also a symptom of our naïveté in spiritual matters.

The real question is, are the spiritual goals of traditional systems, which require accepting the *guru*-disciple relationship real and worthy of our pursuit? If so, can we accept submission to the authoritarianism entailed in these systems? We undergo schooling and education, even though they are riddled with authoritarianism. We sometimes even survive them with our spirit unbroken. It seems that spiritual goals are far more worthy of our wholehearted engagement than other, materialistic matters.

THE GURU

The *guru* is a problem in Western spiritual or quasi-spiritual circles. He or she is generally dismissed as overly authoritarian and as clashing with Western democratic ideals. This problem became trenchant in the 1980s and 1990s with the unsavory exposés of rogue *gurus* from the East and the West. Since I addressed this in my book *Holy Madness* (2006), I will not do so here. Clearly, though, for Westerners to be able to benefit from a *guru*, they must jettison typically Western attitudes and expectations. In other words, we must learn to approach Eastern teachers in terms of the Eastern mind-set and from an exclusively spiritual point of view.

Lest we forget, the "purpose of spiritual practice is to 'deconstruct' our carefully constructed consensus reality so that we can recover the Reality that lies beneath, or beyond, all our signs and symbols" (Feuerstein 2006, 213). This implies that every *guru*, "however gentle and considerate, works toward exploding the disciple's personal universe of meaning" (213). In particular, the guru has the function of undermining our false sense of self, the ego. From the viewpoint of Hinduism, our authentic "I" is the transcendental Self. In Buddhist terms, it is who we are when the dross of desire, greed, anger, and so on has been abandoned. The ego, in the language of spirituality, is our habitual identification with the body-mind, the "I," "me," and "mine." Unless we understand this perspective, we cannot properly relate to a *guru* and the idea of *exercitium spiritualis*.

We must neither elevate the *guru* into a transcendental force without practical efficacy nor make him "one of the guys," thereby accomplishing disabling him in the same way. The middle path is advisable: to see the teacher not as an omniscient and omnipotent god but as a buddha. A *buddha* is someone who has conquered the negative emotions, that is, for whom the passions are no longer blowing (*nirvāna*). This is a hugely important accomplishment in itself, because we can expect real guidance in spiritual matters from such a person. A *guru* may or may not know how to behave in order to secure a job or make millions. But we must realize that this is also not his or her function. In our psychological confusion, we are apt to plead for the *guru*'s help with things in which he is not interested or about which she cannot do much other than advise us to change our life. If we are hoping for energy transmission or psychedelic fireworks from our *guru*, we will ultimately be disappointed, because if we are given these baubles, we will miss out on the transmission of the enlightened consciousness, which is the *guru*'s real gift. But for this, we must be willing to be transformed at the deepest level of our mind and life.

To understand and appreciate the *guru* phenomenon, it is essential that we step beyond scientific materialism, that is, the ideology of scientism. This means, for instance, that we cannot dismiss the subtle experiences, subtle structures, subtle realms, and subtle beings of which traditional spiritual systems speak as delusional or say that *samādhi* is a state of hallucination or superstition. Instead, we must allow the "irrational" and "mythical" features of spirituality into our world of thought—at least as possibilities, if not actualities.

Just as Sri Aurobindo created his Integral Yoga to overcome what he saw as the limitations of the traditional branches of Yoga, he declined to function as a guru and thought that the path to liberation was surrender to the Divine, the inner Guru.

This rings true for many Westerners, who do not want to submit to an outer *guru*. But who is this "inner guide" (*antaryāmin*) of whom the Upanishads speak? How can we be certain that we receive genuine guidance from within? We *cannot*. Therefore, a qualified external teacher is necessary. And *qualified* means the *guru* in whom Awareness is awake; who brims with peace, equanimity, kindness, patience, generosity, and energy; and who has the power of a legitimate tradition behind him or her.

At the same time, we cannot make spiritual progress, regardless of whether we have an external *guru* or not, without being resonant to our own inner needs, our *svabhāva*. This concept, which is central to the ethics of the *Bhagavad-Gītā,* must not be confused with a rigidly prescribed social role. This may have been true in the remote past, but we can also understand it as a role or obligation we have taken on as a result of our integrity or vision. For instance, one person may see a need for discarding caution, because she realizes that she has the inner capacity to become a social activist, even though she can expect nothing but trouble. Many Hindu spiritual leaders of the nineteenth and early twentieth centuries have championed the cause of India's political freedom from the foreign rule of Great Britain—Sri Aurobindo, Mahatma Gandhi, Gangadhar Tilak, Ananda Acharya, and so on.

CHAPTER 18

The Phenomenon of Meditation

> Meditation or contemplation is not a matter of
> belief, dogma, myth, or idea. It is a set of practices
> or experiments in awareness that are performed
> with an enormous amount of rigor.
>
> —KEN WILBER (Shear 2006, xi)

THE HISTORY OF MEDITATION

Meditation is at the core of mystical practice and central to most spiritual traditions around the world. How can we understand it? As John White stated long ago,

[T]he term "meditation" is many things to many people, varying in this or that aspect, depending upon culture, religious traditions, psychological orientation, the individual's purpose, and other factors. It is not the definition but the experience that really matters. (White 1974, xvii–xviii)

Meditation is the principal means to ecstasy (*samādhi*). Ecstasy plays a significant role in the psychotechnologies of the East. The busy Westerner, while intrigued with ecstasy, is generally unwilling to walk the long road to it and prefers the supposed shortcut of psychedelic drugs. In former days, ecstasy was confused with a trance state, and this continues to be a major hurdle in understanding it. At the same time, ecstasy is not the avenue for the West, a point I develop further in chapter 19. I do agree, however, with those who have chosen the path of mindfulness, which is an alternative to the concentrative mind.

Much has been written about meditation, but by far the most extensive and incisive study is a two-volume monograph by Karl Baier (2009) in German. This remarkable history goes back to the *Scala Claustralium* (Guide for the Ordinated) by Guigo II, which dates back to the twelfth century. The Carthusian monk Guigo II was prior of Grande Chartreuse Monastery north of Grenoble in France, and his letter about meditation and the recitation of Christian passages was immensely popular during the Middle Ages. This text, which is based on the spiritual practice of the Desert Fathers, gives us a glimpse into the spiritual *exercitium* in medieval times. For Guigo II, spiritual practice meant the four stages of reading sacred literature, meditating, praying, and contemplating.

Not until the final quarter of the fifteenth century did a new form of meditation come into use, largely thanks to Wessel Gansfort's *Scala meditationis,* which he wrote toward the end of his life and which was adopted a decade later by Johannes Mombaer in his *Rosetum exercitiorum spiritualium et sacrarum meditationum.* Gansfort was instrumental in combining rhetoric with the new devotional approach that connected it with the Arabic-Persian meditation practice of antiquity. The fading away of rhetoric in education in the nineteenth century spelled the decline of that particular form of meditation. There were, of course, many other developments in meditation practice in the centuries after Gansfort, but they all culminated in the crisis of quietism in the late seventeenth century. The argument was between those who used Christian teachings to meditate and those who, like Jeanne-Marie de Guyon, followed a more quietistic ideal.

In the nineteenth century, meditation became associated with mesmerism, a widely influential ideology that gave birth to spiritualism, theosophy, New Thought, and then psychoanalysis and New Age ideology. It also reopened the doors to the magical worldview of esotericism and non-Christian traditions. Created by the Austrian physician Franz Anton Mesmer (1734–1815), mesmerism revolved around the idea that a fluidum filled the entire cosmos and therefore also the human body and that disharmony of this primary element caused sickness. The objective of mesmerism was to restore harmony in the body through appropriate energetic manipulation to remove blockages in the nerve channels. This led to the discovery of suggestion and hypnosis in a medical context.

It was into this pregnant cultural milieu that the Persian translation of the Sanskrit Upanishads—known as *Oupnek'hat*—translated into Latin in 1801–2 by Abraham-Hyacinthe Anquetil-Duperron understandably caused a considerable stir among the intelligentsia. Antequil-Duperron and other scholars saw an inevitable connection between Mesmer's fluidum and the Sanskrit concept of *prāna.* The German scholar Carl Joseph Hieronymus

Windischmann, a professor of philosophy at Bonn University, interpreted the whole of Indian philosophy in the light of mesmerism. The connection between Western occultism and Indian teachings was solidified through the Theosophical Society, which was responsible for translating key scriptures of Yoga, such as the *Yoga-Sūtra* and the *Yoga-Vāsishtha,* into English. The society received a great blow when Swami Dayananda, one of the great reformers of modern Hinduism, resigned from its ranks in 1882.

In 1885, ten years after it was founded, the Theosophical Society eliminated its secret level, and with Helena Petrovna Blavatsky's sudden death in 1891, it went into progressive stasis, though not without first fertilizing the next popular movement: New Thought (also known as Mind Cure and Christian Science). In contrast to theosophy, New Thought—which had attracted roughly one million members in the United States by 1900—was more emphatic about meditative practice (understood mainly as quietism).

Just as theosophy led imperceptibly to New Thought, Mesmerism transformed into suggestion, autosuggestion, and hypnosis. In the early years of psychoanalysis, founded by Sigmund Freud, hypnosis was the central practice by which patients' unconscious was tapped. Subsequently, it was replaced by dream analysis and free association on the psychoanalyst's couch.

MEDITATION RESEARCH

Although we could say meditation research began back in the days when meditation was associated with Mesmerism, I regard it as an interest of the twentieth century. It commenced with the scientific explorations of the nervous system and brain made possible by medical instrumentations such as the electroencephalogram (EEG), the electrocardiogram (ECG), endocrine measurements, and galvanic skin response (GSR) in the 1950s. The scientific concern basically was—and is—to understand the connection between the brain and the mind.

The first research piece to which we can point is Charles Laubry and Therese Brosse (1936). The first research using the EEG was by N. N. Das and H. Gastant (1955). This and similar investigations are mentioned in *Science Studies Yoga: A Review of Physiological Data* (1977) by James Funderburk, a student of Swami Rama of the Himalayan International Institute of Yoga Science and Philosophy in Pennsylvania. Funderburk assembled the medical literature on Yoga research until 1976 (when the acknowledgments were written). Since then, other studies have been reported.[1]

The relevant research is mostly nonreplicable or flimsy. But the main evidence for the distinction between the mind and brain-induced mental activity comes from recent investigations in the field of near-death experience (NDE) research, which is discussed in chapter 20 . When this evidence is considered in conjunction with the research findings on Swami Rama (1925–1996), an advanced adept, who was studied by the Menninger Foundation in Topeka, Kansas, in the 1960s, we have a strong case in favor of the independent existence of the mind and the filtering role of the brain.

MEDITATION TECHNIQUES
AND THE MEDITATIVE STATE

There is a useful distinction between the various techniques of inducing yogic meditation and the resultant altered state of consciousness. Both are called *dhyāna,* which can be derived from the verbal root *dhyai,* "to meditate," and the neuter suffix *ana,* suggesting an action that is in progress; thus, *meditating.* The early Upanishads also use the term *nididhyāsana,* which prompted the South Indian twentieth-century sage Ramana Maharshi, with an eye on the contemporary obsession with bodily poses, to make the following pun: What is the most important *āsana,* or pose? The answer is *nididhyāsana,* which is not a physical *āsana* but "contemplation" (from the intensified verbal root of *ni + di + dhyai*).[2]

The most extensive manual, offering a battery of 112 meditation techniques, is the *Vijnāna-Bhairava.*[3] According to its final stanza, this text belongs to the *Rudra-Yāmala-Tantra* and holds an important place in the Shaivism of Kashmir. It was probably composed in 700–800 C.E. and was mentioned by Abhinavagupta in the tenth century. As the translator explains in his introduction , it subscribes to the *yogaja-mārga* as opposed to the *vivekaja* approach, as is the case with Patanjali and Shankara. The latter proceeds by separation or isolation of *prakriti* from *purusha,* while the former emphasizes union, that is, the connection of *prakriti* to its transcendental source.

YOGA

In the *Rig-Veda,* the earliest Indian "document" that was memorized for millennia before it was committed to writing in medieval times, we see the concept of meditation used in three ways, as defined by Jeanine Miller (1974,

61ff.): mantric meditation; visual meditation (*dhī*), and absorption in mind and heart.

According to Classical Yoga, meditation (*dhyāna*) is the seventh limb of Patanjali's eightfold path. It is preceded by concentration (*dhāranā*) and succeeded by ecstasy (*samādhi*). The former is understood as "one-pointed-ness" (*ekāgratā*), that is, sustained mental focus on a single, ideated object. The term *dhāranā* literally means "holding": We pay continuous attention to the same object. At first, this requires an effort, because the mind naturally wanders, following the senses. Hence, sense control must precede mental concentration. In effect, though, the two processes go hand in hand. When one-pointedness becomes more or less automatic and transforms into "one-flowingness" (*ekatānatā),* the meditative state is reached. The British psychologist John H. Clark astutely observed,

> Meditation is a method by which a person concentrates more and more upon less and less. The aim is to empty the mind while, paradoxically, remaining alert. (Clark 1983, 29)

We have a similar experience when we concentrate on something like a mathematical problem. The difference is that yogic concentration typically has a spiritual purpose and is meant to lead to *samādhi,* which consists of merging mentally with the object:

> Meditation may be said to be a process by which an ordinarily diffused state of mind is brought into focus. The more the dispersion of mind's rays is gathered into a centre, it seems that the more the mind's rays disappear. . . .
> Inasmuch as feelings and emotions are basic to all intellectual processes, meditation is also an approach to the basis of mental life. It proceeds from the more intellectual surface to the emotional substratum. (Guenther 1976, 122)

In medieval times, under the influence of Tantra- and Hatha-Yoga, meditation was generally defined as twelve units of concentration, and ecstasy was explained as twelve units of meditation. This quantification does not altogether make sense, because in Patanjali's *Yoga-Sūtra* (2.45), the attainment or perfection (*siddhi*) of ecstasy is associated with the practice of dedication to the lord (*īshvara-pranidhāna*), that is, with the grace of the *īshvara*. Since we cannot coerce the *īshvara*'s grace, we cannot know precisely when *samādhi* will occur or reach perfection.

In any case, meditation is just the first step in the process of the transformation of the mind; when successful, it leads to the various states of ecstasy. It creates the right condition for the ecstatic consciousness to arise. This is acknowledged in the *scala perfectionis* that is sparsely mapped out in the *Yoga-Sūtra:*

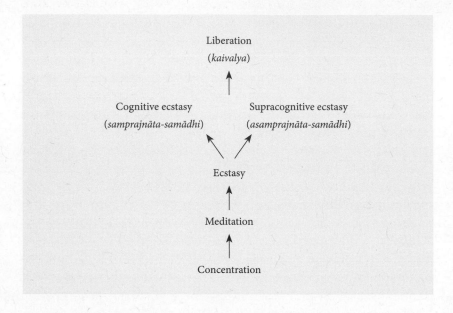

The immediate goal of meditation is *samādhi*. The ultimate goal is liberation, which, in Classical Yoga, is characterized as the "aloneness" (*kaivalya*) of the *purusha*: The spirit wakes up to itself.

BUDDHISM

Meditation is also central in Buddhism. The Buddha was an inveterate and a skilled meditator. In a memorable passage of the *Anguttara-Nikāya* (4), he advised his disciples not to behave like an inexperienced cow that, out of curiosity, explores unknown paths and tries out unknown herbs and waters. More likely than not, such a cow will experience adversity and suffer damage. He himself had abandoned the extremist ascetic approaches, such as willful meditation (that is, clenching of the teeth and forced breath retention) and excessive fasting.

The Buddha judged the meditative attainments of his teachers—Ālāra

Kālāma and Uddaka Rāmaputta—to be limited. Even their lofty states of "no-thing-ness" and "neither-perception-nor-nonperception" fell short of *nirvāna*. He taught that the four *jhānas* with form and the four formless *jhānas* still belonged to the realm of *samsāra,* and they would have to be transcended to attain *nirvāna.* With this, he left behind the entire brahmanical/yogic edifice available to him. He could proclaim that *nirvāna* was, indeed, an unparalleled accomplishment. The four higher or formless *jhānas* were certainly equivalent to various *samādhis* rather than meditation states, but they were not equivalent to liberation.

Vipassanā-bhāvanā, or "insight meditation, which was the Buddha's preferred method and is still the chosen meditative practice of the Theravāda school of Hīnayāna Buddhism, generates insight into the three marks of existence—suffering (*duhkha*), impermanence (*anitya*), and inessentiality (*anātman*). It presupposes a still mind that is produced through *shamatha* ("tranquillity") practice.

In Buddhaghosa's *Visuddhi-Magga* (Pāli; Skt.: *Vishuddhi-Mārga* [Path of Purification], 3.104, 4.22–31), a text of the early fifth century C.E., we find forty topics prescribed for meditation. The Buddha himself apparently made no such stipulations and encouraged his monastics to be a "lamp" unto themselves. But clearly the later monastics found this schema of the forty *kammatthānas* (Pāli, "places of action") useful. These comprise ten devices (Pāli: *kasina*); ten impurities (Pāli: *asubha*); ten recollections (Pāli: *anussati*); four sublime abodes (Pāli/Skt.: *brahma-vihāra*); four formless spheres (Pāli: *arūpāyatana*); perception of the loathsomeness of food (Pāli: *āhāre patikkūla-sannā*); and analysis of the four elements (Pāli: *dhātuv-avatthāna*). All this is discussed at great length in the *Visuddhi-Magga.* In his foreword to the 1976 edition of the two-volume translation by Ñāṇamoli Bhikkhu, Chögyam Trungpa poignantly says,

> The spiritual path is based on working with and training the mind. The example of this is the Buddha himself. Persevering in the practice of meditation, he attained full, complete enlightenment. Enlightenment cannot be attained by magic. It requires exertion and dedication to the path of buddhadharma, the essence and process of which is meditation.
>
> (Buddhaghosa 1976, vi)

Many Westerners are drawn to mindfulness practice. This consists of the continous, nonjudgmental observation of bodily and mental processes, notably breathing, feeling, and thinking. Mindfulness, says Nyanaponika Thera (1962, 24, 26), "is not at all a 'mystical' state." Right mindfulness, the seventh limb of the Buddhist path, entails a "high level of mental clarity." The meditative step came to be elaborated in great detail in Tibetan Buddhism, which since the 1960s has captured the interest of Westerners.

JAINISM

Since the earliest scriptures of Jainism—the *Pūrvas*—have been lost, it is impossible to say how meditation was understood in the early days of this faith. We do, however, know how meditation was taught in later times. Although meditation practice is not widely known in Jaina lay communities, the available texts generally distinguish four modalities: disagreeable (*ārta*), savage (*raudra*), virtuous (*dharma*), and pure (*shukla*, or "white"). In his *Tattvārtha-Sūtra* (9.27) from the first century c.e., Umāsvāti explains meditation as "the restraint of the single-pointed mind (*cintā*) in [the case of one who possesses] the highest steadfastness." Yet the first two types of "meditation" are more like deliberation, as when a person dwells obsessively on a troubling subject. Thus, only the latter two types are said to lead to liberation. While *ārta-dhyāna* is dwelling on an unpleasant subject, *raudra-dhyāna* has the purpose of harming or preserving one's possessions. *Dharma-dhyāna* and *shukla-dhyāna* are characteristic of a transcender.

Meditation is said to last up to one *muhūrta,* which is forty-eight minutes. This notion is also found in the later Hindu Yoga literature. According to one schema, the following twelve legitimate teaching points (*anuprekshā*) are recognized: impermanence, helplessness, the round of rebirths, solitariness, separateness of body and mind, bodily impurity, karmic influx, checking of karma, the world, the difficulty of enlightenment, and teaching of the ritual law.

CHAPTER 19

The Ladder of Ecstasy

> In the state of *samādhi,* the individual ego...
> is absent from the body and the mind,
> and therefore the functions of both the
> mind and the body are not negated.
>
> —HIROSHI MOTOYAMA (1990, 22)

THE PSYCHOLOGY OF MYSTICISM

The term *mysticism,* which became popular in the eighteenth century, is derived from the Greek *mustēs,* describing someone who has been initiated into the mysteries. Generally, it refers to a viewpoint that highlights ecstatic states and theologically favors pantheism or panentheism. As Evelyn Underhill (1961, 82) recognized, it is essentially *practice.* In the language of Yoga, it is essentially the practice of *samādhi* states. This does not occur in a theoretical vacuum. Mysticism is wrapped in philosophical layers of interpretation, although there is also a high state of pure consciousness (see chapter 13).

In the nineteenth century and the first half of the twentieth century, under the impact of materialistic scientism, *samādhi* and other ecstatic states were typically viewed as hysteria, schizophrenia, epilepsy, or (at best) hypnosis or autosuggestion. This was the central flaw of Richard Rösel's (1928), James H. Leuba's,[1] and Pierre Janet's (1926) work. This psychological position was ably reviewed by Ernst Arbman in his impressive three-volume study titled *Ecstasy or Religious Trance.* Arbman (1963, 1:xvi) understands ecstasy as "the total suggestive absorption of the personality and the entire inner conscious life in the object of belief." Taking his cues mainly but not exclusively from Catholic mysticism, he generalizes the evidence on ecstasy. Although Arbman (1963, 3:39–40) says that "ecstasy and the hysteric trance are strikingly alike," he still seriously questions the identity of these two mental states. He agrees that while some ecstatics might manifest psychopathological states, it would be wrong to dismiss ecstasy a priori as such. He concludes that, apart from a few exceptions, "the states of ecstasy...have nothing to do with a psychic abnormality.... Whatever, whenever, and in whatever forms I may appear, religious belief never has the character of a pathological individual insanity...." (1963, 3:383).

HUMAN POTENTIAL

Eventually some psychologists moved away from a psychopathological interpretation of ecstasy and started to regard meditation, ecstasy, and other nonordinary phenomena as an integral part of our human potential. Human potential itself became a viable concept and is mainly tied to the name of the American psychologist Abraham Maslow, who gave psychology a whole new language (see Maslow 1971) and strove for a broad definition of humanness. He associated humanness with self-actualization, or being fully human. He explained self-actualization as the pursuit of what he called B-values (Being-values), such as truth, beauty, goodness, simplicity, or completeness (Maslow, "Theory Z," 1971, 269–95). This includes his so-called peak experiences, or moments of unparalleled happiness or fulfillment. Later on, he accepted U. A. Asrani's contrasting plateau experience, which is the persistent experience of a happy, fulfilled, or enlightened state, as recorded by only a handful of self-actualizers.

With the emergence of first humanistic and then transpersonal psychology—in both of whose formation Maslow played an instrumental role—traditional wisdom and Western science merged.

DEFINING ECSTASY

The early discussions about ecstasy—either from a traditionalist, religious perspective or from the viewpoint of scientific psychology—were centered on Christianity, mostly Catholicism, because the Protestants have always assumed a rather skeptical attitude toward mysticism. Not until the twentieth century was a new element introduced into the study of ecstasy: medical investigations via the electroencephalogram. The early research happened in the 1920s, but it was not until the 1950s that this kind of investigation flourished, largely due to the more widespread use of the electroencephalograph invented in 1924. The EEG, galvanic skin response, temperature, blood pressure, pulse rate, metabolic rate, lactic acid, plethysmographic measurements, and magnetic resonance imaging allowed scientists to get a better understanding of the brain and body as a whole. They found, among other things, that *samādhi* is linked with persistent alpha waves and increased amplitude modulation.

THE CHRISTIAN SCALA PERFECTIONIS

In her fine book on mysticism, Evelyn Underhill (1961, 104) makes the point that the "true mystic...hardly needs a map" on the "stormy sea of the divine." While some mystical virtuosos, even in Christianity, can proceed without a guide or a map, this is rare. Yet, as Underhill notes, the church fathers were busy erecting conceptual scaffolding that the mystic could climb: the theologian and presbyter Clement of Alexandria (c. 150–215 C.E.), who had Origen, the first Christian mystic, as a disciple (condemned as a heretic by the Council of Constantinople in 553); Bishop Irenaeus (c. 125–202 C.E.); Bishop Gregory of Nyssa (335–398 C.E.); Bishop Saint Augustine (354–430 C.E.), who was one of the most influential theologians of Christianity; and Dionysius the Areopagite (late fourth to early fifth century C.E.), author of *The Celestial Hierarchy*. The frameworks erected by these men have sometimes been followed by the Christian mystics, while at other times they have been found too rigid or too rough and have merely caused the mystics uneasiness and anxiety.

Teresa of Avila (1515–1582), a highly accomplished mystic, described with great psychological acumen the stages of the mystical path in her book *Interior Castle*:

> Mansion 1 (touched by grace but beset by many "venomous" things, which do not allow the soul to see the goodness of the "king" in the seventh chamber; this difficulty must be overcome by prayer, self-knowledge, and confidence in the king's goodness); mansion 2 (still troubled, the soul seeks to obey God, moves forward, and attempts to practice "recollection"); mansion 3 (the great obstacle is vainglory and the demands of ordinary life, but active love is stronger; the soul moves on motivated by silence and hope); mansion 4 (the king dispenses his favors at will; the soul must abandon thinking and cultivate love); mansion 5 (here the soul is betrothed to the king; bliss is experienced, but the soul knows it must work on love); mansion 6 (the soul delights in God's proximity but has a powerful yen for uniting with him completely); mansion 7 (the soul enters God and enjoys his presence in "immense silence" just as God enjoys the presence of the soul). (Peers 1974)

The Hindu sages, in contrast to the Christian mystics, were fond of such maps, and always found new ways to express the stages of the path. They also offered succinct definitions of the *samādhi* state. Thus, in the *Yoga-Sūtra* (3.3), Patanjali explains, "[When] nothing but the object is shining forth [in] that [meditation], [and when the mind is] as it were void of [its] own form, [that is known as] ecstasy." Yoga also recognizes a state of pure consciousness beyond all cognitive processes. The term *samādhi* is often reserved for this higher state, which is known as *asamprajnāta-samādhi* (or in Vedānta, *nirvikalpa-samādhi*), that is, transconceptual ecstasy.

THE LADDER OF HINDU AND JAINA YOGIC ECSTASIES

The classic map of *samādhi* states can be found in Patanjali's *Yoga-Sūtra* (especially 1.18, 1.42–44, 1.47, and 3.3). From this text, we can reconstruct the following six-step scaffolding:

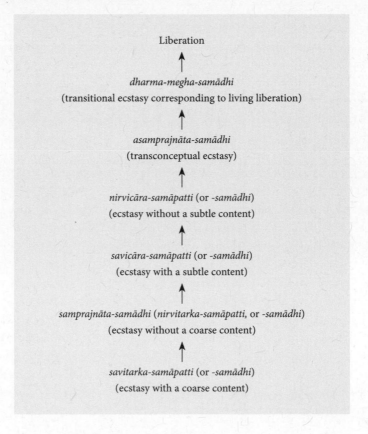

Liberation

↑

dharma-megha-samādhi
(transitional ecstasy corresponding to living liberation)

↑

asamprajnāta-samādhi
(transconceptual ecstasy)

↑

nirvicāra-samāpatti (or *-samādhi*)
(ecstasy without a subtle content)

↑

savicāra-samāpatti (or *-samādhi*)
(ecstasy with a subtle content)

↑

samprajnāta-samādhi (*nirvitarka-samāpatti*, or *-samādhi*)
(ecstasy without a coarse content)

↑

savitarka-samāpatti (or *-samādhi*)
(ecstasy with a coarse content)

The scholar Vācaspati Mishra (*Tattva-Vaishāradī* 1.17) adds four more steps after *nirvitarka*, because he regards *ānanda* (bliss) and *asmitā* (I-am-ness) as cognitions that—like *vitarka* and *vicāra*—can make the contents of higher-level ecstasies. This is explicitly rejected by Vijnāna Bhikshu (*Yoga-Vārttika* 1.46). But everyone agrees that, in contrast to the *samprajnāta-samādhi* or conceptual ecstasy, the transconceptual ecstasy is necessarily singular. It occurs when the mind is totally empty of all contents, and there is not even the vision of discernment (*viveka-khyāti*) at the highest level of *nirvicāra-samāpatti*.

It is important to understand that the cognitive acts in *samprajnāta-samādhi* are not ordinary thought processes (*vritti*). *Samādhi* only ensues when the *vrittis* have been silenced and all discursive thinking has stopped. The *vitarkas* and *vicāras* are spontaneous insights relating to the coarse or (in the latter case) subtle object of meditation.

ECSTATIC STATES IN BUDDHISM

In Buddhism, *jhāna* (= *dhyāna*) is the term used for *samādhi*. Four *jhānas* with form (*rūpa*) and four formless varieties are recognized (see table on page 200).

Liberation

↑

Eighth *jhāna*
(the state of neither perception nor nonperception,
naivasamjnā-naivāsamjnā-bhāva, that corresponds to
asamprajnāta-samādhi)

↑

Seventh *jhāna*
(the experience of nothing at all)

↑

Sixth *jhāna*
(the experience of infinity of consciousness)

↑

Fifth *jhāna*
(the experience of infinity of space)

↑

Fourth *jhāna*
(the state marked by even-mindedness; loss of *sukha,* or "joy")

↑

Third *jhāna*
(the state marked by equanimity; loss of *prīti,* or "delight")

↑

Second *jhāna*
(the state marked by loss of discursive thinking and appearance
of serenity; continuation of *prīti* and *sukha*)

↑

First *jhāna*
(the state marked by detachment from sense desires,
accompanied by discursive thought;
appearance of *prīti* and *sukha*)

CHAPTER 20

Paranormal Abilities, Psychotropic Drugs, and Yogic Discipline

> From the perspective of yoga and the classical Indian tradition, the cognitive anomalies claimed by parapsychologists... are no anomalies at all.
>
> —K. RAMAKRISHNA RAO (2010, xi–xii)

THE SCIENTIFIC INVESTIGATION OF THE PARANORMAL

Parapsychology, still under the rubric of "psychical investigation," was ushered in as a scientific discipline in the nineteenth century with the inquiries of Frederic W. H. Myers, a philosopher, psychologist, and poet. His interest in psychical research was born in 1869 after a conversation with the esteemed Cambridge philosopher Henry Sidgwick during a stroll under a starlit sky. In 1882, Myers cofounded the Society for Psychical Research (SPR) in London. His principal work, *Human Personality and Its Survival of Death,* a large tome, was published posthumously in 1903. Myers died in 1901 at the age of fifty-eight, one year after the demise of his friend and collaborator Sidgwick. They were both primarily and passionately concerned with the survival of death; as K. R. Rao (2010, 263) remarked, "In a sense parapsychology is a by-product of survival research." This means parapsychology grew out of our natural desire to lift the curtain from the mystery that follows life.

In 1871, the distinguished physicist Sir William Crookes encountered his first "psychical" phenomena, and he started to devote himself to the scientific study of what was then known as spiritualism. A fellow of the influential Royal Society since 1863, the discoverer of thallium, an inventor of scientific devices, and a recipient of various prestigious medals, Crookes was widely expected to reveal spiritualism for the humbug many people thought it was, but he turned out to become a stalwart champion of "spiritual" phenomena.

In the first quarter of the twenty-first century, we sadly have to note that despite undeniable successes, parapsychology has yet to impress mainstream scientists as a legitimate scientific discipline. Departments of parapsychology are rare and, if they exist, often have to contend with considerable peer pressure, funding problems, and small-time political intrigue. A good example is the case of the Center for Frontier Sciences, which was founded by Beverly Rubik in 1987 and had a short span of existence at Temple University in Philadelphia, Pennsylvania.

In the meantime, some psychological and parapsychological investigations were conducted by the Institute of Noetic Science, a nonprofit membership organization that was founded in 1973 by the Apollo 14 astronaut Edgar Mitchell and the investor Paul N. Temple. The institute, whose president is currently Marilyn M. Schlitz, was set up to investigate phenomena related to consciousness and healing that lie at the fringe of science.

ENHANCED SENSORY CAPACITIES

Yoga is shot through with paranormal elements that deserve proper investigation. Thus far, few scientists have turned their attention to the rich paranormal evidence and lore of Yoga. This may well have to do with the fact that the world has few experts trained in parapsychology. This field does not promise young students respectable positions with hefty salaries, which undoubtedly affects their eventual career choices.

Parapsychology, taught at only a few Western and Eastern universities, is a reasonably young scientific discipline that is surrounded by controversy. This is not a statement about the validity of parapsychology as a proper scientific discipline but a statement about the current scientific paradigm, which does not know how to handle phenomena that contradict its materialistic bias.

Be that as it may, paranormal phenomena exist, and Yoga is replete with them. Surprisingly, only a handful of Indian publications have spoken to this side of Yoga. The most noteworthy is K. R. Rao's *Yoga and Parapsychology: Empirical Research and Theoretical Studies* (2010). Rao, who has authored a dozen books and nearly two hundred research papers, is far from being unknown in American parapsychological circles, because in the early 1960s, he worked with J. B. Rhine at the Parapsychology Laboratory at Duke University in North Carolina and later served as the executive director of Rhine's Foundation for Research on the Nature of Man. His interests are wide-ranging, and he is currently the chairman of the Indian Council of Philosophical Research in Delhi. He thus brings to the interest in parapsychology a rich background in both experimental investigation and theoretical inquiry.

In his recent anthology, Rao makes the point that parapsychology in India and the West is associated with two distinct orientations that are tied to the different perspectives on science in general as approached in either part of the world. As Rao sees it, science in India is not strictly separated from spirituality but is pursued as a complementary discipline. In contrast, science as pursued in the West views itself in opposition and antagonistic to spirituality. For Rao (2010, 2), this means that parapsychology is bound to be practiced in the West as a "study of anomalies" rather than as a "science with a specific subject matter."

In his book *The End of Materialism: How Evidence of the Paranormal Is Bringing Science and Spirituality Together*, the noted American psychologist Charles T. Tart (2009, 290) made this pertinent observation: "[T]he problem is not a conflict between science per se and spirituality, but between *scientism* and spirituality." Scientism is an ideology based on science—an ideology that is essentially a belief system, not unlike religion.

It was J. B. Rhine at Duke University who, as early as 1927, vigorously introduced the experimental study of paranormal phenomena. In more than 140 experiments, he tirelessly demonstrated that psi (or paranormal) phenomena are not merely triggers or fantasies but real, if elusive. In his book *Extra-Sensory Perception*, Rhine explained,

> It is to be expected, I suppose, that these experiments will meet with a considerable measure of incredulity and, perhaps, even hostility from those who presume to know, without experiment, that such things as they indicate simply cannot be! But this inevitable reactionary response to all things new and strange, which is as old as the history of science, already shows many signs of decline, as the scientific world turns a "scientific attitude," one of open-minded but cautious inquiry, toward the facts. Even so short a period as the last ten years has been one of marked transition. (Rhine 1934, 2)

In the intervening years, many more experiments and meta-analyses have confirmed Rhine's findings. Yet the credibility of parapsychology in scientific circles cannot be said to have noticeably increased, because those circles are significantly steeped in scientism rather than science. As *Science* magazine sarcastically stated back in 1955 (in an article by the chemist G. R.

Price), we can either accept or reject parapsychology (see Mishlove 1975, 111). The same author judged Rhine's results to be miraculous, and since miracles do not happen, dismissed Rhine as a liar. This is still the position of mainstream scientists if they venture to think about paranormal reports at all.

Scientists, who are as human as the next person, are reluctant to accept that their model of the universe is basically wrong. Even to suggest this here will predictably raise hackles. Nevertheless, psi phenomena clearly show— and large-scale deceit of thousands of researchers is hardly an explanation— that the unshakable laws of science are little more than probabilities and that the observer is perhaps not as neutral as we would like to believe. But this is not the place to argue in favor of paranormal phenomena, which has not had much success thus far. If the scientific discipline of quantum physics, which is often questionably invoked to explain psi phenomena, cannot dislodge the Newtonian paradigm on which scientism leans, parapsychology—which is usually considered only as a quasi-scientific discipline—certainly will not. The anomalies will continue to pile up until the current scientific paradigm finally collapses. Then a new paradigm will come into vogue.

In the context of this book, we will simply presume that parapsychology is a legitimate scientific discipline and that paranormal phenomena do exist. As Frits Staal observes,

> How many of these miracles or which miracles, if any, have really taken place we do not know. There are responsible scholars who accept some, and equally responsible [but biased] scholars who reject all. (Staal 1975, 154)

Paranormal abilities are certainly well known in Yoga where they are con- sidered not as "anomalies" but as a normal, if generally undesired, by-prod- uct of the yogic process (see Lindquist 1935).

We can tell from the prominence given to paranormal abilities in Patan- jali's classical vade mecum, the *Yoga-Sūtra,* that they are an integral aspect of Yoga. This is disturbing only to those who would like to regard Yoga as a purely rational philosophical enterprise. But, in fact, the philosophical schools of India—with the exception of the materialistic school of the Cār- vakas and the naturalistic system of Vaisheshika—have from the beginning adopted a spiritual orientation that integrates the paranormal with soterio- logical (liberative) teachings.

Not only are paranormal phenomena well-known in Yoga, they have also been tentatively classified. Patanjali discussed them in the third chapter of his work, which he—or more likely a later editor—titled *vibhūti-pāda,* or "chapter on the manifestations." Perhaps this term was taken from the *Bhagavad-Gītā,* where it means "choicest manifestation" of an aspect of the world, which was understood as the god Krishna's "lower nature." More commonly, the paranormal abilities are called *siddhis,* or "accomplishments," which are regarded as inferior to the eight great accomplishments, or perfections, of enlightenment.[1]

From the *Yoga-Sūtra* (3.37), we learn that Patañjali considered certain paranormal abilities to be obstacles (*antarāya*) to *samādhi.* These extrasensory abilities, such as divine sight and divine hearing, are attributed to the "divine sense faculties" (*divya-indriya*). The word "divine" (*divya*) does not refer here to any godly being, realm, or quality but simply to paranormal activity that looks godlike to the ordinary mind, because the mind cannot explain it. These powers, which many *yogins* possess but are not supposed to use, were thought to flash out in "illuminations" (*prātibha*). They have rightly been considered to be obstacles to the attainment of ecstasy, because they involve the senses. To reach *samādhi,* the senses must be disabled through the practice of sensory inhibition, or *pratyāhāra.* Paranormal processes were never meant to be dismissed tout court.

GODLIKE POWERS

Some people, especially followers of Vedānta, who are particularly critical of paranormal skills, often overlook the fact that the so-called *ashta-siddhis,* or "eight powers," are not regarded as obstacles. In fact, they spontaneously arise as a result of enlightenment, or liberation. In other words, the *yogin* is essentially a thaumartugist, a potent, godlike being. According to the *Yoga-Bhāshya* (3.45), the eight powers are as follows:

1. Miniaturization (*animan*): the paranormal ability to shrink oneself to the size of an atom (*anu*). The *Yoga-Bhāshya-Vivarana* (3.45) by Shankara Bhagavatpāda states that by means of *animan,* one can become more subtle than the subtle and hence can no longer be seen.
2. Magnification (*mahiman*): the paranormal ability to expand to a vast size. In his *Tattva-Vaishāradī* (3.45) commentary on the *Yoga-Sūtra,* Vācaspati Mishra explains this as the capacity to become as large as an elephant, mountain, town, and so on.

3. Levitation (*laghiman*): the paranormal ability to become, in the words of the *Tattva-Vaishāradī* (3.45), weightless "like the tuft of a reed."
4. Extension (*prāpti*): the paranormal ability to bridge great distances instantly. The *Yoga-Bhāshya* (3.45) suggests that by means of this power, the *yogin* can touch the moon with his fingertips.
5. Irresistible will (*prākāmya*): the paranormal ability to realize one's will. The *Yoga-Bhāshya* (3.45) gives the example of being able to dive into solid earth as if it were liquid.
6. Mastery (*vāshitva*): the paranormal ability to demonstrate complete control over the material elements (*bhūta*) and their products or, as the *Yoga-Bhāshya-Vivarana* (3.45) claims, control over all worlds.
7. Lordship (*īshitritva*): perfect mastery of the subtle causes of the material world, which makes the *yogin* godlike.
8. Fulfillment of all desires (*kāmāvasāyitva*): the paranormal ability to will into being whatever one sees fit. The *Yoga-Bhāshya* (3.45) makes it clear that the adept's will does not go against the will of the creator-deity (*īshvara*); thus, as the *Yoga-Bhāshya-Vivarana* (3.45) further explains, the adept does not make fire cold, because he respects the preestablished order of things.

These eight powers encompass a wide range of paranormal abilities and were probably conceptualized as a set gradually over a long period of time.

Yoga recognizes many other paranormal abilities that play an important role, especially in the tradition of Tantra, which is often seen as separate from Yoga but can also be regarded as a major branch of Yoga (which is my preference). Tantra is steeped in magic, and a well-known group of six paranormal abilities is frequently cited in the Tantric literature. Thus, the sixteenth-century Bengali adept Krishnānanda Vidyāvāgīshvara mentions the following (standardized) set in his *Tantra-Sāra*:

- Pacification (*shānti*): the paranormal ability to pacify any being
- Subjugation (*vashīkarana*): the paranormal ability to bring others under one's complete control and make them subservient like slaves
- Stoppage (*stambhana*): the paranormal ability to completely immobilize another being or render a situation ineffective
- Eradication (*uccātana*): the paranormal ability to destroy someone at a distance

- Causing dissension (*vidveshana*): the paranormal ability to create discord or enmity among people
- "Death-ing" (*mārana*): the paranormal ability to kill someone at a distance by the mere power of one's mind

Except perhaps for the first ability, these practices amount to black magic and fall short of the lofty yogic ideal of nonharming. Nevertheless, they have been deployed for thousands of years, and even today it is possible to find *tāntrikas* in India who, for a handful of rupees, will use their magical skills to harm others. Occasionally, in the courts of India, an unfortunate judge has to try a case that involves black magic. It is even conceivable that some legal cases in the Western world that supposedly involve "mind control" of Eastern cult victims entail the undue exercise of paranormal abilities. However, this is difficult to prove. At any rate, this is not the way of high Tantra, which upholds inner freedom and the spiritual upliftment of others.

In its introduction to the Western hemisphere, the paranormal arsenal of Yoga acted as a chief attractor for the prominent occult Western league. As Karl Baier (2009, 121–22) explains, the French writer and practitioner of magic A. L. Constant (alias Eliphas Levi), coined the terms *esoterics* and *occultism* and was the first to become interested in Yoga. He regarded India as the place of ancient traditions and, without mentioning Yoga by name, wrote about typically yogic exercises, notably breath control and concentration. Under the inspiration of Eliphas Levi, Helena Petrovna Blavatsky (the cofounder with Henry Steel Olcott of the Theosophical Society in 1875) and Aleister Crowley ("The Beast") explored Yoga's occult legacy in the last quarter of the nineteenth century.

The Theosophists seriously endeavored to gain a better understanding of Yoga by delving into its literature. The society commissioned native Indian scholars to translate the the *Shiva-Samhitā* (by C. Vasu, 1884); the *Yoga-Sūtra* (by M. N. Dvivedī, 1890); the *Yoga-Vāsishtha* (by V. L. Mitra, 1891); the *Hatha-Yoga-Pradīpikā* (by S. Iyangar, 1893); the *Yoga-Sāra-Samgraha* (by G. Jha, 1894); the *Bhagavad-Gītā* (by Annie Besant, 1894); the *Gheranda-Samhitā* (by C. Vasu, 1895), the *Jīvanmukti-Viveka* (by G. Jha, 1897); and other Sanskrit works. While Levi saw in Yoga a magical system that served the stupefaction of the Indians who sought flight into catalepsy (*samādhi*) and could not be recommended to Western seekers, Blavatsky recognized it correctly as a spiritual tradition.

The Theosophical Society was instrumental in bringing Yoga to Western audiences. In 1904, the second-generation theosophist William Quine Judge translated and commented on Patanjali's text, and his work indirectly enticed other theosophists such as Alice Bailey (1927),[2] Ernest Wood (1948), I. K. Taimni (1961), and Rohit Mehta (1975) to follow suit. In 1907, Rama Prasad discussed Patanjali's Yoga in his book *Self-Culture,* and two decades later, Charles W. Leadbeater (one of the leaders of early theosophy) published his immensely successful illustrated book *The Chakras: A Monograph.* In the preface, Leadbeater (1927, v) made this statement, which epitomizes the Theosophical Society's fascination at the time with the occult: "When a man begins to develop his senses, so that he may see a little more than everybody sees, a new and most fascinating world opens before him, and the chakras [*cakra*] are among the first objects in that world to attract his attention."

But sensory enhancement is not necessarily the most intriguing of Yoga's paranormal feats. A particularly fascinating *siddhi* is leaving one's own body and entering another; this is referred to in the *Yoga-Sūtra* (3.38 and 3.43) and, according to Yoga cognoscenti, is a lost art:

bandha-kārana-shaithilyāt pracāra-samvedanāc ca cittasya para-sharīra-āveshah (3.38) "By relaxing the causes of bondage and by the knowledge of going forth, the mind's entrance (*āvesha*) into the body of another [human or non-human being is achieved]."

bahir-akalpitā vrittir mahā-videhā tatah prakāsha-āvarana-kshayah (3.43) "The nonimaginary movement [called] 'the great disembodied' [occurs] outside [the body]. By that, the dwindling of the covering of the [inner] light [is effected]."

The first aphorism is intelligible in principle. The "causes of bondage" are the karmic fetters that tie us to our physical body. It is clearly a description of what is known in parapsychology and occultism as an out-of-body experience (OBE). But the second aphorism needs some explanation. A "nonimaginary movement" (*akalpitā vritti*) would be an actual mental process happening in the subtle body, outside the material body. Thus, it would not be merely an instance of ESP. Patanjali failed to tell us how entry into another body, which is a common folkloristic feat, is accomplished. We may assume that this was deemed possible and was not just fictional.

Out-of-body experiences were vigorously pursued and first described in great detail by Sylvan Muldoon (1929). In his book, which was coauthored with Hereward Carrington, he presented literally hundreds of his own out-of-body experiences. A decade before this, Carrington published his book *Modern Psychical Phenomena* (1919), in which he reported on investigations conducted by the French researcher Charles Lancelin. A somewhat more scientific approach was first taken by Robert Crookall, who wrote *The Study and Practice of Astral Projection* (1966), *Out-of-the-Body Experiences* (1970), and *Case-Book of Astral Projection* (1972). Around the same time, Robert A. Monroe published his self-experiments in the fascinating book *Journeys Out of the Body* (1971). In the late 1960s, the renowned psychologist Charles Tart turned his attention to the investigation of OBEs (see Tart 1974, 349ff.; see also the extensive survey of OBEs by Green 1973; Alvarado 2000; and Cohen and Phipps 1979). Out-of-body experiences can be deliberately induced and may be studied profitably in conjunction with near-death experiences, which were investigated by the prominent Dutch cardiologist Pim van Lommel (2010), many of whose patients reported this phenomenon after coming out of anaesthesia. His research, which was published in the prestigious British medical journal *The Lancet* (van Lommel et al., 2001), showed that at least 88 percent of the near-death accounts were completely accurate and only 10 percent contained some error, while 3 percent were completely wrong. In light of this, he concluded that such experiences could not be mere hallucinations. As far as I know, those who have deliberately induced out-of-body experiences have never reported an instance of entering another body.

We could dismiss the yogic claim that it is possible to enter another's body off the cuff, but this would lack all scientific merit. However, if we give credence to this paranormal feat, we must assume that the *yogins* knew what they were talking about, which is reasonable and applies to all other *siddhis* as well.

Many of the ecstatic "constraints" (*samyama*) indicate a correlation between certain bodily (microcosmic) parts and macrocosmic features, such as the relationship between the solar plexus area (or *manipura cakra*) and the sun. This corroborates the correlations given in the Western occult or hermetical tradition and requires scientific study.

PSYCHOTROPIC DRUGS

The relationship between drug-induced experiences and altered states of consciousness has been recognized since ancient times. When we look at India, we see the earliest references to the use of hallucinogenic substances in the archaic *Rig-Veda* (10.61.13), which some scholars dated back to more than four thousand years ago.[3] In the 1970s, research on so-called mind-altering drugs made its debut, and in a short time—partly due to Aldous Huxley (1979)—hallucinogenic substances became widely available for consumption by people looking for entertainment and an escape from ordinary life. The widespread use of such drugs is held to be one of today's serious social problems. In his popular book *The Politics of Ecstasy,* first published in 1968, Timothy Leary, who was a professor of psychology at Harvard University, argued that everyone should "turn on, tune in, drop out." When Ram Dass (Richard Alpert) learned that his Indian *guru* Neemkaroli Baba had taken huge doses of LSD without experiencing any reaction to it, he resolved to dedicate himself fully to meditation and the yogic path.

Charles Tart, one of the early experimenters, based much of his book *States of Consciousness* (1975a) on drug-induced altered states. In 2011, the American psychoanalyst James Fadiman, who has been involved in psychedelic research since the 1960s, published a book titled *The Psychedelic Explorer's Guide.*[4]

Most *sādhus,* who must not be confused with *yogins,* smoke hashish. Hashish smoking is common in some "yogic" groups, such as the Nāga Babas (or naked ascetics). Since they also cultivate meditation, their hashish habit is not considered antagonistic to their spiritual purposes. Rather, they generally see the relaxation state derived from the substance as a means of deepening their meditative discipline (see Hartsuiker 1993 and Rampuri 2010). In the absence of any research into this controversial custom, I will abstain from commenting on it, other than to state that mainstream Yoga looks askance at the use of mind-altering substances of any kind. Instead, it favors an approach that focuses on the powers of the mind in the opus of transformation.

At the same time, we must acknowledge that the *Yoga-Sūtra* includes one aphorism (4.1) that points to *oshadhi* as a means of generating paranormal powers. This Sanskrit term is perhaps best translated as "herb" here, denoting a substance, probably a herbal concoction, that is known to have a paranormal effect. The classic *oshadhi* was the mysterious "divine" soma, which was widely enjoyed in a ritual context in Vedic times. R. Gordon Wasson (1972) wrongly identified it with the fly agaric mushroom, an opinion endorsed by the American Sanskritist Wendy Doniger. Admittedly, the references in the Vedic literature are inconclusive. However, the *Rig-Veda* describes the soma plant as having hanging branches (1.9.1, 9.79.4) for "fingers" *kṣipaḥ*), having more than one branch (*párvan*), and being a leafless creeper that is sweet and milky. Wasson's interpretation is certainly imaginative, but it does not account for all native descriptions.

The plant, which is reported to have grown on mountain slopes, was compressed and filtered, and the resulting juice was then mixed with milk and other liquids to yield the soma draft (*madhu*) that had mind-altering properties. It was not only poured ritually into the sacred fire, but it was also imbibed by the sacrificers, for it was thought to remove sin; encourage truth; bring protection against wickedness and bad omens; bestow the paranormal ability to kill with a glance; and yield health, longevity, and even immortality. When drunk in moderation, the soma draft inspired poetry; when drunk in excess, as happened especially in late Vedic times, it produced intoxication. The best overview of beliefs and rituals about soma is given by the German scholar Alfred Hillebrand in *Vedic Mythology* (see Hillebrand 1990, especially vol. 1, 121–332). This thorough work is scarcely known today by those popularizers who claim expertise on the subject.

Indian alchemy (*rasāyana*) knows of many other substances that have, or claim to have, a paranormal effect. That even Patanjali, or a later editor or interpolator, felt obligated to mention *oshadhi* in a serious book on Yoga is a sign that in those days hallucinogenic drugs were familiar in yogic circles as a means of acquiring paranormal abilities. The fact that the Buddha did not forbid the acquisition of *siddhis* but only their display to laypeople would seem to confirm the same.[5]

NEUROSCIENCE AND PARANORMAL ABILITIES

In the 1960s, neuroscience turned to God, looking for the infinite Divine in the brain box. This approach culminated in the article "Toward a Psychobiology of Transcendence: God in the Brain" by Arnold J. Mandell (Davidson and Davidson 1980, 379–434). In the 1980s, Stanley Koren invented what is known as the "God Helmet," which experimental subjects wear on their heads. It generates fluctuating, weak magnetic fields. Apparently, many subjects report sensing a "presence" that some associate with God. In a way, this controversial device epitomizes the new materialistic scientific discipline of neurobiology.

When archatheist Richard Dawkins of Oxford University tried on the God Helmet, he did not have the mystical experience for which he had hoped. Apparently, his temporal lobe was relatively insensitive to magnetic fields. Dawkins was greatly disappointed, even though a mystical experience would not have convinced him of God's existence.

BUDDHISM AND JAINISM

I will refrain from discussing the Buddhist and Jaina evidence separately, because it is very similar to the Hindu data. Mircea Eliade (1973) mentions the six or seven "superknowledges" (*abhijnās*) of Buddhism and makes reference to Étienne Lamotte (1944 and 1949), as well as Charles de la Vallée Poussin (1931).

The Buddhists recognize *iddhis* (Pāli for Skt. *siddhis*), *riddhis*, and the previously mentioned *abhijnās* (Pāli: *abhinnas*), which include the divine eye, divine hearing, knowledge of another's mind, and recollection of previous lives. It is noteworthy that Buddhism maintains that spiritual practitioners can reach enlightenment purely through wisdom (*prajnā*) and do not necessarily need to go through *samādhi, samāpatti,* and the paranormal abilities. This "Protestant" antimystical attitude is characteristic of the "dry saints." This makes sense, because spiritual progress is, after all, primarily a matter of profound wisdom and perfect inner renunciation. The critical issue is whether these two mental qualities are easily forthcoming without the experience of the various ecstatic states. Profound wisdom has, by the way, little in common with the rational mind, which is easily ensnared in the ideology of scientism rather than being committed to open-minded, unbiased science; the former is likely to dismiss something it does not understand instead of researching it without prejudice and at the risk of discovering inconvenient facts.

Buddhism looks suspiciously at paranormal powers. They certainly should not be displayed, as this merely boosts one's ego. If Buddhism is ambivalent toward them, Jainism has a definitely negative attitude and regards the *siddhis* as unworthy of pursuit. It is even ambiguous about the omniscience (*kevala-jnāna*) attributed to *siddhas* or arhats and makes it clear that the freed being, or *jina,* only "knows" the soul.

CHAPTER 21

Death and the Art of Dying

> Death really reminds us how little we know,
> and yet how important it is to try to understand.
>
> —CHARLES T. TART (1997, 172)

Death is not, to put it mildly, deemed a subject for polite dinner conversation. In fact, we tend to shun the topic. As Ignace Lepp explains, most people in our Western civilization consider death a scandalous injustice:

> Even when we know well in advance that someone close to us is mortally ill, his death always comes to us as something "unbelievable and paradoxical." (Lepp 1969, 41)

Our attitude contrasts significantly with that of the ancients, who thought of death as part of life. In classical times, they spoke of the *ars moriendi,* the art of dying, as a skill to be honed and not an accident that happens without the possibility of conscious input. Erasmus of Rotterdam recommended that the best preparation for a good death is a good life. The Hundred Years War and the Black Death, which together decimated the population of Europe, made the theme of a good death a popular subject in the Middle Ages. The *ars moriendi* was medieval Christianity's answer to this pressing matter. It arose in the early to mid-fifteenth century C.E.

Going back much further, the Yoga masters of old regarded *how* a person died as vital. This was first explained in the *Bhagavad-Gītā* (8.5, 8.10):

> And he who in the last hour, having released the body [and while] remembering Me alone, goes forth—he goes to My state-of-existence; there is no doubt of this.

> [T]hat [*yogin*], at the time of going forth [that is, at death], with unmoving mind, yoked by devotion and by the power of Yoga, directing the life

213

force properly to the middle of the eyebrows, comes to that supreme divine Spirit.

These stanzas are spoken by the God-man Krishna, who is the "supreme divine Spirit" who alone should be remembered. From stanza 8.13, we know that the dying *yogin* should also repeat the syllable AUM (symbolizing the Divine). This repetition is to be done with the mind focused on the crown of the head, which is the proper exit point for the departing spirit.

More than two millennia later, Hatha-Yoga connected death with the wasting of semen (*bindu*). Thus, the *Hatha-Yoga-Pradīpikā* (5.120–28), a text that can be placed in the middle of the fourteenth century C.E., elucidates,

The *bindu*, [which ordinarily] drops into the lap of a woman, should be raised upward through practice, and one's *bindu* having moved should be protected after raising it upward.

By falling, the *bindu* leads to death. By concentrating the *bindu*, it [becomes] enlivening. So long as the *bindu* is stabilized in the body, how can there be fear of death (*kāla*)?

The *bindu* is twofold; it is said to be red and white. The white, they say, is semen (*shukla*). The red is called menstrual fluid (*mahārajas*).

Rajas, [which] resembles red lead, is located at the place of the sun. When there is a merging with the *bindu*, then the body becomes divine.

The *bindu* is Shiva; *rajas* is Shakti. The *bindu* is the [inner] moon; *rajas* is the [inner] sun. Through the union verily of both, one attains the supreme state.

The semen is connected with the [inner] moon and *rajas* is joined with the [inner] sun. The *bindu* is located at the place of the moon. The union (*aikya*) of both is difficult to accomplish.

By stimulating the air through the [conscious] movement of the Shakti when *rajas* is in the space [at the crown of the head], it goes to union (*aikatva*) with the *bindu*. Then the body becomes divine.

He who knows that *shukra* is connected with the [inner] moon [and] *rajas* is joined with the [inner] sun is a knower of Yoga.

The semen of a human being is dependent upon the mind, while life is dependent upon the semen. Therefore, semen and *rajas* should be preserved with effort.

This passage continues in the same vein. The gist is clear: One should arrest the flow of the semen by arresting the flow of the mind. This is accomplished by raising the *kundalī-shakti* from the lowest psychoenergetic center to the crown of the head. Thus, according to this Tantric process, the adept of Yoga defeats death, for the ascending *kundalī* or *kundalinī* "cheats time" (*Hatha-Yoga-Pradīpikā* 5.3).

A good death is one that prepares the mind for tackling the death process and what is to come. Aldous Huxley, a self-actualizer, clearly agrees in his last novel, *Island* (1962).

In the second half of the twentieth century, the art of dying was revived through the scientific study of dying and the findings of thanatology. This interest started with Raymond Moody's daring book *Life After Life* (1975), which was followed by numerous other publications on the subject by different writers (see, for example, Stevenson 1966; Ring 1980; Doore 1990; Bailey and Yates 1996; Ring and Cooper 1999; Schwartz and Simon 2002; and van Lommel 2010). With the epochal discovery that some near-death experiences occur when the brain and nervous system are fully disabled—that is, when the patient is clinically dead—we can indeed boldly declare, as Charles T. Tart (2009) has done, the end of materialism.

DEATH AND YOGA

In the *Rig-Veda*, which has been dated conservatively to about 1500 B.C.E. but may have been written millennia earlier, we find a worldview whose eschatology, in contrast to later Hinduism, consists of a two-tier concept of the afterlife: heaven (*svar*) and hell (*tamas*, "darkness"), the latter of which does not appear to be emphasized. Liberation was thought to take place in the company of the gods and ancestors in heaven, who were immortal (the latter thanks to the rituals performed by their surviving descendants). Although some scholars interpret certain Vedic hymns as evincing the doctrine of rebirth, the *Rig-Veda* does not seem to refer to this teaching (see, for example, Reat 1990). The *Rig-Veda* speaks often of a "birth" into the luminous heaven, which has wrongly been interpreted as a case of rebirth.

In Upanishadic times, liberation was considered a state sui generis, beyond the heavenly or godly realms (*loka*). Those who failed to gain liberation were doomed to spend time in the cyclic existence (*samsāra*) of either heaven or hell before they were reborn in the earth realm to be given another opportunity at aspiring to liberation. This teaching is associated with the doctrine of the two ways—the *pitri-yāna* ("vehicle of the forefathers") and the *deva-yāna* ("vehicle of the gods"), where the former term refers to the pathway to reincarnation. The two vehicles are mentioned in the *Rig-Veda* (10.88.15), but probably without reference to rebirth.

The yogic teachings about death and dying are surrounded by secret knowledge in a circle of peers. These signs of death, or omens, are called *cihna* or *arishta* in Sanskrit. They are made possible by the interconnection of the mind and the outside world to which *yogins* and *yoginīs* pay great attention. Such signs are also connected with the birth of a master, significant teachings, *samādhi*, initiations, or liberation.

Patanjali's *Yoga-Sūtra* (3.22) mentions knowledge of death in its chapter on the paranormal abilities of Yoga. Later, in the manuals of Svara-Yoga ("Yoga of the Breath"), we find an assortment of omens for all kinds of purposes other than death. We can see, however, that death is of signal importance for a Yoga adept, because he or she can suitably prepare for this moment. Traleg Kyabgon Rinpoche, the Tibetan-born director of the Kagyu E-Vam Buddhist Institute in Melbourne, Australia, says,

> When the signs are all there that death can no longer be averted, we shouldn't indulge in self-deception and fixate on false hopes that we'll somehow be revived. At this point it's extremely important that we maintain a very clear mind and prepare ourselves for death. (Traleg 2007, 138)

DEATH IN BUDDHISM

The Buddha's hagiography tells how, as a young prince, he saw an old man, a sick person, and a corpse. Recognizing these signs of the changing and ephemeral nature of life prompted him to renounce his comfortable life and aspire to gain spiritual liberation, the deathless reality. In his discourses, he often brought up death. For instance, in the *Devatā-Saṃyutta* (16) of the *Saṃyutta-Nikāya,* he affirmed that no one can escape death but that it can be conquered. The way beyond death is the Buddha's famous eightfold path.

The *Prajñā-Pāramitā* literature of Mahāyāna Buddhism continued the attitude toward death found in the Pāli canon. The decisive difference between the two approaches is that the bodhisattva endeavors to attain liberation so that all beings can overcome suffering and death.

Dying is a fine art in Tibetan Buddhism, which arose from the Mahāyāna teachings, as is well-known from the *Bardo Thödol* (Tib.: *bardo'i thosgrol*), the Book of the Dead, ascribed to the great adept Padmasambhava (c. eighth century). His instructions are read to the recently deceased person to help him or her recall the spiritual disciplines practiced during life. In his foreword to Robert A. F. Thurman's *The Tibetan Book of the Dead: Liberation through Understanding in the Between* (1993, xvii), His Holiness the Dalai Lama states that this "is one of the most important books our civilization has produced."

The Buddhist scholar Reginald Ray writes in the *Secret of the Vajra World,*

> The subject of death and dying occupies a central place within Tibetan Buddhism. This centrality derives from the fact that in Buddhism, and particularly in Tibetan tradition, death and life are not seen as opposed realities or even as separate from one another. To live is to experience death continuously; there is no such thing as life without the constant presence and reality of death. Death is, moreover, the key to life. Without an open and confident relation to death, one cannot live a full and meaningful life.... Tibetan Buddhism is about nothing more or less than learning the practice of dying in order to live in a true and authentic way.
>
> (Ray 2001, 329ff.)

There exists an extensive literature on this subject in Tibetan, and the so-called Tibetan Book of the Dead, which has been translated many times, is at the summit of this body of literature. This text is concerned with the in-between state (*bardo*) just before rebirth takes place. It is both a reliable map and a guide to the opportunities of achieving liberation while in the after-death existence. There are six such states: the stretch from birth to death, the dream state, meditation, the death process, the in-between state of hallucinations, and the search for rebirth.

THE ART OF DYING IN JAINISM

Jainism is famous for its practice of *sallekhanā*, that is, the voluntary discipline of fasting to death. Given Jainism's emphasis on nonharming (*ahimsā*), this probably strikes us as peculiar. But we need to understand it as a rigorous discipline that is in keeping with the severe mind-set of much of Jainism. When a monastic or layperson is nearing the end and feels that control over his or her mind is slipping away, he or she may essentially commit suicide by strict fasting until death sets in. At this stage, a layperson may take the *mahāvrata* vows that are intended for monastics. It is important to die in a pure manner, meaning while in *samādhi*. One does not have to be absolutely decrepit to undertake *sallekhanā*, though old age is one of the legitimate causes for fasting to death. Looking forward to a quick death in order to end one's suffering is an impure motive, and a mendicant will instruct a layperson taking the *mahāvrata* vows accordingly. The vows cannot be rescinded, and therefore laypeople tend to wait until death is inevitable.

CHAPTER 22

Postmortem Freedom and Living Liberation

> The *jīvanmukti* ideal is one of the greatest contributions
> that India has made to the religious thought of the world.
>
> —CHACKO VALIAVEETIL (1980, xi)

EARLY TEACHINGS

India's greatest contribution to the world's spirituality is undoubtedly the ideal of perfect freedom (*mukti* or *moksha*) before and after death. This contrasts with the traditional religious notions of heaven (a state of everlasting beatitude in the company of angels, or *devas*) and hell (a state of unceasing terror and suffering in punishment for a sinful life). The freedom that awaits an accomplished Yoga adept is freedom from both pleasure and pain, from knowledge and ignorance, and from any kind of form, limitation, or change.

The ideal of spiritual freedom was first formulated in the *Atharva-Veda* and the early Brāhmanas, the ritual texts appended to the Vedic hymnodies. In the early Vedic era (see *Rig-Veda* 1.89.8ff.), the ordinary person reasonably wished for a full hundred autumns lived on earth in happiness, health, and wealth. The sage, however, looked forward to living in the company of the immortal deities after death in a realm of unexcelled joy (see *Rig-Veda* 9.113.9ff.). Then, in late Vedic times, the ideal of total spiritual freedom after death began to be put forward as the summum bonum of life. In the later Hindu schema of the four legitimate goals of human life (called *purusha-arthas*), liberation always stands at the apex of this value pyramid. In ascending order, the four goals, or values, are material welfare (*artha*), pleasure (*kāma*), moral virtue (dharma), and spiritual freedom. Those who find the pursuit of the first three values limiting are qualified to engage the kind of spiritual practice that in the short or long run will yield spiritual freedom.

The *Vājasaneyi-Samhitā*, or White *Yajur-Veda* (31.18), states that only someone who knows "him"—the *purusha*—escapes the realm of death. A similar declaration can be found in the *Atharva-Veda* (10.8.44), which is probably contemporaneous. In the *Shata-Patha-Brāhmana* (10.5.4.15), we can also read the following: Since the Self contains all desires, no desire for any specific thing can sway it. Neither asceticism (*tapas*) nor the relinquishment of action but only the realization of the Self can lead to spiritual freedom beyond heaven, hell, and cyclic existence (*samsāra*). Hence the Self (*ātman*) is equivalent to freedom.

The general idea appears to have been that upon attaining Self-knowledge (*ātma-jnāna*), or realizing the Self, an adept would achieve total freedom in the hereafter, although some scriptural passages suggest that he or she might have to undergo one or two more births to consume all the karma that is already in motion (see Shankara's commentary on the *Brahma-Sūtra* 3.4.51). This makes little sense, since liberation is typically thought to imply the exhaustion of all karma. Clearly, at the time of the Brāhmanas, the concept of liberation was still crystallizing in the minds of the sages. This does not, however, suggest that liberation is a mere concept, though it naturally requires conceptual language to be expressed.

In the early to mid-seventh century C.E., the sage Gaudapāda—Shankara's teacher's teacher—articulated the ideal of liberation in the here and now (see *Māndūkya-Kārikā* 4.89). Some writers have wrongly assumed that this was also the first time this concept was articulated. In fact, we find it discussed at least one millennium earlier in the *Bhagavad-Gītā* (2.54), when Prince Arjuna asks his *guru*, the God-man Krishna,

How does [he who is] steadied in gnosis (*sthita-prajna*) speak? How sit? How move about?

The adept who is steadied in gnosis is liberated while yet embodied. The ideal of living liberation suggested itself by—and is logically consistent with—the kind of plateau state realized long ago by the great Yoga masters, such as Yājnavalkya and his famous disciple King Janaka. They did not merely dip into the glorious freedom of the Self on rare occasions; they lived permanently *as* the Self. This recognition is coherent with the idea that, according to Hinduism, the Self is the inalienable essence of everything, and therefore the unenlightened state is illusory. This is clearly formulated in Gaudapāda's *Māndūkya-Kārikā*, which teaches the Noncontingent Yoga (*asparsha-yoga*). Here we have the first exposition of the philosophy of radical nondualism (or Kevalādvaita), which was clearly inspired by Buddhism but must not be confused with it. Self-realization is not an innovation but is simply due to removing obscurations in the mind; by cleansing the mind, we can realize that the Self has always been our true nature. The Self is not brought into existence through any specific effort, but it reveals its *eternal* presence whenever we polish the mirror of the mind. As the *Māndūkya-Kārikā* (4.29) asserts, the Self is ever unborn, so liberation has no beginning but is always the case (4.30).

When the Sanskrit texts speak of Self-*knowledge*, they always mean Self-*realization*, or being the Self without the intervention or intrusion of any mental filters or constructs. The same is true of the phrase *ātma-anu-bhāva*, or unmediated Self-*experience*. In this sense, Self-realization is not an attainment, or accomplishment; it is always the case. Only from the perspective of the individual mind does Self-realization appear to be an actual event occurring in historical time, with a before-and-after condition. Self-realization pertains exclusively to the mind, not the Self.

Because the Self does not confront any objects, Yājnavalkya was able to say—rather dramatically—to his wife, Maitreyī, that all consciousness (*sam-jnā*) in the Self-realized sage ceases after death. The consciousness he had in mind is the conventional consciousness made up of a subject (the ego) facing multiple objects. This unique conversation is recorded in the *Bri-hadāranyaka-Upanishad* (2.4.1ff.; especially 2.4.12–4.5.13).

The same Upanishad (4.4.7) quotes a declaration that speaks of liberation as immortality, which consists of realizing the Absolute (*brahman*) "here [and now, while still embodied]" (*atra*). This is one of the first mentions of living liberation. Ever since, Hindu philosophers and sages have championed or sought to explain this apparently paradoxical condition: The liberated being is continuously present as the nondual Reality and yet is active in the world of seeming duality—eating, drinking, defecating, urinating, speaking, listening, thinking, reading, and so on. How is this possible? Well over two thousand years ago, Arjuna was perplexed about this, and Krishna patiently answered his question (2.70–71):

Just as the waters enter the ocean, full and of unmoving ground, so all desires enter him who attains peace [but] not the desirer of desires.

That man who, forsaking all desires, moves about devoid of longing, devoid of [the thought of] "mine," without ego-sense—he approaches peace.

In consonance with Buddhism, the high state described by Krishna is one in which desire and the sense of "I" and "mine" have become extinct. Indeed, the *Bhagavad-Gītā* often speaks of brahma-*nirvāna,* or "brahmic extinction." This phrase has the specific connotation of "extinction in the world-ground," the matrix of psychocosmic existence (elsewhere known as *prakriti-pradhāna*). According to verse 2.72, when the Yoga adept is able to maintain this elevated disposition through the process of death, he or she enters brahmic extinction, which is the lower form of liberation (see 18.54–55). The higher form is being in the perennial presence of Krishna, who is the Godhead rather than an individual deity or its human emissary.

The liberated being, whose mind is completely stabilized, distinguishes him- or herself from others primarily in that the psychic forces and structures that commonly handicap or bind people are no longer present or have binding power over the mind. The classic example is the God-man Krishna himself. He is traditionally deemed to be a full *avatāra,* or "divine descent." At the same time, he is seen to have many human traits in the *Mahābharata* epic that tells his story and his history-making role.

MEDIEVAL TEACHINGS

Non-*advaita* teachers of Vedānta like Bhāskara, Yādavaprakāsha, Shrīkantha, and Nimbārka maintained that liberation is possible only after the demise of the body-mind. In other words, liberation is always *videha-mukti.* As long as we live in the world of multiple phenomena, there can be no true freedom.

Following Gaudapāda, Shankara thought that living liberation is possible, though he makes the point in his commentary on the *Brahma-Sūtra* (4.1.15 and 19) that even upon embodied liberation, fructifying karmas continue to ripen, just as a potter's wheel keeps on revolving for a while even when it is no longer activated; both definitely come to a full stop eventually. This type of karma is known as *prārabdha,* or "commenced." Because an enlightened adept, like everyone else, is subject to accidents and illness in principle, it is easy to assume that he or she is not yet liberated, but this would be wrong. We should, however, expect that a being who is liberated while still embodied meets with such occasions calmly and fearlessly. When Ramana Maharshi (1879–1950), who is widely hailed as a liberated adept, developed cancer in one arm; he simply shrugged it off. On the insistence of his disciples, he finally agreed to have an operation that he endured painlessly without anaesthetic. The cancer grew back faster than anyone had expected.

The disciples became fearful for Ramana's life and typically wondered what they would do without him when he died. He promptly reminded everyone, "Where could I possibly go?"[1]

Using the *Bhagavad-Gītā* as a guide but teaching a radical philosophical idealism, the *Yoga-Vāsishtha* of the ninth century also promulgates the ideal of living liberation. In Swami Venkatesananda's fine abridgment of this gargantuan text, we can read Sage Vasishtha's explanation to Prince Rāma (3.9.4ff.):

> He who, while living an apparently normal life, experiences the whole world as an emptiness, is a Jīvanmukta. He is awake but enjoys the calmness of deep sleep; he is unaffected in the least by pleasure and pain. He is awake in deep sleep; but he is never awake to this world. His wisdom is unclouded by latent tendencies. He appears to be subject to likes, dislikes and fear; but in fact he is as free as the space. He is free from egotism and volition; and his intelligence [*buddhi*] is unattached whether in action or inaction. None is afraid of him; he is afraid of none. He becomes a Videhamukta when, in due time, the body is dropped. (Venkatesananda 1993, 47)

The *jīvanmukta*'s life is indeed only apparently "normal" or "ordinary." His or her calmness is palpable, and his or her freedom from egotism is self-evident to everyone. Above all, the *jīvanmukta* manifests an unbiased friendliness (*maitrī*) toward all. He or she truly cares for the welfare of all others and will not fail to be directly helpful if possible. His or her disposition is, in religious terms, one of blessing.

We see the same characteristics in an accomplished bodhisattva who, in order to benefit others in ways that really matter, aspires to attain enlightenment as swiftly as possible. As an enlightened being, he or she willingly postpones ultimate liberation (*parinirvāna*), which is analogous to the Hindu ideal of postmortem emancipation. The Buddhist bodhisattva ideal was demonstrated by the Buddha himself, who, after realizing enlightenment, resolved to teach others the way to the same realization instead of simply exiting the world in favor of liberation. Even Shankara admits this possibility in his commentary on the *Brahma-Sūtra* (3.32), but he supposes that one would have to gain the authority (*adhikāra*) to return to the phenomenal world. It is not clear how this authority comes about.

The *Yoga-Vāsishtha*, which was clearly inspired by Buddhism, was very influential in Sanskrit-speaking Hindu circles. It impacted the fourteenth-century Vedānta scholar and Yoga practitioner Vidyāranya, among others, who quotes profusely from this text (in its abridged version) in his *Jīvanmukti-Viveka*. As the title of the latter work suggests, Vidyāraṇya pays close attention to the ideal of living liberation. Quoting a verse from the *Laghu-Yoga-Vāsishtha* (5.90), he defines this condition as follows:

> He is called a *jīvanmukta* for whom the empirical world ceases to exist, and becomes stably [present like the all-pervasive] ether-space.

The liberated being continues to see and respond to the world of multiplicity, but he or she sees through it—that is, regards it as "empty" (*shūnya*)—and thus is not caught up in it like everyone else who is not yet enlightened. The *jīvanmukta* is not driven by desire or sheer karmic reactivity (or unconscious motivations). Such a being inevitably stands out from the crowd, and most people would see him or her as a saint or profoundly good person. There is, however, no intention on his or her part to manifest either excellence or ordinariness.

The late medieval *Avadhūta-Gītā* is a Vedānta tract of 271 verses distributed over eight chapters and attributed to the Self-realized and divinized adept Dattātreya. It extols the paradoxical life of the *jīvanmukta* who, following Tantra, acts unconventionally in order to teach the wisdom of nonduality. The *Avadhūta-Gītā* (7.1–3, 7.9, 7.15, 8.6–9) effectively captures the raison d'être and behavioral traits of this kind of teacher:

> Immersed in pure, stainless equilibrium (*samarasa*), he abides, naked, in an empty place, [following] the path free from merit [and] demerit, [his] neck draped with rags [picked up from] the road.

> Characterized as devoid of aim [or] aimlessness, [as] skillfull [but] devoid of [either] attention [or] inattention, purified [and made] stainless [by] the absolute Reality (*tattva*), how can the *avadhūta* [engage in] discussion [or] dispute?

> Free from entanglement in the fetters of hope, controlled [and] devoid of purifying conduct, tranquil [and] thus free from all, [the *avadhūta*] possesses pure, stainless Reality.

> [The *avadhūta*] is a *yogin* without union (*yoga*) [or] separation (*viyoga*); [he] is an enjoyer without enjoyment [or] lack of enjoyment; thus he moves about slowly, with [his] mind transformed by innate bliss.

The letter *a* [in *avadhūta*] signifies that he exists always in bliss, free from the bond of hope, unblemished in the beginning, middle, [and] end.

The syllable *va* signifies that he exists in the present devoid of [unconscious] traits and with salubrious speech.

The syllable *dhū* signifies that [his] limbs are gray from the dust [of the road], [he] is well, [with his] mind cast off, released from concentration [and] meditation.

The syllable *ta* signifies that the thought of Reality is stabilized by him [who is] devoid of thought and action, released from [spiritual] darkness (*tamas*) [and] the ego.[2]

Similar sentiments are expressed in the *Siddha-Siddhānta-Paddhati*, a medieval text ascribed to Nityanātha. One verse (6.19) states that the *avadhūta* "delights in the world through play (*līlā*)," which is a reference to the crazy-wisdom adept's playful and unpredictable conduct. Another verse (6.20) indicates that he sometimes walks about nude and acts "like a demon"; at other times, he seems like a king or an upright citizen. His spontaneous purpose is to manifest the nondual Reality and awaken others to it. I have written at length about this type of adept in my book *Holy Madness* (2006), using both medieval and modern examples.

In Shankara's eyes, the *jīvanmukta*—contrary to the *avadhūta*'s unconventional behavior—does not go to the extreme of flouting established tradition. His pupil, Sureshvara, holds the same view. This is evident, for instance, from verses 4.62–63 of his *Naishkarmya-Siddhi* (seventh century C.E.?[3]):

If [someone who is] awakened to the truth of nonduality were to do as he pleases, what would be the difference between seers of Reality and dogs, [who] eat what is impure?

Sureshvara rightly points to the *Bhagavad-Gītā* (4.19ff.), which argues that an adept has neither desire nor motive and therefore, by implication, would never act out of self-will. This does not, of course, imply that the *avadhūta*'s unconventionality is egoic. The Avadhūta tradition, which is affiliated with the Dattātreya cult, assures us otherwise.

JĪVANMUKTI IN VEDĀNTA AND CLASSICAL YOGA

As already indicated, the idea of living liberation goes back to very early times. In the Upanishads, we can distinctly see the tendency to distinguish Self-knowledge from postmortem liberation, and we may understand the former as indicating living liberation. This is well articulated in the *Katha-Upanishad* (6.4):

> If one were able to know it [that is, the Self] here prior to the body's dissolution, one would become fit for embodiment in [any of] the created realms.

The Sanskrit of this verse is not clear. It seems to be saying that upon Self-knowledge, there is no compulsion to embody in a specific realm or world. Instead, the person endowed with Self-knowledge can manifest anywhere or nowhere.

The *brahman*-knower is as good as immortal. As, again, the *Katha-Upanishad* (6.15) affirms,

> When all the knots of the heart are severed, then a mortal becomes immortal. This is the instruction.[4]

In the seventh or eighth century, Shankara repeatedly considered the topic of liberation in his various commentaries, especially the one on the *Chāndogya-Upanishad* (6.14.2) and the *Brahma-Sūtra* (4.1.15). He used the term *jīvanmukta* (the adept enjoying living liberation) only once, in his commentary on the *Bhagavad-Gītā* (6.27), but he did not refer to *jīvanmukti* by name. He was, however, patently in favor of living liberation. He never described precisely how this state might manifest, although he predictably saw the enlightened adept as a renouncer (*samnyāsin*). He obviously relied on the empirical evidence of his teacher and others who, in his eyes, had attained this high state.

Shankara's elder contemporary Mandana Mishra, who was an early Advaita Vedānta teacher and the author of the *Brahma-Siddhi*, seems to have used the term *jīvanmukti*, as did Shankara's own disciples and later followers. In the eleventh and twelfth centuries, Rāmānuja—Shankara's principal opponent—commented on the concept of *jīvanmukti* from the viewpoint of his Vishishtādvaita system. In his commentary on the *Brahma-Sūtra* (1.1.4), he explains that, contrary to Shankara's position, the individual being and the world are real and not merely illusory. Living liberation is impossible even if a *yogin* knows Reality, and actual liberation can occur only after death.

The issue of how someone could be embodied and simultaneously enjoy spiritual liberation or enlightenment is discussed at some length in post-Shankara Vedānta works. One of the earliest instances in which the term *jīvanmukti* is prominently used is in the *Yoga-Vāsishtha,* referred to earlier. The classic discussion of this concept is by Vidyāranya in his *Jīvan-mukti-Viveka,* which presents a yogic type of Vedānta. Vidyāranya sought to integrate Advaita philosophy with Patanjali's eight-limbed path of Yoga.

While Shankara and many of his followers emphasized the importance of traditional knowledge, Vidyāranya felt that living liberation is gained by three means: knowledge of the Real (*tattva-jnāna*), "destruction" of the mind (*mano-nāsha*), and annihilation of the unconscious traits (*vāsanā-kshaya*). This triad should ideally be cultivated simultaneously. Knowledge of the ultimate Reality alone is not enough. The *yogin* must also ensure that the mind is held in perfect abeyance, and this is accomplished by eradicating the unconscious traits that, as the *Yoga-Sūtra* explains, give rise to renewed mental activity. Knowledge of *brahman* on its own makes a *yogin* a *brah-man*-knower and not a *jīvanmukta.* This differs significantly from the beliefs of Shankara and those who follow him closely. As Andrew O. Fort puts it in his valuable monograph *Jīvanmukti in Transformation,*

> To Vidyāraṅya, a *paramahamsa yogin* (that is, *jīvanmukta*) combines the best qualities of the knower and the *yogin:* a mere *yogin* does not have knowledge of the real and desires supernatural powers like flying; a mere *paramahamsa,* while knowing reality (*brahman*), spurns Vedic injunctions and prohibitions (*vidhi-niṣedha*). A *paramahamsa yogin,* however, neither desires powers nor disregards injunctions.... Thus, this *yogin* still follows both the Vedantic and the yogic paths. He removes ignorance (of non-duality) by realizing the meaning of the great sayings (*mahāvākya*) and removes impressions (*vāsanās*) arising from ignorance by repeated yogic practice.... Only together can these paths bring eternal awakening (*nitya-bodha*). (Fort 1998, 109)

The traditions of Classical Sāmkhya and Classical Yoga make statements that seem to allow the possibility of living liberation. Thus, Īshvara Krishna's *Sāmkhya-Kārikā* (67) employs the image of the potter's wheel when mentioning *prarābdha-karman,* that is, the karma that is in motion. Later Sāmkhya, which has a decidedly Advaita Vedāntic slant, confirms this position on *jīvanmukti*. Thus, the *Sāmkhya-Sūtra,* authored anonymously (probably in late medieval times), discusses living liberation in aphorisms 3.77–84.

Patanjali's *Yoga-Sūtra* (4.29–30) has two aphorisms that suggest—but do not conclusively demonstrate—that living liberation was entertained by this Yoga adept. Gerald J. Larson (1969) regards Classical Yoga as a new school of Sāmkhya. If true, it would not be quite so strange to attribute the ideal of living liberation to Patanjali, since it is a Sāmkhya ideal. But as with Classical Sāmkhya, the problem is that the sharp split between Self (*purusha*) and Cosmos (*prakriti*) does not logically allow the possibility of *jīvanmukti*. Some scholars, however, interpret the *Yoga-Sūtra* along these lines anyway (see, for example, Whicher 1998; Chapple 1996; and Fort and Mumme 1996, 115–34).

The *Yoga-Sūtra* (3.55 and 4.34) has two definitions of *kaivalya*. The first one may refer to the ideal of living liberation: "Aloneness [results] when equal purity [exists] between *sattva* [and] Spirit. Finis." Certainly, the Sanskrit commentaries on the *Yoga-Sūtra* unquestioningly subscribe to the ideal of living liberation, though they do not discuss it in any detail. Sri Ramana Maharshi, himself an enlightened sage, has this to say:

> Unless *prarabdha*[*-karma*] is completely exhausted the ego will be rising up in its *pure* form even in *jivanmuktas.* (Ramana and Ramananda 1955, 245)

Prārabdha-karma is karma in progress; therefore, the identification with the body-mind can spring up again. Only when *prārabdha-karma* is entirely exhausted is the state of a *jīvanmukta* ensured. There is thus no safety unless the Self is realized; all other spiritual attainments can be lost. We ought to take the testimony of Ramana Maharshi seriously, because as a Self-realizer, he went beyond living liberation, which requires that a sage dip periodically into *nirvikalpa-samādhi* (or *asamprajnāta-samādhi*) to purify the mind.

JĪVANMUKTI IN JAINISM

As we have seen in expounding the fourteen stages of the Jaina path to perfection, the *sayogi-kevalin* stage marks someone who has reached omniscience but is still endowed with an active body. This is equivalent to living liberation. At this stage, karma is produced but does not stick to the person, which is contrary to Ramana Maharshi's understanding. It is at this stage that the *tīrthānkaras,* the great teachers of Jainism, impart the doctrinal knowledge.

The next and final stage of *ayoga-kevala* is of very short duration and leads to *nirvāna*, which is understood as the state of a perfected adept (*siddha*).

LIBERATION IN BUDDHISM

In Buddhism, the ideal of *jīvanmukti* is embodied in the Buddha himself, who, according to tradition, attained *nirvāna* while still alive. The ideal is also illustrated by the figure of the enlightened bodhisattva who works untiringly for the welfare of all others. This notion is central to the "Great Vehicle," or Mahāyāna, that emerged as a branch of the Buddhist culture in the centuries just before the Common Era.

In the tradition of Mahāyāna Buddhism, a fully enlightened being has three "bodies": *dharma-kāya, sambhoga-kāya,* and *nirmāna-kāya.* Only the first body is real, while the other two are regarded as phantoms—an idea that crystallized at the time of the first council a century after the earthly life of the Buddha. The *sambhoga-kāya,* or "enjoyment body," is an illusory appearance of the *dharma-kāya* at the subtle level, and the *nirmāna-kāya* appears at the coarse level that is accessible to human perception. Thus, the Mahāyānists believe that Gautama the Buddha only apparently strove for *nirvāna* and only apparently attained it. They understand him as a mere apparition who taught others the way to spiritual freedom.

For the Theravādins, this illusionism is a controversial philosophical teaching that goes counter to the tangible historical reality of the Buddha. Some modern scholars regard this as a doctrinal development that effectively deifies the Buddha. As Sangharakshita rightly observed,

> Within the context of a non-theistic religion the concept of deification has no meaning. The Buddha claimed to be a fully enlightened human being, superior even to the gods, and as such He has invariably been regarded....
>
> No deification of an originally "merely human" teacher ever having taken place, we must also dismiss as impertinent the several theories according to which the Buddha was in reality an ethical teacher like Socrates or Confucius, a rationalist, a humanist, a social reformer, and so on. (Sangharakshita 1980, xxvi–xxvii)

Psychologically, the *tri-kāya* doctrine is an eminent teaching, because it affirms that we—the average individual—are not really deluded, and our spiritual ignorance is not really as abysmal as some would have us believe.

• Rather, we all have or are Buddha nature. Our nature is thus inherently noble and free, and we are called to awaken to this intrinsic nobility and freedom even in this lifetime. Instead of wallowing in mud, we are beings of sheer luminosity. Acknowledging this in any therapeutic intervention inevitably defines the relationship of therapist and patient in a significantly different way from the professional routine.

TULKUHOOD IN TIBETAN BUDDHISM

Importantly, in the Tibetan Vajrayāna tradition, bodhisattvas may happily reincarnate at various levels of existence to aid the denizens of those realms. They are known in Tibetan as *sprulkus* (pron. *tulkus*)—a term meaning "reincarnation"; they are identified reincarnations of particular adepts.[5] The criteria of identification are not entirely clear, so history is full of *tulkus* who were nominated by fiat to play this role either for political or spiritual reasons rather than be called to demonstrate moral, intellectual, and spiritual qualifications as the genuine continuations of their supposed predecessors. Today, with *tulkus* apparently being born outside of Tibet, including in Western countries, the problem of identifiying a literal reincarnation is formidable. Great *tulkus,* about whose qualifications in terms of conduct, wisdom, and inner authority there is no doubt, are usually identified at a very young age (if not before their birth) by high lamas, notably by the Dalai Lama, the Tai Situpa (the supreme head of the Nyingma branch of Vajrayāna), or the Karmapa (the supreme head of the Kagyu branch). Given that Buddhism denies that the personality is anything but a bundle of factors (*skandha*) without a permanent identity, a larger problem concerns how a reincarnation of a previous individual is at all feasible. Reginald Ray offers the following clarification:

[T]he tülku phenomenon makes no sense as long as one remains within a theoretical framework that insists on the unity of the person and its substantial and indivisible existence. However, when this belief is called into question, other possibilities can be entertained. Then we can imagine a life, a mode of being, that is infinitely more expansive and responsible to this realm of reality, such as it may be, that we inhabit. (Ray 2001, 383)

This observation is all the more pertinent when we consider that the Tibetans allow for a *tulku* to incarnate in more than one personality simultaneously; some *tulkus* are traditionally said to have incarnated in up to a thousand beings at the same time, which confirms the materialist's suspicion that the *tulku* phenomenon is little more than pious fantasy. But this kind of partiality shatters when we consider the undoubted moral integrity of the Tibetan masters and teachers. If we cannot muster modesty in such matters, we ought to at least suspend judgment, as demanded by scientific "objectivity." We also ought to realize that this is a self-imposed stricture that amounts to a cognitive, emotional, and indeed cultural limitation.

Living liberation and the *tulku* phenomenon are unquestionably a great paradox, which mysteriously links a transcendental state with the empirical world. Thus, at the core of yogic philosophy and psychology is an apparently irresolvable paradox. The Indian traditions have failed to resolve it, and our own "scientific" worldview certainly offers no plausible resolution either. Yet the *tulku* phenomenon is worthy of extensive consideration. I have gone through the mental exercise of applying quantum theory, which I understand only imperfectly, to this situation. But I had to conclude that a truly transcendental noumenon requires a fundamental shift (or *saltus*) to be "realized." This implies that full liberation cannot involve the mind. However hard we may try, our intellect has to accept defeat. I was thrilled to learn that in his book *The End of Materialism* (2009), Charles T. Tart arrived at the same conclusion.

Yoga does, however, admit of a highly refined state of mind that resembles transcendence and has traditionally been treated as being transcendental from a practical standpoint. This state has been interpreted in various ways, which all inevitably involve the paradox already mentioned. That paradox is entailed in the notion that *buddhi*, the higher mind, can appear as lucidly as the transcendental Self.[6]

Theoretically, we can either reject or accept this position. Regardless of our preference (or bias), the path to spiritual freedom will inevitably unfold itself and prove us either right or wrong. Sooner or later, we will come to a point where all our biases will be exposed and challenged. We can then either cling to or jettison them. Only the latter option will be reasonable if we want to engage Yoga with due judiciousness.

PART FOUR

Analysis and Relevance

Toward a Western Yoga

> Utterly free from all concepts,
> the great wisdom dwells in the body,
> it encompasses all things.
>
> —SAMBHUTI (=*Samputa-Tantra*)
> JAMGÖN KONGTRÜL THE GREAT (1995, 30)

In this book, I have attempted to look at yogic or Yoga-like features in various Indian traditions. This has sometimes proved awkward. But a comparative framework commended itself and should be useful. Many psychological elements are prominent in modern psychology but are of relative unimportance or altogether absent in Indian thought and culture. I have demonstrated, however, that Indian thought—be it Hindu, Buddhist, or Jaina—has a distinct advantage over contemporary psychology when it comes to the issue of spiritual freedom and the path to freedom. The Indian sages are able to look back on the collective (empirical) wisdom of a hundred generations. Carl Jung saw the difference very clearly when he admitted,

> I do not apply yoga methods in principle, because in the West, nothing ought to be forced on the unconscious.... On the contrary, everything must be done to help the unconscious to reach the conscious mind and to free it from its rigidity. (Jung 1978, 85)

In *Psychology and Religion*, Jung (1958a, 537) noted cautiously, "No insight is gained... by imitating methods which have grown up under totally different psychological conditions." The conditions about which he was speaking were those of India, and the methods he had in mind were those of Yoga. Jung believed that the West would eventually produce its own Yoga based in Christianity.

Some of his followers thought that Jung's own psychotherapeutic method of active imagination was at least gesturing toward such a Western Yoga. Unfortunately, Jung seems to have kept this therapeutic technique quiet from the larger public.

This was contrasted with the body-oriented therapies that emerged after the 1960s, in particular Eugene T. Gendlin's Focusing approach (1981). This method was taken up and developed further by Peter A. Campbell and Edwin M. McMahon, coauthors of *Bio-Spirituality* (1985). Campbell and McMahon used Focusing (or what I call here somatic concretion)[1] in regard to a biologically anchored spirituality, not necessarily Christianity.

A decade into the twenty-first century, many people are alienated from Christianity and have no connection to it; many have adopted Buddhism, Hinduism, or some other tradition; many are simply secular nonbelievers. In the previous century, Jung and Gebser still thought that Christianity would have a role to play in the emerging spirituality. As someone who became estranged from the Christian faith at a young age, I doubted this back in the 1960s; in 2011, when I am writing this book, I question Christianity as the emerging religious denomination even more.

I am, however, struck by the eminent applicability of the method of somatic concretion, or Focusing, and I see it as the main alternative to *samādhi* and the most viable route to enlightenment for the Westerner who has left all isms behind. In fact, I am so impressed with Focusing that I plan to study this method with the Canadian psychologist Esther Stenberg. Eugene Gendlin (1981, 59–71) mapped out the following six steps:

1. *Clear a space:* Is your body open to a round of focusing? Just relax and let the body answer! What is between you and feeling fine? Whatever issues come up, put them aside for now.
2. *Felt sense:* What does your body tell you when you select one of the issues or problems you set aside? Allow yourself to feel the confusion or lack of clarity in the felt sense.
3. *Get a handle:* What one word, phrase, symbol, or image does the felt sense suggest? The felt sense necessarily has many parts, but there is a total feeling to it, which is what you seek to cultivate.
4. *Resonate:* Go back and forth between the word/phrase/image and the felt sense until you know you have a perfect match. If the felt sense changes, allow this to happen.
5. *Ask:* What do I dislike/hate/etc. most about the problem? Wait for the

felt sense to answer. When no answer is forthcoming, ask yourself, What's the worst about the felt sense? What should happen? Let your body answer!

6. *Receive:* Welcome the felt sense. Don't let your own critical voice or that of another interrupt.

Really allow the felt sense to speak. Be careful to avoid labelling things! The felt sense comes from the body and not from the conceptual mind, which is an incorrigible critic. Allowing the body to speak is an acquired skill. When answers come quickly, they are apt to be from the mind, and they are not empowered to transform. Somatic concretion is not just bodily sensation. It is feeling the identified problem with the body. This requires the middle path: we neither run away from the problem (and usually into the conceptual mind) nor fall into it and become it.

We distance ourselves from the problem, and the distance is all in our feeling. While we witness the problem in all its inchoate feeling force, we do not wallow in suffering. Campbell and McMahon (1985, 5) understood that by tapping into the body's feeling mode, we have a "humane valuing process." We need no longer rely on the mental right or wrong but now have a means—the *felt* "meaning," the *felt* "truth," or the *felt* "direction"—by which we can evaluate from a deeper sense. As Campbell and McMahon also saw, this can be the way to a nondoctrinal faith.

This is psychological integration that also integrates our world. This has been superbly explained by Michael Washburn in what may be the most poetic passage in his book:

The integrated world is a world of exquisite beauty because, like the garden of delight, it is charged with a plenipotent energy that, as an attracting energy, renders the world irresistibly inviting and that, as an amplifying energy, intensifies perceptual qualities in pleasing ways.... The energy that enlivens the integrated world is a radiant and soothing energy, an energy that makes the world gleam with sparkling, gentle light. The integrated world is resplendent through and through. It is a glorified world. (Washburn 2003, 194)

Hindu, Buddhist, and Jaina Yoga

These three forms of Yoga—Hindu, Buddhist, and Jaina—are not merely specific spiritual traditions spawned on Indian soil; they are embedded in whole cultures with their own distinct moral and spiritual teachings, art, architecture, and social organization. There are many overlaps but also significant divergences. For instance, in the area of social organization, Buddhism does not subscribe to the caste system, which is a hallmark of Hinduism (though by no means all Hindu traditions accept or support it) and which is not accepted by Jainism, though actual living practice is different.

Yoga is commonly understood to be an aspect of Hinduism. However, both the term and the concept (in the sense of spiritual practice) are also widespread in Buddhism and are used in Jainism as well. Thus, it makes little sense to compare Yoga and Buddhism or Jainism unless we define Yoga more narrowly as the particular philosophical system known as *yoga-darshana,* as expounded in Patanjali's *Yoga-Sūtra* and its extensive commentaries.

In the broadest sense, Yoga is simply spiritual practice, or spirituality. It is India's version of what has long been known as mysticism in Christianity, kabbalah in Judaism, and Sufism in Islam. Hinduism and Buddhism, as well as Jainism, are all yogic *cultures,* or traditions. That is to say, these cultures are spiritual at heart: they acknowledge and promote the age-old ideal of liberation (*moksha*), however it may be conceived. Yoga has, from the beginning, been a liberation teaching (*moksha-shāstra*), and as such has shaped Hinduism, Buddhism, and Jainism.

Hinduism is the name given to a particular developmental phase of the complex civilization that originated in India more than eight millennia ago and that has since spread throughout the world. Buddhism is not, as is widely thought, an offshoot of Hinduism but of the Indic civilization. Yoga is the Indic civilization's unique contribution to humankind.

Many Western Yoga students confuse Yoga with Hinduism and typically pitch it against Buddhism. Many more Westerners confuse Yoga (that is, the yogic poses) with physical exercise and see in Buddhism a path of meditation. But the opposition of Yoga-Hinduism versus Yoga–Buddhist meditation is ill-conceived.

Yoga is common to both cultural traditions and forms their spiritual essence. Yoga must not be reduced to a mere system of physical exercises; it clearly offers many spiritual methods and approaches, especially meditation. It makes no sense to say, as is often heard, that Yoga has no meditation practice and that one must therefore resort to Buddhist meditation. Yoga has a wide variety of meditation techniques that include Buddhist, Hindu, and Jaina practices.

During the past two and a half millennia or so, Hinduism, Buddhism, and Jaina have been in dialogue with one another, and each cultural tradition has incorporated elements from the others. It has even been said that the disappearance of Buddhism from India was largely due to the fact that Shankara and his school of Advaita Vedānta, or nondual metaphysics, so successfully assimilated Buddhist ideas that Buddhism lost its foothold with regard to the dominant Hindu culture. The Muslim invasion of Northern India was, however, a more decisive factor.

There has traditionally been far less tension between Hinduism and Jainism, since most Jaina adherents regard themselves as Hindu or as not being in conflict with Hinduism. At times, the dialogue between Hindu and Buddhist Yoga has been doctrinaire and fierce indeed, but when we look at the great teachers and teachings, we also find much common ground. To those of us in the West who are not mired in religious ideology and have imbibed a cosmopolitan outlook, the doctrinal squabbles among the Indic traditions are of little relevance. We hunger for practices that can nourish us spiritually and, in our pragmatist approach, are willing to regard their theoretical underpinnings with open-mindedness.

Since the mid-1960s, I have endeavored to make Hindu Yoga accessible to my fellow Westerners. I have focused on such key scriptures as the *Yoga-Sūtra* (see Feuerstein 1989, 1996, and 2011b) and the *Bhagavad-Gītā* (see Feuerstein 2011a) but have also translated or commented on other, less well-known (in the West) Yoga texts.[1] I brought many of them together in my book *The Yoga Tradition*, and in that volume, I furnished a broad overview of the history of Hindu, Buddhist, and Jaina Yoga.

In my scholarly work thus far, I have been less concerned with Buddhist Yoga, which from the beginning of my career, I felt had received considerable attention from preceding scholars. Certainly over the past two decades, there has been an increasing preoccupation with Buddhist Yoga in the form of Tibetan Buddhism. What is more, the custodians of the Tibetan Buddhist heritage have shown a great willingness to impart the esoteric practices underlying their sacred texts to Westerners. In the case of Hindu Yoga, this is no longer possible to the same extent, though there are still masters capable of imparting the full range of practices and expounding the teachings of specific schools, such as Shrī Vidyā, Kaula, Nātha, and Kashmiri Shaivism.

Compared to Hindu and Buddhist Yoga, Jaina Yoga is a sealed book for Western spiritual seekers, who may not even have heard of it. Yet it has its own distinct path and practices that are kept alive by a few adepts and definitely deserve to be better known. However, only a few Jaina texts are available in English, and studying this tradition, which is based on the Prakrit languages (especially Ardha Magadhi), is therefore difficult.

From the vantage point of our own time, we can look on the incredibly complex and diversified heritage of Yoga and appreciate its unique significance for the human race. The adepts of Yoga have blazed trails to summits that at present we see only through a glass darkly but that we sense are of utter relevance to our human destiny. As we delve into the yogic heritage, we encounter a breathtaking wealth of ideas and practices. Yet at the bottom of it all are a handful of universal truths that, once we have recognized them, can become powerful agents of transformation for us. Equipped with that recognition, we can engage any form of Yoga or any specific practice with efficiency and tolerance.

A Survey of the Literature on Yoga Psychology

It may be helpful to other researchers investigating the connection between Yoga and psychology to provide an overview of work done so far by surveying the available literature. Over the years, I have had the opportunity to either inspect (in libraries such as those of the School of Oriental and African Studies in London, the School of Oriental Studies in Durham, or the British Museum in London) or acquire and work with most of the books mentioned in this survey. I have not seen all of the articles, though. I have not included the majority of the many publications on Transcendental Meditation, because a number of researchers have questioned the validity of the investigations. I will proceed chronologically to provide a sense of how the field has slowly emerged.

First to address psychological issues in the context of Indian philosophy was Paul Deussen's masterful scholarly work *Das System des Vedānta*, first published in **1883**. This tome was translated into English by Charles Johnston and published in 1912 as *The System of Vedānta* by Open Court Publishing (Chicago). It included a seventy-page section titled "Psychology or the Doctrine of the Soul," in which Deussen reviewed the psychological position of this system focusing on the Indian sources and ignoring any possible parallels to the West. Admittedly, the work was published before Sigmund Freud and psychoanalysis had achieved renown. Deussen, who was possibly inspired by the psychospiritual work of Gustav Fechner (*Über die Seelenfrage,* 1861), also provided a translation of the *Yoga-Sūtra* of Patanjali in his *Allgemeine Geschichte der Philosophie* (*General History of Philosophy*), 1, 3 (Leipzig: Brockhaus, 3rd ed., 1920, S. 511–43), first published in 1894.

Although Freud did not pay any attention to Indian philosophy, in 1927 he became fleetingly interested in mystical experiences in response to a letter from his friend Romain Rolland, a well-known writer and the author of *La vie de Ramakrishna* (1929). Freud, for whom this experience was little more than an illusion, politely dismissed Rolland's notion of an "oceanic feeling" as the source of religion. As a mystical Catholic, Rolland stood in sharp contrast to Freud, who was committed to smashing any illusions he recognized as such. Yet, paradoxically, he seems to have had a lifelong curiosity about mystical experiences. In *Das Unbehagen in der Kultur* (1930), Freud confessed,

> I cannot discover this "oceanic" feeling in myself. It is not easy to deal scientifically with feelings.... I may remark that to me this seems something rather in the nature of an intellectual perception, which is not, it is true, without an accompanying feeling-tone, but only such as would be present with any other act of thought of equal range. From my own experience I could not convince myself of the primary nature of such a feeling. But this gives me no right to deny that it does in fact occur in other people. (Freud and Strachey 1961, 12)

Rightly or wrongly, much has been made psychoanalytically of Freud's relationship with Rolland. What is for certain, however, is that by rejecting the notion of an oceanic feeling, he missed the opportunity to see the real ground behind mysticism. It was left to his disciple Carl Jung to attempt to understand the Indian philosophical heritage and to locate such experiences in the collective unconscious.

After Deussen, came William James's perennially readable *The Varieties of Religious Experience* (London and Bombay: Longmans, Green & Co.) in **1902**. This book was based on his Gifford Lectures.

Then, in **1911**, came Evelyn Underhill, who in her well-known book *Mysticism* included a chapter titled "Mysticism and Psychology" (1961, 44–69). Apart from referring to a handful of psychologists (notably William James, Edwin Diller Starbuck, James Bissett Pratt, and Edouard Récéjak), Underhill only remarks that the field of mysticism has suffered severely at the hands of the "new psychologists."

In **1914**, the first edition of Caroline Rhys Davids's significant monograph *The Birth of Indian Psychology and Its Development in Buddhism* (London: Luzac & Co., 1936; first published as *Buddhist Psychology*) was published in the Quest series. The opening sentence of the editor's statement reads, "One of the most marked signs of the times is the close attention that is being paid to psychological research, the results of which are being followed with the greatest interest by an intelligent public, and the continued advance of which promises to be one of the most hopeful activities of modern science" (Rhys Davids 1936, vii). Rhys Davids was keenly aware of the psychological implications of her field and the widespread mistaken idea that psychological observation started with the pre-Socratics. In the 1936 version of her book, she included five chapters on psychology in the *Nikāyas*, the books of the Pāli Canon—a total of more than one hundred pages.

In **1927**, Carl Jung furnished a psychological commentary on the widely read *The Tibetan Book of the Dead* by Walter Evans-Wentz. In a letter to Caroline Rhys Davids, he modestly called his forays into Buddhism "pre-studies," which is how we ought to regard them. (See Rhys Davids 1936, 7n1.)

In **1928**, Richard Rösel's *Die Psychologischen Grundlagen der Yogapraxis* (The Psychological Foundations of Yoga Practice; Stuttgart, Germany: Kohlhammer Verlag) was published.

In **1930**, Girindrasekhar Bose delivered a presidential address titled "Indian Thought of Psychology" at the Indian Philosophical Congress.

In **1932**, Sigurd Lindquist's book *Die Methoden des Yoga* (The Methods of Yoga; Lund, Sweden: Ohlsson) saw the light of day. Lindquist approached Yoga from the viewpoint of hypnosis, which was popular in those days. In the same year, Pathak published *The Heyapaksha of Yoga*, which was originally his master's thesis at Ahmedabad University (1931) and has a foreword by Sarvepalli Radhakrishnan.

Lindquist applied the hypnotic perspective in his monograph on the paranormal abilities of Yoga, which was published in **1935** under the title *Siddhi und Abhiññā: Eine Studie über die klassischen Wunder des Yoga* (Siddhi and Abhiññā: A Study of the Classical Miracles of Yoga; Uppsala, Sweden: Uppsala Universitets Arsskrift).

The British psychotherapist Geraldine Coster was the first to write about the implications of Yoga theory and practice from a psychotherapeutic perspective in her widely read book *Yoga and Western Psychology: A Comparison* (London: Oxford University Press, **1934**), which was reissued with only slight changes by Oxford University Press in 1971. It still makes for helpful and fascinating reading. Her treatment is based on Patanjali's *Yoga-Sūtra* and, though somewhat dated, is still a valuable discussion of Yoga psychology.

In the same year, Jadunath Sinha published *Indian Psychology* (London: Kegan Paul and Co., 1934).

In **1936**, the British Buddhologist Caroline Rhys Davids published the revised and expanded version of her 1914 study *Buddhist Psychology*.

In 1939, Sarvepalli Radhkrishnan in his *Eastern Religions and Western Thought* dwells on ecstatic experiences arguing that "[e]cstasy is not the only way to spirititual life" (Radhkrishnan 2007, 79). He continues,

It is often a perversion of mysticism rather than an illustration of it. As there is a tendency to mistake it for spiritual life, we are warned against it. The spiritual mystics the world over regard ecstasy, visions, auditions as things to be avoided and of secondary importance. They are the anomalies of the life of mystics from which they sometimes suffer and are the results of an imperfect adaptation to a changed inner world.

Radhakrishnan pointed to Arjuna's cosmic vision in the *Bhagavad-Gītā* (chapter 11) indirectly spurring him on to not merely catch a glimpse of the divine Krishna but actually to enter his immense being by practicing the Yoga imparted by the God-man.

The first edition of Surendranath Dasgupta's *Philosophical Essays,* which contained a nineteen-page chapter titled "Yoga Psychology," was published in 1941 and based on a talk given at an open meeting at the Quest Society in 1921. The author ended by saying, "If we do not believe the testimony of the Yogin, there is probably no way for us either to prove or disprove its [*prajñā's*] reality" (Dasgupta [1941] 1990, 197).

This was also the year the German psychoanalyst Franz Alexander published his article "Buddhistic Training as an Artificial Catatonia" (*Psychoanalytic Review* 18[1941]:129–45) and his book *The Scope of Psychoanalysis* (New York: Basic Books).

In 1946, Swami Akhilananda's readable *Hindu Psychology: Its Meaning for the West* (Boston: Branden Press) was published.

The following year, H. P. Mehta completed a master's thesis titled "Psychoanalytic Representation of a Phase of Iranian Religion" at Nagpur University.

In 1953, R. K. Rai completed a master's thesis on "Jung and Indian Thought" at the Benares Hindu University in Varanasi.

This was followed two years later by L. B. Tripathi's master's thesis called "Human Personality: Indian Approach" at the same university.

Another decade passed before Indologist E. Abegg published his small but expertly crafted introduction to the field, *Indische Psychologie* (*Indian Psychology*; Zurich: Rascher-Verlag, 1955).

In the same year, M. L. Mehta published his "Jain Psychology", which was a doctoral dissertation at the Benares Hindu University, and N. S. N. Shastri published his article "Trends of Psychological Research in India" in the *Indian Journal of Psychology.*

Three years later, Johann W. Hauer published his important book *Der Yoga: Ein indischer Weg zum Selbst* (Yoga: An Indian Way to the Self; Stuttgart: Kohlhammer Verlag, 1958), which was the reworked and greatly expanded second edition of his book *Der Yoga als Heilsweg* (Yoga as a Liberating Path), first released in 1932. Hauer had been educated as a Protestant missionary, but in 1933, he left the church and explored a "free" religion. In 1922, he had published his brilliant monograph *Die Anfänge der Yogapraxis im alten Indien* (The Beginnings of the Practice of Yoga in Ancient India), which was based on his 1917 dissertation.

Although Hauer has many interesting things to say about Yoga and depth psychology, he has been all but ignored by the academic establishment because of his idealistically based support of the Nazi party; apparently he sided with the moderates. Even though his affiliation with national socialism is to be regretted and his establishment of a nationalistic religious movement—the German Faith Movement—was misguided, there is no excuse for the wholesale neglect of his scholarship, which should be judged in its own right. If he is deemed one of the black sheep in the history of Indology, then this should be noted and lamented but not used as a justification for condemning his work as a whole. I realize that for many people this is a knotty moral issue, and my own standpoint comes mainly from the Buddhist value of kindness (*maitrī*), which surely includes forgiveness, especially after such a long time.

The year 1958 saw the publication of H. Kelman's "Zen and Psychotherapy" in *Psychologia* (1[1958]:219–28) and K. Sato's "Psychotherapeutic Implications of Zen" in *Psychologia* (1[1958]:213–18). This year also heralded W. Van Dusen's articles "Wu-wei, No-mind, and the Fertile Void in Psychotherapy" in *Psychologia* (1[1958]:253–56) and "Zen and Western Psychotherapy" in *Psychologia* (1[1958]:229–30).

In 1959, R. Marsh submitted his doctoral dissertation titled "A Comparative Analysis of the Concept of Individuality in the Thought of C. G. Jung and Sri Aurobindo" to Pacific University through the American Academy of Asian Studies. The 1959 issue (no. 2) of the German magazine *Yoga* contained the first part of Henri Birven's article "Yoga und Psychoanalyse" (Yoga and Psychoanalysis). Erich Fromm's "Psychoanalysis and Zen Buddhism" appeared in the same year in *Psychologia* (2[1959]:79–99).

R. C. Rao submitted a doctoral dissertation called "Development of Psychological Thought in India" at the Mysore University in **1960,** and L. A. Singh published his article on "Volition: A Viewpoint in Indian Psychology" in the *Proceedings of the International Congress of Psychology.*

The same year saw Tomio Hirai's "Electroencephalographic Study on Zen Meditation (Zazen): EEG Changes During the Concentrated Relaxation" in *Folio Psychiatrica et Neurologia Japonica* (62[1960]:76–105).

Hans Jacobs's *Western Psychotherapy and Hindu Sādhanā* (London: George Allen & Unwin, **1961**) has a broader compass than Coster's pioneering book, including a trenchant and acerbic critique of the approaches by Freud and Jung. Also in **1961**, Dietrich Langen published *Archaische Ekstase und asiatische Meditation mit ihren Beziehungen zum Abendland* (Archaic Ecstasy and Eastern Meditation with its Relation to the Occident; Stuttgart: Hippokrates Verlag).

In the same year, Rider & Co. in London released Anagarika Govinda's book *The Psychological Attitude of Early Buddhist Philosophy,* and Pantheon Books in New York published Alan W. Watts's book *Psychotherapy East and West.*

In the same year, W. Van Dusen published "LSD and the Enlightenment of Zen" in *Psychologia* (4[1961]:11–16).

In **1964,** S. P. Atreya submitted a doctoral dissertation on "Personality in the Light of Yoga" to Benares Hindu University at Varanasi. The following year, R. K. Rai's doctoral dissertation on "Jung and Indian Thought" was submitted to the same university. In the same year, S. P. Srivastava submitted his doctoral dissertation on "Indian Psychology with Special Reference to the Structure and Development of the Human Personality" to Agra University. R. Prince and C. Savage had their paper "Mystical States and the Concept of Regression" published in *Psychedelic Review* (8[1964]:59–75), and it was later republished in John White's *The Highest State of Consciousness* (New York: Doubleday, 1972).

The year **1966** saw the publication of Alan W. Watts's "Asian Psychology and Modern Psychiatry" in the *American Journal of Psychoanalysis* (13[1966]:25–30).

In **1967,** Wilhelm Bitter, a professor of neurology at the University of Stuttgart, presided over a congress called "Abendlandische Therapie und ostliche Weisheit" (Occidental Therapy and Eastern Wisdom). The contributions were published a year later by Klett Verlag under the same title. The book includes essays called "Autogenic Training and Yoga," "Jung's Analytical Psychology and Indian Wisdom," and "On the Psychology and Symbology of Tantric Yoga." The various contributions are interspersed with helpful dialogues among the participants.

In the same year, *The Journal of Humanistic Psychology* carried D. Sinha's article "Integration of Modern Psychology with Indian Thought," and J. S. Neki's "Yoga and Psychoanalysis" appeared in *Comprehensive Psychiatry* (8[1967]:160–67).

S. K. Pande published his essay "The Mystique of Western Psychotherapy and Eastern Interpretation" in the *Journal of Nervous and Mental Diseases* (168[1968]:425–32).

A year later, R. E. A. Johansson published his important book *The Psychology of Nirvana* (New York: Anchor Books).

In 1970, Theodore Xenophon Barber published *LSD, Marihuana [sic], Yoga, and Hypnosis* (Chicago: Aldine). Also in 1970, Lal A. Singh published the two volumes of his *Yoga Psychology* (Varanasi, India: Bharatiya Vivya Prakashan). This work is a collection of conference papers and essays. In the same year, R. K. Wallace and H. Benson's paper "The Physiology of Meditation" appeared in *Scientific American* (February 1970: 85–90).

In 1971, Abraham Maslow published his seminal work *The Farther Reaches of Human Nature* (New York: Viking Press), which bridged the gulf between psychology and Eastern spiritual disciplines.

At the same time, the noted British psychotherapist James Hillman wrote a psychological commentary to Gopi Krishna's *Kundalini: The Evolutionary Energy in Man* (London: Robinson & Watkins). This book has an introduction by the eminent American scholar Frederic Spiegelberg (Stanford University).

This year also saw the release of Claudio Naranjo and R. E. Ornstein's *On the Psychology of Meditation* (New York: Viking) and of W. N. Pahnke's "The Psychedelic Mystical Experience in the Human Encounter with Death" in *Psychedelic Review* (11[1971]:3–21). R. W. Fischer also published his important essay "A Cartography of the Ecstatic and Meditative States" in *Science* (174[1971]:897–904).

The year 1972 saw the publication of I. Veith's "Zen Psychotherapy" in *Behavior Today* (January 24, 1972: 3).

In 1973, I. K. Taimni published *Glimpses into the Psychology of Yoga* (Adyar, India: Theosophical Publishing House), but this book focuses on metaphysics rather than psychology and has a theosophical slant. In this year, Padmasiri De Silva also published *Buddhist and Freudian Psychology* (Colombo, Sri Lanka: Lakehouse Investments Ltd.).

In **1974**, John White published his anthology *What Is Meditation?* (New York: Anchor Books/Doubleday), which contains several essays that are relevant to the Yoga/psychology theme.

Of importance to the study of Yoga is Walter Bromberg's *From Shaman to Psychotherapist* (Chicago: Henry Regnerey Co., **1975**).

In **1976,** Peter P. Coukoulis published his *Guru, Psychotherapist, and Self* (Marina del Rey, Calif.: DeVorss & Co.). This is a comparative study of the *guru*-disciple relationship from a Jungian perspective.

The same year saw the publication of Kenneth R. Pelletier and Charles Garfield's *Consciousness: East and West* (New York: Harper Colophon Books), as well as the important book *The Kundalini* by the open-minded psychiatrist Lee Sannella (San Francisco: Deakin), reissued in 1992 in a revised edition as *The Kundalini Experience* (Lower Lake, Calif.: Integral Publishing). J. M. Davidson also published his article "The Physiology of Meditation and Mystical States of Consciousness" in *Perspectives in Biology and Medicine* (19[1976]:345–79).

In **1977,** Daniel Goleman published *The Varieties of Meditative Experience* (New York: Irvington), which included an entire section (part 4) titled "The Psychology of Meditation."

The two volumes of Inder Pal Sachdeva's *Yoga and Depth Psychology* (Delhi: Motilal Banarsidass) came out in **1978**. Also in this year, Princeton University Press published the book *Psychology and the East* by Carl G. Jung. The essays in this selection date from the 1920s and later.

Just one year later, in **1979,** psychologist John Welwood released *The Meeting of the Ways: Explorations in East/West Psychology* (New York: Schocken Books). This anthology contains contributions by Tarthang Tulku, Chögyam Trungpa, Robert Ornstein, Medard Boss, and its editor, John Welwood.

In **1980,** Lati Rinbochay published *Mind in Tibetan Buddhism* (London: Rider) with an introduction by Elizabeth Napper.

The year **1982** marked the publication of Eliot Deutsch's *Personhood, Creativity and Freedom*. Deutsch was a professor of philosophy at the University of Hawaii, and this book contains much material that is relevant to a psychological study of Indian philosophy.

In **1983,** Nathan Katz edited *Buddhist and Western Psychology* (Boulder,

Colo.: Prajñā Press). The anthology has an introductory essay by Chögyam Trungpa, in which he states, "I have been impressed by some of the genuine strengths of western psychology" (7).

In **1988,** Edwina Pio published her *Buddhist Psychology: A Modern Perspective* (New Delhi: Abhinav Publications).

N. Ross Reat's fascinating and informative book *Origins of Indian Psychology* (Berkeley, Calif.: Asian Humanities Press) was published in **1990.** In the same year, Terry Clifford published *Tibetan Buddhist Medicine and Psychiatry* (York Beach, Me.: Samuel Weiser); Hiroshi Motoyama put out his *Toward a Superconsciousness: Meditational Theory and Practice* (Berkeley, Calif.: Asian Humanities Press); and transpersonal psychologist Bonnie Greenwell published her *Energies of Transformation: A Guide to the Kundalini Process* (Saratoga, Calif.: Shakti River Press).

In **1991,** Georg Feuerstein published the first edition of *Holy Madness* (New York: Paragon House), in which he described and analyzed, in balanced fashion, the radical teaching style of "rascal *gurus*." A revised and expanded edition followed in 2006 (Prescott, Ariz.: Hohm Press).

In the same year, M. C. Jackson submitted a doctoral dissertation titled "A Study of the Relationship between Psychotic and Spiritual Experience" to the University of Oxford.

The two volumes of U. A. Asrani's *Yoga Unveiled* (Delhi: Motilal Banarsidass) were published in **1993.** Another important work that year was the anthology edited by Roger Walsh and Frances Vaughan, *Paths beyond Ego* (Los Angeles: J. P. Tarcher/Perigee). This book includes significant essays by Mark Epstein, Stan Grof, Jack Kornfield, and Kenneth Ring, as well as supportive section introductions by the editors.

The year **1995** saw the publication of the important book *The Selfless Mind* by Peter Harvey (London: RoutledgeCurzon).

In **1996,** Carl G. Jung's *The Psychology of Kundalini Yoga* was published by Princeton University Press. This book contains lectures delivered in 1932 at the Eranos symposium in Ascona, Switzerland.

Also in 1996, the British psychiatrist Anthony Storr tackled the *guru* syndrome in *Feet of Clay.* He included in his analysis figures like Jim Jones, David Koresh, Carl Jung, and Sigmund Freud. Given Storr's psychiatric bias, the book, though fascinating, focuses on delusions, illusions, hallucinations, obsessions, mental breakdowns, and so on.

The year **1999** saw the release of Eugene d'Aquili and Andrew B. Newberg's book *The Mystical Mind: Probing the Biology of Religious Experience* (Minneapolis: Fortress Press). This is a groundbreaking study on the neurophysiology of religious experience.

In 2000, Padmasiri De Silva published *An Introduction to Buddhist Psychology* (Houndmills, England: Palgrave Macmillan), and Marvin Levine published *The Positive Psychology of Buddhism and Yoga* (London: Routledge). The latter book considers the important traditions of Buddhism and (Hindu) Yoga together.

In 2001, A. S. Dalal published his edited anthology *A Greater Psychology: An Introduction to the Psychological Thought of Sri Aurobindo* (New York: J. P. Tarcher/Putnam). This 425-page tome has a foreword by Ken Wilber and an introduction by Arabinda Basu.

Also in 2001, we have the publication of Judith Harris's *Jung and Yoga: The Psyche-Body Connection* in the series *Studies in Jungian Psychology by Jungian Analysts* (Toronto: Inner City Books).

Harold Coward's *Yoga and Psychology,* published by SUNY Press in 2002, is an excellent introduction to this wide-ranging topic. Psychotherapists may find his treatment slanted toward Indological concerns.

In 2005, Tashi Tsering published *Buddhist Psychology* (Somerville, Mass.: Wisdom Publications).

In 2006, Mark Unno edited *Buddhism and Psychotherapy* (Boston: Wisdom Publications). Rob Preece wrote *The Psychology of Buddhist Tantra* (Ithaca, N.Y.: Snow Lion Publications).

In 2007, Don Salmon and Jan Maslow published *Yoga Psychology and the Transformation of Consciousness* (New York: Paragon House). The authors approached their subject matter from the viewpoint of clinical psychology on one hand and of Sri Aurobindo on the other. Although this book is full of interesting facts and opinions, it does not evince much acquaintance with Yoga other than the Integral Yoga of Sri Aurobindo.

This was also the year that Mark Epstein published his perspicacious *Psychotherapy without the Self: A Buddhist Perspective.*

In 2010, Tao Jiang's excellent *Yogācāra Buddhism and Modern Psychology* (Delhi: Motilal Banarsidass) was published.

Most of the relevant books do not tend to mention materials on parapsychology, which is integral to traditional Yoga. The present book addresses this and other gaps.

East and West in Antiquity

Since the modern interest in Yoga's psychology is closely associated with the general reception of Yoga in the West, I will briefly review the West's encounter with the thought and culture of India. The critical term is *philosophy,* which for a long time included psychology; even today the two are closely related fields of inquiry, providing philosophy is understood in a broader sense.

The story starts with the ancient Greek "cosmologists" such as Thales of Miletus (flourished early sixth century B.C.E.), Anaximander (a pupil of Thales's), Anaximenes (mid-sixth century B.C.E.), and Diogenes of Apollonia (early fifth century B.C.E.), who were concerned with understanding how the cosmos functions. Aristotle, for one, considered Thales to be the first philosopher. The phrase supposedly was originally used by Plato's pupil Heraclides Ponticus. But some ancient authorities remember Pythagoras of Samos as the first to have declared himself to be a *philos sophias,* or "lover of wisdom." A philosopher was understood to be someone who cultivates *sophía*—a term generally translated as "wisdom," though entailing more than the English equivalent suggests. It also denotes carefulness and mastery.

In the fourth century B.C.E., Alexander the Great's military exploits in India (327–325 B.C.E.) brought the Mediterranean civilization in touch with that Eastern culture. Thanks to the Greek scholar and Cynic Onesicritus, who served as Alexander's historian, we have an interesting account of the "natives" and some of their religious ideas. In his travelogue, he speaks about the gymnosophists ("naked sages"). The Greek knowledge of their thinking was, however, rather flawed, because Onesicritus had to rely on the assistance of three translators speaking various languages.

Alexander's military campaign in the East certainly was the beginning of a cultural encounter between the two hemispheres, laying the foundations for Greek cosmopolitanism, and the emperor probably thought so himself. At any rate, we must drop the Eurocentric preconception that antiquity was marked by cultural isolation. On the contrary, we have good reason

to assume that travelers (usually merchants) undertook lengthy and difficult journeys to cross the permeable national borders, bringing with them
more than material things. Two good examples of this are Scylax and Cte-
sias, Greeks who visited India nearly two centuries prior to Alexander but
offered rather fantastic travel accounts that mythologized the foreign land
and said nothing about its philosophical font.

Plato and Aristotle, as well as the historian Herodotus, freely admitted the
influence of the Orient upon Greek thought. The renowned church father
Eusebius of Caesarea (c. 263–339 C.E.) referred to a tradition credited to
Aristoxenus (flourished c. 300 B.C.E.), according to which an Indian visited
Athens to question Socrates about his philosophy. Apparently, he did not
think much of the philosopher's approach, because it left out the Divine.
This, one imagines, would have appealed to the Christian Eusebius.

For the Greeks, the Indian sages exemplified the highest virtues of the
philosophical life that they themselves sought. The Greeks admired the
sages' apparent immunity to pain and discomfort, as well as their disinterest
in pleasure and what the Greeks saw as their contempt of death.

They had their high opinion confirmed in the figure of the Indian sage
who accompanied Alexander's party on its homeward march. They had
named him Kalanos (or Karanos), apparently because he would call out
"*Kāle!*" when meeting someone. Some have interpreted this as being an
invocation of the goddess Kālī, but this is unlikely, as the vocative of Kālī
is still Kālī. It makes more sense to assume that *kāle* was the locative of
the Sanskrit word *kāla,* meaning "at the right time." The Greeks were both
impressed and shocked when Kalanos calmly ascended a pyre to immolate
himself, presumably "at the right time"—an act witnessed by the entire army.

The most comprehensive account of Alexander's campaign in India, the
Indika, was completed several decades after the emperor's death. It was written by Megasthenes, who spent several years at the court of Candragupta,
emperor of the Maurya dynasty, at his capital Pātaliputra (modern Patna).
Though Megasthenes was clearly sympathetic toward Indian culture, his
account of Indian thought is marred by the fact that, as a typical Greek
resistant to learning a foreign language, he insisted on reporting through
the conceptual filter of his mother tongue. Thus, the Indian deity Indra (or
Krishna) was rendered as Heracles, while the deity Shiva was equated with
Dionysus. Megasthenes's interest was more in the ethical and ascetic domain
of India's spirituality than in its philosophical aspects. He opined that the
Brahmins were already familiar with the theories that the Greek philoso-

phers were formulating. His *Indika* proved a key source of reference about things Indian with many of his contemporaries and subsequent generations of thinkers, not least Christian thinkers like Saint Ambrose (340–397 C.E.) and Hippolytus (flourished third century C.E.).

In the early centuries of the Common Era, the idea of the Oriental origin of philosophy gained momentum and was promoted by men like the neo-Pythagorean miracle worker Apollonius of Tyana (flourished c. 100 C.E.); Philostratus the Athenian (c. 172–250 C.E.), who wrote a hagiography of Apollonius that made him out to be a Christ-like figure; Plotinus's pupil Porphyry (c. 232–304 C.E.); and Porphyry's miracle-working pupil Iamblichus "the divine" (c. 270–330 C.E.), who had Emperor Julian (ruled 361–363 C.E.) as a disciple. Plotinus (205–270 C.E.), the highly influential founder of Neoplatonism, is thought to have joined the military campaign of Gordian III in order to learn about Persian and Indian philosophy firsthand. This ambition was frustrated when the emperor was assassinated.

Plotinus's teacher, Ammonius Sakkas (c. 175–242 C.E.), has often been stamped as a spokesman of Indian wisdom. His epithet, Sakkas, has been interpreted as a derivative of *shākhya,* which would mark him as a follower of the Buddha. While this hypothesis is intriguing and not entirely without merit, the fragments that have survived of Ammonius's teaching are inconclusive. Born a Christian, he converted to Hellenism, more particularly the philosophical syncreticism of Alexandria.

Perhaps more promising is the evidence of early gnosticism, and the ancient world's quest for the Eastern origins of Mediterranean philosophical thought in particular points to the Christian gnostic Bardesanes of Edessa (flourished c. 200 C.E.). Tradition has it that he lived at the court of King Abgar IX of Edessa, which relocated to Armenia after the city's conquest by the Romans in 216 C.E. He is even said to have visited India, though this may be nothing more than a faulty memory about a more believable tale that had him discussing philosophical matters with a delegation from India.

A visit to India is, however, far more likely for the Persian gnostic Mani (216–276 C.E.); elements of Buddhism are definitely superimposed on his teaching of Manichaeism, which even includes the name of the Buddha. Mani hailed from Mesopotamia, which was then ruled by the Persians. He joined his father's Jewish Christian sect going back to the prophet Elchasaios, and when he left this sect at the age of twenty-four, only his father and two disciples stayed with him. But under the early patronage of the royal house of Persia, the spread of Manichaeism was destined to be fast and furious. Its ecumenical/syncretistic orientation also ensured wide appeal. In 241 C.E., Mani journeyed to India and apparently converted the Buddhist king Tūrān Shāh, though it is not clear precisely what wisdom Mani himself gained from this journey. It is known, however, that he considered himself to be the future Buddha Maitreya, one in a line of many.

The first authority to demonstrate a modicum of knowledge about Indian philosophy was the church father Hippolytus in the early third century C.E. His work *Elenchos,* which was written to refute all the heresies of the time, suggests that he was familiar with certain concepts from the Upanishads. The French Indologist and physician Jean Filliozat has daringly speculated that Hippolytus had the *Maitrī-Upanishad* as a reference. As Wilhelm Halbfass, whose *India and Europe* provides the foundation of the present section, summarized,

> The Hellenic confidence in philosophy, theory and the autonomy of human reasoning gave way to a great readiness for accepting sacred tradition and divine inspiration. In a sense, the curiosity of the classical period turned into readiness for self-transformation.
>
> Among the traditions of the Orient, India rises to greater significance after the campaign of Alexander. Yet, this does not lead to a systematic exploration. In spite of extensive contacts, the factual knowledge of Indian religion and philosophy remains very limited. (Halbfass 1988, 20)

Looking at India, we find that the long-lasting European flurry of interest in its culture and philosophical teachings, and even Alexander's so-called conquest, left no noticeable impact. In the West, the triumphant emergence of Christianity out of the cultural-philosophical melee of the early centuries of the Common Era barred any deeper contact with India's wisdom heritage.

The pipeline to Indian culture was, however, not entirely cut off. During the Middle Ages, the originally Buddhist legend of Barlaam and Josaphat was widely circulated as a Christian tale, but without the least knowledge of its actual origins. The same was true of the well-known collection of fables known as Bidpai, which had its origins in the Sanskrit text known as the *Pancatantra* (Five Books) and was translated first into Persian and then into Arabic. There is even a strong resemblance between this collection and *Aesop's Fables,* written in Greek. Emerging in the twelfth century, the legend of Prester John (Presbyter Johannes) was in vogue until the seventeenth century. The legend was somehow mixed up and boosted by the also wildly popular romantic version of Alexander's short-lived military campaign in India. The kingdom of this imaginary Christian hero figure was conveniently located in far-away phantasmagoric India. The spell of the Greek and Roman conceptual overlay on the West's image of India as a land full of strange and miraculous things continued well into the nineteenth century. It is still one of the sources of misunderstanding about India's philosophical world.

The first accurate portrayal of Indian culture and thought came from an unexpected direction: the Muslim scholar and genius Ibn al-Bīrūnī (973–1048 C.E.). He was a leading astronomer, mathematician, and geographer of his day. Uniquely, al-Bīrūnī suspended any ideological limitations imposed by Islam and strove to understand India and the Indians correctly, and to this end, he even learned Sanskrit. Among other things, he translated Patanjali's *Yoga-Sūtra* and an as-yet-unidentified commentary into Arabic.

Despite al-Bīrūnī's fame and the great scholarship shown in his *Kitāb al-Hind* (Book on India), his work was essentially ignored by his own people. Only at the beginning of the fourteenth century C.E. was al-Bīrūnī's contribution appropriately honored by being used in Rashīd ad-Dīn's monumental history of East and West (titled *Jāmi' at-tawārīkh*, or Gatherer of Stories).

Where al-Bīrūnī endeavored to be accurate without immersing himself in risky philosophical-theological comparisons between Islam and Hinduism, the seventeenth-century Muslim ruler Dārā Shukōh—a great grandson of Emperor Akbar—actively sought to make Hinduism look legitimate in the eyes of Islam. In his work *Majma' al-baĥrain* (Mingling of the Oceans), he attempted to harmonize Hinduism and Islam and argued that Hinduism is basically monotheistic and that prophets have also appeared outside the fold of Islam. He paid for this intellectual broad-mindedness with his life. With the approval of the Islamic orthodoxy, his brother Aurangzeb condemned him as a heretic and ordered him executed.

Dārā Shukōh's legacy has survived, however. In 1657, he published an Arabic translation of fifty Upanishads under the title *Sirr-i Akbar* (The Great Secret). It was his Persian rendering of this text that, at the beginning of the nineteenth century C.E., prompted Anquetil Duperron to prepare a Latin translation under the title *Oupnek'hat,* which inaugurated the modern scholarly and popular interest in Indian philosophy. It is surely an ironic twist of fate that a member of the Muslim ruling elite in India, which exercised great intolerance and cruelty over its Hindu subjects, should have served as an effective bridge between East and West.

By comparison, the intellectual efforts of Christian missionaries from the sixteenth century on have been largely ineffectual in creating a road of communication to India, primarily designed as they were to propagate Christianity among the Hindus and not to understand them for their own sake. Missionaries who had a genuine interest in understanding and reporting on the worldview of the "heathens" met with clerical disapproval and even suppression of their work. The German Bartholomaeus Ziegenbalg (1682–1719) was one of these unfortunate mavericks. Apart from his Tamil grammar, which was published in 1716, his work was buried by the church authorities. Whatever scholastic merits might attach to some of the missionaries' works, they are by and large tarnished by self-interest. The Jesuits even went so far as to produce a forgery—the so-called *Ezourvedam*—which they scandalously hoped to employ (but did not) in their conversion of Hindus. One of the victims of this forgery was Voltaire, who when writing his *Encyclopédie* relied exclusively on this text for information about India.

The Christian missionary spirit overshadowed even the cradle of Indology and once marked this scholarly discipline as a vividly biased Eurocentric enterprise. The pioneers of this enterprise included Heinrich Roth (1620–1668), one of the first Europeans to learn Sanskrit; Hermann Gundert (1814–1893), translator of the New Testament into Malayam; Karl Graul (1814–1864), the editor of the four-volume *Bibliotheca Tamulica;* Heinrich August Jaeschke, author of a *Grammar of the Tibetan Language;* Ernst Trumpp (1828–1885), translator of the *Adi-Granth;* Ferdinand Kittel (1832–1903), compiler of the *Kannada-English Dictionary;* Rudolf Hoernle (1841–1918), author of *A Comparative Grammar of the North Indian Vernaculars;* Joseph Dahlmann (1861–1930), well-known for his work on the *Mahābharata* and Buddhism; and Hermann Francke (1870–1930), who translated parts of the Bible into Tibetan.

The earliest literature dealing with Yoga consists of rudimentary "ethnographies" and travel reports (such as those of Jean-Baptiste Tavernier, Jean de Thevenot, Pierre Sonnerat, François Bernier, John Fryer, Pallebot de Saint Lubin, Reginald Heber, and August de Boeck in the seventeenth and eighteenth centuries). Few books in the ethnography genre had the quality of Ibn al-Bīrūnī's *Kitāb al-Hind.* The travelogues generally focused on so-called yogic miracles that confirmed the long-standing image of India as a land of the extraordinary, strange, and sometimes bizarre.

In the twentieth century, books like Richard Schmidt's *Fakire und Fakirtum* (1907) and Baptist Wiedenmann's *Die indischen Fakire* (1920) did much to stimulate the popular imagination in the West, which then prompted physicians to take an interest in yogic—or more precisely, fakiristic—feats. While Schmidt's illustrated work is more substantial and well informed and even includes his translation of the *Gheranda-Samhitā,* he is careful to distinguish the yogi from the fakir. Wiedenmann singles out the sensational and mysterious, and he also produced volumes on the practice of magic, occultism, and breath control.

Sober and more reliable were the scholarly works of William Jones (1746–1794), Charles Wilkins (1749–1836), and H. T. Colebrooke (1765–1837), who endeavored to make India's cultural-philosophical heritage accessible via the original Sanskrit texts. Jones's founding of the Asiatic Society of Bengal in 1784 was an especial milestone in the "objective" study of India. Remarkably, the first philosophical (in the broadest sense) text to be translated into English was Wilkins's *Bhagavad-Gītā* in 1785. By its own testimony, this scripture is both a *yoga-shāstra* ("Yoga text") and a *dharma-shāstra* ("text on ethics").

A triadic grouping of psychological disciplines was suggested by A. S. Dalal, who distinguished between lateral, depth, and height approaches in contemporary psychology. The first ten of the fifteen disciplines mentioned in chapter 3 would fall under lateral psychology; the eleventh through thirteenth disciplines could be viewed as depth psychology; and the last two would make sense as height psychology. Depth psychology, parapsychology, and transpersonal psychology are closest to the basic approach and concerns of Yoga. Integral psychology stands on its own in both purpose and scope. It is a bridging discipline that allows us to integrate the various psychological approaches among themselves but also with other scientific disciplines, all under an overarching philosophical agenda of integration. It is clearly a bold and ambitious project, but it is also one that has become possible only in our time. Its necessity is hardly questionable. Some critics of integral psychology challenge the possibility or desirability of constructing a comprehensive system like Ken Wilber's. Yet, so long as the system has a system-transcending quality built into it, as envisioned by the Swiss cultural philosopher Jean Gebser (1985), it is difficult to find fault with such an approach.

Notes

Preface

1. The first edition was published in 1847. See also Georg Feuerstein's e-book *The Yoga-Sūtra: A Nondualist Interpretation* (2011b).

Introduction

1. My inquiries about Assagioli among psychotherapists yielded no results.
2. James Fadiman, PhD, personal communication with the author, September 2010. It appears, however, that these two intellectual titans never met in person.
3. In the Sanskrit language, the concept of philosophy is captured in the phrase *adhyātma-vidyā*, or "science of the soul."
4. For more on Tantra, see my book *Tantra: The Path of Ecstasy* (Boston: Shambhala Publications, 1998). See also the more academic synopsis *History of the Tantric Religion* (New Delhi: Manohar, 1992) by N. N. Bhattacharyya and the excellent overview *Hindu Tantric and Śākta Literature* (Wiesbaden: Harrassowitz, 1981) by Teun Goudriaan and Sanjukta Gupta.
5. "The Holy Men of India," an introduction written for Heinrich Zimmer's *Der Weg zum Selbst,* 1944, reprinted in C. G. Jung (1978), 185.
6. Swami Yogeshananda, *Six Lighted Windows: Memories of Swamis in the West,* 2nd ed. (Hollywood, Calif.: Vedanta Press, 1997).
7. See Robert Love (2010).
8. Crowley 1939. Crowley's book was reprinted in 1991 and 1994 by New Falcon Publications.
9. For a more balanced point of view from the perspective of a Yoga teacher, see Tom Pilarzyk (2008).
10. Two footnotes from the original text have been omitted.
11. See, for example, Mark Epstein (2007). See also Mark Epstein, "The Deconstruction of the Self: Ego and 'Egolessness' in Buddhist Insight Meditation," *Journal of Transpersonal Psychology* 20 (1988):61–69.

CHAPTER 2 The Reality of Suffering

1. See, for example, Schweitzer 1961.
2. There is no direct mention of the karma and rebirth doctrines in the Vedas. In his book *Origins of Indian Psychology* (1990), N. Ross Reat looked at all the adduced verses but—and I agree—found all of them unconvincing. Yet we cannot assume that only because a secret teaching is not mentioned in these orally transmitted texts, it was not known in the Vedic culture.
3. See *Sangiti-Sutta* 33.1.11(29).
4. This phrase is also found in the *Yoga-Sūtra* (1.37) and refers to a being who is free from passion.
5. See Garfield 1995, 26: "Someone is disclosed by something. / Something is disclosed by someone. / Without something how can someone exist? / Without someone how can something exist?"
6. *Vedanā-Samyutta-Sutta* (21ff.) in the *Samyutta-Nikāya* (36).
7. All this has been insightfully explained by Nagapriya (2004).
8. "While the possibility of cellular memory from the earliest stages of our lives may stretch the boundaries of our imagination, it is by no means the greatest challenge posed by transpersonal experience. It is not unusual for people in nonordinary states of mind to accurately portray material that precedes their conception or to explore the world of their parents, their ancestors, and of the human race" (Grof 1993, 118).
9. Reincarnation, or rebirth, was empirically investigated by Ian Stevenson (1966), mostly on the basis of children who seemed to remember bits and pieces of an earlier life.

CHAPTER 3 Psychocosmological Matters

1. Such as in "What Is Yoga?" www.traditionalyogastudies.com, 1997. This essay is now included in Feuerstein 2003.

CHAPTER 4 Of Paradigms, Models, and Participatory Reality

1. Cited in Mishlove 1975, 95.

CHAPTER 5 Mind and Its Layers, States, Structures, and Functions

1. Vidyāranya also rejects the notion that the Self's luminosity is reflected in the

higher mind (8.35–36). He argues that it is the Self that is reflected and that the *cid-ābhāsa* is an unnecessary intermediate concept.

2. See S. N. Dasgupta (1975, vol. 2, 251n2). He speculates that there are two Vidyāranyas: one who composed the *Panca-Dashī,* and the other who composed the *Jīvanmukti-Viveka.*

CHAPTER 7   The Sensory Apparatus

1. See, for example, *Samyutta-Nikāya* 5.196. It is not surprising that the earliest definition of *yoga* is "the steady holding (*dhāranā*) of the senses" (see *Katha-Upanishad* 3.2.11). The same text (1.3.3–1.3.4) proffers the metaphor of the body being a chariot, the senses taking the place of the horses, and the lower mind being the reins.

2. But see the suggestive work by Subhash Kak (2002).

CHAPTER 9   The Emotive Side of Yoga

1. This text extends at least from 2.1 to 2.27 and is to be demarcated from the *yogānga* text, which runs from 2.28 to 3.8.

CHAPTER 10   The Subtle Body

1. For an early treatment of the subtle body, see C. W. Leadbeater's illustrated volume *The Chakras* (1927), which examines the topic from the eclectic viewpoint of theosophy. More recently, the subtle body has been graphically surveyed by Maureen Lockhart (2010) and Cyndi Dale (2009). The most detailed account of the *cakras* and *prāna* channels can be found in Shyam Sundar Goswami (1999).

2. The will to dedicate oneself to the liberation of all beings is a major aspect of the bodhisattva path of Mahāyāna Buddhism. It corresponds to the Hindu *kundalinī.*

CHAPTER 11   The Serpent Power

1. David Gordon White (1996, 79) translates the term *kubjikā* as "contracted one, ... an alloform of the hathayogic *kundalinī*."

2. One can very tentatively see in the term *kunamnamā* ("she who is bent") an early version of the *kundalinī.*

3. This section uses some of the material found in my review essay "Kundalinī

According to Pandit Gopi Krishna," *Bulletin of the Yoga Research Center* 4 (Winter 1980):31–38.

4. Gopi Krishna (1979) not only awakened interest in the *kundalinī*, he also inadvertently slanted the West's understanding in light of his unorthodox experience.

CHAPTER 12 Knowledge, Wisdom, Gnosis

1. Georg Feuerstein, "Wisdom: The Indian Experience and Perspective," in *The World's Great Wisdom,* ed. Roger Walsh (Albany, N.Y.: SUNY Press, 2013). With prior permission from SUNY Press.

2. An arhat is a spiritual practitioner who is enlightened and in whom the passions are extinguished.

CHAPTER 13 Pure Awareness

1. Based on the testimony of Yoga masters like Irina Tweedie (personal communication) and Neemkaroli Baba, I am inclined to think that drug-induced altered states do not necessarily represent genuine mystical experiences. But see Fadiman 2011 for the opposite view.

2. At the end of this revered text, there is a list of teachers in the Yājnavalkya lineage. The esoteric knowledge was transmitted (*sampratti,* "transmission") from father to son, and Yājnavalkya was preceded by no fewer than ten individuals (not counting the clearly mythological Vāc, Ambhinī, and Āditya), which can be reckoned as comprising a period of roughly 220 years.

3. I am following the dating proposed in Hajime Nakamura (1990).

4. See, for example, *Sarva-Vedānta-Siddhānta-Sāra-Samgraha* (826).

5. *na + eva + samjnā + na + eva + asamjnā.*

CHAPTER 14 The Invariable Witness and the Variable Self

1. See, for example, Wilber 2000a, 91. It is clear from Wilber's discussion that ego is a polysemous concept.

2. The two outstanding sages, who are remembered by name, are Uddālaka Āruni (*Brihadāranyaka-Upanishad* 6.3.1ff.; *Chāndogya-Upanishad* 6.1.2–6.16.3) and his illustrious disciple Yājnavalkya (see *Brihadāranyaka-Upanishad* 2.4.1ff.; 3.1.3ff.; 3.2.1ff.; 3.4.1–3.7.23; 3.9.1ff.; 4.1.1–4.5.15). There also was King Ajātashatru (*Brihadāranyaka-Upanishad* 2.1.1ff.); King Janaka (*Brihadāranyaka-Upanishad* 4.2.8ff.); King Ashvapati Kaikeya (*Brihadāranyaka-Upanishad* 5.11.5–5.24.5);

the female sage Gārgī (*Brihadāranyaka-Upanishad* 3.8.1ff.); and the sage-bard Nārada (*Chāndogya-Upanishad* 7.1.3–7.26.2). Of the many mythological and metaphoric accounts, we have utterances like, "There was nothing in the beginning; this was covered by Death" (*Brihadāranyaka-Upanishad* 1.2.1); "Speech is *brahman;* this is its lord" (*Brihadāranyaka-Upanishad* 1.3.20); "In the beginning was only the Self in the shape of a person (*purusha*); looking around, he saw nothing but the Self" (*Brihadāranyaka-Upanishad* 1.4.1); "*Brahman,* verily was this in the beginning. It knew itself only as 'I am *brahman*'; hence it became all" (*Brihadāranyaka-Upanishad* 1.4.10); "He said: 'The person who is seen in the eye, he is the Self'; this one is immortal; this one is *brahman*" (*Chāndogya-Upanishad* 4.15.1); and so on. Of the exceedingly few metaphysical accounts, we have statements like, "The Self [is best described as] 'not this, not that' (*neti neti*); [it is] incomprehensible, for it cannot be comprehended" (*Brihadāranyaka-Upanishad* 4.4.22); "There the eye does not go, speech does not go, nor does the mind go. We do not know, we do not understand how this [supreme Reality] can be taught" (*Kena-Upanishad* 1.3); and "The knowing [Self] is not born, does not die, nor does it cease to be at any time; ever unborn, it is always eternal, primordial; it is not slain when the body is slain" (*Katha-Upanishad* 1.2.18). There is, however, one passage in the ancient *Brihadāranyaka-Upanishad* (2.3.1) that speaks of the two forms (*rūpa*) of *brahman*—one formed (*mūrta*) and the other unformed (*amūrta*). The former is mortal, while the latter is immortal. Interestingly, the air and atmosphere are deemed unformed, while the *purusha,* who contains the unformed breaths and ether-space, is formed and mortal. Hence the importance of the breath in the actual process of liberation.

3. In the era slightly after the *Katha-Upanishad* (c. 400 B.C.E.), there was the *Bhagavad-Gītā,* followed by the *Shvetāshvatara* (c. 300 B.C.E.), certain didactic portions of the *Mahābharata* (c. 100 B.C.E.–100 C.E.), Bādarāyana's *Brahma-Sūtra* (c. 100–200 C.E.), grammarian and poet Bartrihari's *Vākya-Padīya* (c. 450–500 C.E.), and Gaudapāda's *Māndūkya-Kārikā* (flourished c. 650 C.E., based on Shankara's date).

4. See Deikman 1983, 94: "The most important fact about the observing self is that it is incapable of being objectified."

CHAPTER 15 The Transformative Path

1. For example, Jīva Gosvāmin, *Shat-Sandarbha,* Sanskrit edition, sixteenth century, 541.

2. See, for example, the *Brihadāranyaka-Upanishad* 2.4.5 and 4.5.6.
3. S. N. Dasgupta (1975, 232) assigns this text to the seventh or eighth century, while some scholars place it several centuries later.
4. See the *Aggivacchagotta-Sutta* of the *Majjhīma-Nikāya*. This challenging teaching is perhaps best grasped from the perspective of Mahāyāna Buddhism, which equates all things with *nirvāna*.

CHAPTER 16 The Yoga of Sound and Dance

1. See, for example, Naranjo and Ornstein 1972, Odajnyk 1993, Adiswarananda 2003, Bodhipaksa 2003, Gardner-Nix and Hall 2009, and Kaplan 2010.
2. Swami Radha (1911–1995) reminisced that her teacher, the renowned Swami Sivananda, said to her, "Learn some Indian dance and learn to spiritualize the body. Learn to create and bring back that spiritual point in the consciousness of the cells of the body. Make the body a spiritual tool."

CHAPTER 17 Authority and Discipleship

1. *Individuation* is the authentic process of growth in an individual that leads to psychic wholeness and social integration.
2. In a 1935 letter, quoted in Storr 1996, 85.

CHAPTER 18 The Phenomenon of Meditation

1. See, for example, Motoyama 1978a. See also Thomas J. McFarlane, "EEG Correlates of Stages of Meditative Quiescence: A Pilot Study" (2000); 2004, www.integral science.org/EEGmeditation.html; Tomio Hirai, *Psychophysiology of Zen* (Tokyo: Igaku Hoin Ltd., 1974); Donald B. Lindsley, "Psychological Phenomena and the Electroencephalogram," *EEG and Clinical Neurophysiology* 4 (1952):442–56; Peter Fenwick, "Meditation and the EEG," in *The Psychology of Meditation, ed. Michael A. West (New York: Clarendon Press and Oxford University Press, 1987); and Dean H. Shapiro, Jr., and Roger Walsh, eds., *Meditation: Classic and Contemporary Perspectives* (Piscataway, N.J.: Transaction Publishers and Rutgers, 2008).
2. See *Talks with Sri Ramana Maharshi* (Tiruvannamalai, India: Sri Ramanasramam, 1994).
3. See Jaideva Singh, trans., *Vijnānabhairava or Divine Consciousness: A Treasury of 112 Types of Yoga* (New Delhi: Motilal Banarsidass, 1979).

CHAPTER 19 The Ladder of Ecstasy

1. See James H. Leuba, *The Psychology of Religious Mysticism* (New York: Harcourt, Brace, 1925).

CHAPTER 20 Paranormal Abilities, Psychotropic Drugs, and Yogic Discipline

1. These are known as the *ashta-siddhis* ("eight powers"), explained in the next section.
2. Alice Bailey (1880–1949) was formally affiliated with the Theosophical Society until 1919, when she founded her own organization at a time when theosophy had come under sustained public attack.
3. For an early date of the *Rig-Veda,* see Feuerstein et al. 1995.
4. With 23.3 million Americans aged twelve and over having used LSD in 2006, Fadiman's advice on safe use is to be welcomed. Of course, it is debatable whether publications of this kind do not entice the public to experiment with drugs.
5. The reason for this injunction was probably that the display of paranormal abilities inflated the ego that was to be transcended on the path to *nirvāna*.

CHAPTER 22 Postmortem Freedom and Living Liberation

1. *Talks with Sri Ramana Maharshi: Three Volumes in One*, 9th ed. (Tiruvannamalai, India: Sri Ramanasramam, 1994).
2. Each of the last four verses explaining the word *avadhūta* is replete with word play. Thus, in verse 8.6, the letter *a* is echoed in *āsha* ("hope"), *ādi* ("beginning"), and *ānanda* ("bliss").
3. This date is based on Shankara having lived in the sixth to seventh century and not, as customarily thought, in the late eighth to early ninth century C.E. (see Nakamura 1990).
4. The last sentence seems to mark the end of the original Upanishad or a section of it. The verses that follow would therefore be interpolated or appended.
5. The best discussion about *tulkus* can be found in Ray 2001, 374–425.
6. For instance, in *sūtra* 3.55 in *Yoga-Sutra* of Patanjali's work.

EPILOGUE Toward a Western Yoga

1. I have borrowed the term *concretion* from Jean Gebser, who understood this

as the main feature of the arational-integral consciousness, which he thought was emerging in his era. It makes the luminous origin virtually concrete, as the "uncreate light." In somatic concretion, the feelings held in and by the body are rendered concrete.

APPENDIX 1 Hindu, Buddhist, and Jaina Yoga

1. Most of these translations are as yet unpublished.

References

Abhinavagupta. 1989. *A Trident of Wisdom: Translation of Parātrīśikā-Vivarana.* Translated by Jaideva Singh. Albany, N.Y.: SUNY Press.

Adiswarananda, Swami. 2003. *Meditation and Its Practices: A Definitive Guide to Techniques and Traditions of Meditation in Yoga and Vedanta.* Woodstock, Vt.: Skylight Publications.

Aiyar, K. Nārayānaswami, trans. 1980. *Thirty Minor Upanishads.* El Reno, Okla.: Santarasa Publications.

Akhilananda, Swami. 1946. *Hindu Psychology: Its Meaning for the West.* Foreword by Edgar Sheffield Brightman. Introduction by Gordon W. Allport. Boston: Branden Press.

Alvarado, C. S. 2000. "Out-of-Body Experiences." In *Varieties of Anomalous Experience: Examining the Scientific Evidence,* ed. E. Cardena, S. J. Lynn, and S. Krippner, 183–218. Washington, D.C.: American Psychological Association.

Arbman, Ernst. 1963. *Ecstasy or Religious Trance: In the Experience of Ecstatic and from the Psychological Point of View.* 3 vols. Uppsala, Sweden: Scandinavian University Books.

Aronson, Harvey. 2004. *Buddhist Practice on Western Ground: Reconciling Eastern Ideals and Western Psychotherapy.* Boston: Shambhala Publications.

Asrani, U. A. 1993. *Yoga Unveiled.* 2 vols. New Delhi: Motilal Banarsidass.

Assagioli, Roberto. 1973. *The Act of Will.* New York: Viking.

———. (1965) 1993. *Psychosynthesis: A Manual of Principles and Techniques.* New York: Arkana/Penguin.

Aurobindo, Sri. 1955. *The Synthesis of Yoga.* Pondicherry, India: Sri Aurobindo Ashram.

———. 1964. *On the Veda.* Pondicherry, India: Sri Aurobindo Ashram.

———. 1976. *The Life Divine.* Pondicherry, India: Sri Aurobindo Ashram.

———. (1915) 1991. *Rebirth and Karma.* Wilmot, Wis.: Lotus Light Publications.

Avalon, Arthur [also John Woodroffe]. (1919) 1974. *The Serpent Power: The Secrets of Tantric and Shaktic Yoga.* New York: Dover Publications.

Baier, Karl. 2009. *Meditation und Moderne.* 2 vols. Würzburg, Germany: Königshausen and Neumann.

Bailey, Alice. 1997. *The Light of the Soul: The Yoga-Sutras of Patanjali.* New York: Lucis Publishing.

Bailey, Lee Worth, and Jenny L. Yates. 1996. *The Near-Death Experience: A Reader.* New York: Routledge.

Ballantyne, James R. 1885. *The Sānkhya Aphorisms of Kapila with Illustrative Extracts from the Commentaries.* 3rd ed. London: Trübner & Co.

Barnes, J. A. 1994. *A Pack of Lies: Towards a Sociology of Lying.* Cambridge: Cambridge University Press.

Batchelor, Stephen. 1994. *The Awakening of the West: The Encounter of Buddhism and Western Culture.* Berkeley, Calif.: Parallax Press.

Beauregard, Mario, and Denyse O'Leary. 2007. *The Spiritual Brain: A Neuroscientist's Case for the Existence of the Soul.* New York: HarperCollins.

Benor, Daniel J. 2002. *Spiritual Healing: Scientific Validation of a Healing Revolution—Professional Supplement.* Vol. 1. Foreword by Larry Dossey. Southfield, Mich.: Vision Publications.

Bentov, Itzhak. 1988. *Stalking the Wild Pendulum.* Rochester, Vt.: Destiny Books.

Bharati, Veda, Swami. 1986. *Yoga-Sūtras of Patañjali with the Exposition of Vyāsa: A Translation and Commentary.* Vol. 1, *Samādhi-pāda.* Honesdale, Pa.: Himalayan International Institute of Yoga Science and Philosophy of the USA.

"Bhavanga." *Wikipedia.* Wikimedia Foundation, April 27, 2013. http://en.wikipedia.org/wiki/Bhavanga.

"Bhavanga-citta." *The Dhamma Encyclopedia RSS.* www.dhammawiki.com/index.php?title=Bhavanga-citta.

Bodhipaksa. 2003. *Wildmind: A Step-by-Step Guide to Meditation.* Birmingham, England: Windhorse Publications.

Broughton, Richard S. 1991. *Parapsychology: The Controversial Science.* New York: Ballantine Books.

Buddhaghosa. 1976. *The Path of Purification: A Classic Textbook of Buddhist Psychology.* Translated by Ñāṇamoli Bhikkhu. Berkeley, Calif.: Shambhala Publications.

Callahan, David. 2004. *The Cheating Culture: Why More Americans Are Doing Wrong to Get Ahead.* Orlando, Fla.: Harvest Books/Harcourt.

Campbell, Peter A., and Edwin M. McMahon. 1985. *Bio-Spirituality: Focusing as a Way to Grow.* Chicago: Loyola University Press.

Cardeña, Etzel, Steven J. Lynn, and Stanley Krippner. 2000. *Varieties of Anomalous Experience: Examining the Scientific Evidence.* Washington, D.C.: American Psychological Association.

Carrington, Patricia. 1978. *Freedom in Meditation*. New York: Anchor Books.

Carus, Paul. 1894. *The Gospel of the Buddha: According to Old Records*. Chicago: Open Court Publishing.

———. 1897. *Buddhism and Its Christian Critics*. Chicago: Open Court Publishing.

Cary, Henry Francis, ed. 2006. *The Poetical Works of Alexander Pope*. London: Routledge.

Chalmers, David J., ed. 2002. "Consciousness and Its Place in Nature." In *Philosophy of Mind: Classical and Contemporary Readings*, edited by D. J. Chalmers. Oxford: Oxford University Press.

Chapple, Christopher. 1986. *Karma and Creativity*. Albany, N.Y.: SUNY Press.

———. 1990. "The Unseen Seer and the Field: Consciousness in Samkhya and Yoga."In *The Problem of Pure Consciousness: Mysticism and Philosophy*, edited by Robert K. Forman, 53–70. New York: Oxford University Press.

———. 1996. "Living Liberation in Sāmkhya and Yoga." In *Living Liberation in Hindu Thought*, edited by Andrew O. Fort and Patricia Y. Mumme. Albany, N.Y.: SUNY Press.

Chaudhuri, Haridas. 1975. *Integral Yoga: The Concept of Harmonious and Creative Living*. Foreword by Pitirim A. Sorokin. London: George Allen & Unwin.

Chaudhuri, Haridas, and Frederic Spiegelberg, eds. 1960. *The Integral Philosophy of Sri Aurobindo: A Commemorative Symposium*. London: George Allen & Unwin.

Clark, John H. 1983. *A Map of Mental States*. London: Routledge & Kegan Paul.

Cohen, J. M., and J. F. Phipps. 1979. *The Common Experience*. New York: St. Martin's Press.

Conze, Edward. 1967. *Thirty Years of Buddhist Studies*. Oxford, England: Bruno Cassirer.

———. 1975. *The Large Sutra on Perfect Wisdom with the Divisions of the Abhisamayālankāra*. Berkeley: University of California Press.

Crowley, Aleister. 1939. *Eight Lectures on Yoga*. Dallas: Sangreal Foundation.

Dale, Cyndi. 2009. *The Subtle Body: An Encyclopedia of Your Energetic Anatomy*. Boulder, Colo.: Sounds True.

Das, N. N., and H. Gastant. 1955. "Variations de l'Activité Electrique du Cerveau, du Coeur et des Muscles Squelettiques au Cours de le Méditation et de l'Extase Yogique," *EEG*, Suppl. 6:211–19.

Dasgupta, S. N. (1922) 1975. *A History of Indian Philosophy*. Indian ed. 5 vols. Cambridge: Cambridge University Press.

———. (1941) 1990. *Philosophical Essays*. New Delhi: Motilal Banarsidass.

Dasgupta, Shashi Bhushan. 1974. *An Introduction to Tantric Buddhism*. Berkeley, Calif.: Shambhala Publications.

Deikman, Arthur J. 1983. *The Observing Self: Mysticism and Psychotherapy*. Boston: Beacon Press.

De Michelis, Elizabeth. 2004. *A History of Modern Yoga: Patañjali and Western Esotericism*. London: Continuum.

Doidge, Norman. 2007. *The Brain That Changes Itself: Stories of Personal Triumph from the Frontiers of Brain Science*. New York: Viking Penguin.

Doore, Gary. 1990. *What Survives? Contemporary Explorations of Life after Death*. Los Angeles: J. P. Tarcher.

Drengson, Alan. 1995. *The Practice of Technology: Exploring Technology, Ecophilosophy, and Spiritual Disciplines for Vital Links*. Albany, N.Y.: SUNY Press.

Dumoulin, Heinrich, and John C. Maraldo, eds. 1976. *The Cultural, Political, and Religious Significance of Buddhism in the Modern West*. New York: Collier Books.

Eccles, John, and Daniel N. Robinson. 1985. *The Wonder of Being Human: Our Brain and Our Mind*. Boston: Shambhala Publications and New Science Library.

Eliade, Mircea. (1951) 1972. *Shamanism: Archaic Techniques of Ecstasy*. Princeton, N.J.: Princeton University Press.

———. (1954) 1973. *Yoga: Freedom and Immortality*. Princeton, N.J.: Princeton University Press.

Engler, Jack. 2006. "Promises and Perils of the Spiritual Path." In *Buddhism and Psychotherapy Across Cultures: Essays on Theories and Practices*, edited by Mark Unno, 17–30. Boston: Wisdom Publications.

Epstein, Mark. 2007. *Psychotherapy without the Self: A Buddhist Perspective*. New Haven, Conn.: Yale University Press.

Erikson, Erik. 1950. *Childhood and Society*. New York: W. W. Norton.

Evans, John. 1986. *Mind, Body and Electromagnetism*. Longmead, England: Element Books.

Fadiman, James. 2011. *The Psychedelic Explorer's Guide: Safe, Therapeutic, and Sacred Journeys*. Rochester, Vt.: Park Street Press.

Fechner, Gustav Theodor. 1848. *Nanna: Über das Seelenleben der Pflanzen*. Leipzig: Leopold Voss.

Feuerstein, Georg. (1979) 1989. *The Yoga-Sūtra of Patañjali: A New Translation and Commentary*. Rochester, Vt.: Inner Traditions International. Also published as an e-book 2011.

———. 1992. *Wholeness or Transcendence? Ancient Lessons for the Emerging Global Civilization.* Burdett, N.Y.: Published for the Paul Brunton Philosophic Foundation by Larsons Publications.

———. (1980) 1996. *The Philosophy of Classical Yoga.* Rochester, Vt.: Inner Traditions International.

———. 1998. *The Yoga Tradition: Its History, Literature, Philosophy, and Practice.* Prescott, Ariz.: Hohm.

———. 2003. *The Deeper Dimension: Theory and Practice.* Boston: Shambhala Publications.

———. (1990) 2006. *Holy Madness: Spirituality, Crazy-Wise Teachers, and Enlightenment.* Revised and expanded ed. Prescott, Ariz.: Hohm Press.

———. 2007. *Yoga Morality: Ancient Teachings at a Time of Global Crisis.* Prescott, Ariz.: Hohm.

———. 2011a. *The Bhagavad-Gītā: A New Translation.* With Brenda Feuerstein. Boston: Shambhala Publications.

———. 2011b. *The Yoga-Sūtra: A Nondualist Interpretation.* E-book. www.traditionalyogastudies.com.

Feuerstein, Georg, Subhash Kak, and David Frawley. 1995. *In Search of the Cradle of Civilization.* Wheaton, Ill.: Quest Books.

Fields, Rick. 1986. *How the Swans Came to the Lake: A Narrative History of Buddhism in America.* Boston: Shambhala Publications.

Ford, Charles V. 1999. *Lies! Lies!! Lies!!!: The Psychology of Deceit.* Washington, D.C.: American Psychiatric Press.

Forman, Robert K. 1990. *The Problem of Pure Consciousnes: Mysticism and Philosophy.* New York: Oxford University Press.

Fort, Andrew O. 1998. *Jīvanmukti in Transformation: Embodied Liberation in Advaita and Neo-Vedanta.* Albany, N.Y.: SUNY Press.

Fort, Andrew O., and Patricia Y. Mumme. 1996. *Living Liberation in Hindu Thought.* Albany, N.Y.: SUNY Press.

Frankl, Victor. 1959. *Man's Search for Meaning: An Introduction to Logotherapy.* Boston: Beacon Press.

———. 1965. *The Doctor and the Soul: From Psychotherapy to Logotherapy.* 2nd ed. New York: Alfred A. Knopf.

———. 1967. *Psychotherapy and Existentialism: Selected Papers on Logotherapy.* New York: Washington Square Press.

———. 1969. *The Will to Meaning: Foundations and Applications of Logotherapy.* New York and Cleveland: The World Publishing Company.

———. (1948) 1985. *The Unconscious God.* New York: Washington Square Press.

——. 1997. *Man's Search for Ultimate Meaning.* Cambridge, Mass.: Perseus Books.

Fredrickson, Barbara L. 2009. *Positivity: Top-Notch Research Reveals the 3-to-1 Ratio That Will Change Your Life.* New York: Three Rivers Press.

Freud, Sigmund. (1900) 1961. *Die Traumdeutung* [*The Interpretation of Dreams*]. Frankfurt, Germany: G. B. Fischer.

——. 1976. *Introductory Lectures on Psychoanalysis, Standard Edition.* Vol. 16. New York: W. W. Norton.

Freud, Sigmund, and James Strachey. 1961. *Civilization and Its Discontents.* New York: W. W. Norton.

Ganguly, Swati. 1992. *Treatise in Thirty Verses on Mere-Consciousness.* New Delhi, India: Banarsidass.

Gardner-Nix, Jackie, and Lucie Costin-Hall. 2009. *The Mindfulness Solution to Pain: Step-by-Step Techniques for Chronic Pain Management.* Oakland, Calif.: New Harbinger.

Garfield, Jay L., trans. 1995. *The Fundamental Wisdom of the Middle Way: Nāgārjuna's Mūlāmadhyamnakakārikā.* New York and Oxford: Oxford University Press.

Gebser, Jean. 1985. *The Ever-Present Origin.* Athens, Ohio: Ohio University Press.

Gendlin, Eugene T. 1981. *Focusing.* 2nd ed. New York: Bantam Books.

Gerzon, Robert. 1997. *Finding Serenity in the Age of Anxiety.* New York: Macmillan.

Gharote, M. L., Parimal Devnath, and Vijaykant Jna. 2007. *Hathatat[t]vakaumudī.* Lonavla, India: Lonavla Yoga Institute.

Gharote, M. L., and Parimal Devnath, eds. and trans. 2001. *Hathapradīpikā.* Lonavla, India: Lonavla Yoga Institute.

Glossary of Buddhist Terms. http://dharma.ncf.ca/faqs/glossary.html.

Goddard, Dwight. 1981. *The Buddha's Golden Path.* 2nd ed. Santa Fe, N.M.: Sun Books.

Gonda, Jan. 1963. *The Vision of the Vedic Poets.* The Hague: Mouton.

Goswami, Shyam Sundar. (1980) 1999. *Layayoga: The Definitive Guide to the Chakras and Kundalini.* Rochester, Vt.: Inner Traditions International.

Green, Celia. 1973. *Out-of-the-Body Experiences.* New York: Ballantine.

Grof, Stanislav. 1993. *The Holotropic Mind.* With Hal Zina Bennett. New York: HarperCollins.

Guenther, Herbert V. 1976. *Philosophy and Psychology in the Abhidharma.* Berkeley, Calif.: Shambhala Publications.

Halbfass, Wilhelm. 1988. *India and Europe: An Essay in Understanding.* Albany, N.Y.: SUNY Press.

Hanson, Rick. 2009. *Buddha's Brain: A Practical Neuroscience of Happiness, Love, and Wisdom.* With Richard Mendius. Oakland, Calif.: New Harbinger.

Hartsuiker, Dolf. 1993. *Sādhus: India's Mystic Holy Men.* Rochester, Vt.: Inner Traditions International.

Harvey, Peter. 2004. *The Selfless Mind: Personality, Consciousness and Nirvana in Early Buddhism.* London: RoutledgeCurzon.

Hillebrand, Alfred. (1891) 1990. *Vedic Mythology.* Translated by Sreeramula Rajeswar Sarma. New Delhi, India: Motilal Banarnsidass. 2 vols.

Hooper, Judith, and Dick Teresi. 1986. *The 3-Pound Universe.* New York: Macmillan.

Huxley, Aldous. 1962. *Island: A Novel.* New York: Harper.

———. 1979. *The Doors of Perception* and *Heaven and Hell.* London: Granada Publishing and Triad Panther Books.

Investigations: A Research Bulletin of the Institute of Noetic Sciences 7 (1988):22–26.

Jacobs, Hans. 1961. *Western Psychotherapy and Hindu Sâdhanâ: A Contribution to Comparative Studies in Psychology and Metaphysics.* London: George Allen & Unwin.

James, William. 1890. *Principles of Psychology.* New York: Henry Holt.

———. 1902. *Varieties of Religious Experience.* New York: Longman, Greens & Co.

———. 1909. "The Final Impressions of a Psychical Researcher." *The American Magazine* (October).

———. (1902) 1961. *Varieties of Religious Experience: A Study in Human Nature.* New York: Collier MacMillan.

Jamgön Kongtrül the Great. 1995. *The Light of Wisdom.* Root text *Lamrim Yeshe Nyingpo* by Padmasambhava. Boston: Shambhala Publications.

Janet, Pierre. 1926. *De l'angoisse à l'extase: Études sur les croyances et les sentiments.* Paris: F. Alcan.

Jayatilleke, Kulatissa Nanda, and Ninian Smart. 1975. *The Message of the Buddha.* New York: Free Press.

Jiang, Tao, ed. 2010. *Yogācāra Buddhism and Modern Psychology.* New Delhi: Motilal Banarsidass.

Jigme Lingpa, Patrul Rinpoche, and Getse Mahāpandita. 2006. *Deity Mantra and Wisdom: Development Stage Meditation in Tibetan Buddhist Tantra.* Translated by Dharmachakra Translation Committee. Ithaca, N.Y.: Snow Lion Publications.

Jung, Carl Gustav. 1933. *Modern Man in Search of a Soul.* New York: Harcourt, Brace & World.

———. 1939. *The Integration of the Personality.* New York: Farrar & Rinehart.

———. (1929) 1978. *Psychology and the East.* Princeton, N.J.: Princeton University Press.

———. 1958a. *Psychology and Religion: West and East.* New York: Pantheon.

———. 1958b. *The Relations of Psychotherapy to Soul Care/Seelsorge.* Zurich: Rascher Verlag.

Kabat-Zinn, Jon. 1990. *Full Catastrophe Living: Using the Wisdom of Your Body and Mind to Face Stress, Pain, and Illness.* Preface by Thich Nhat Hanh. Foreword by Joan Borysenko. New York: Delta Books.

Kafatos, Minas C., and Thalia Kafatou. 1991. *Looking In, Seeing Out: Consciousness and Cosmos.* Wheaton, Ill.: Quest and Theosophical Publishing House.

Kak, Subhash. 2002. *The Gods Within: Mind, Consciousness and the Vedic Tradition.* New Delhi: Munshiram Manoharlal.

Kaplan, Jonathan S. 2010. *Urban Mindfulness: Cultivating Peace, Presence and Purpose in the Middle of It All.* Oakland, Calif.: New Harbinger Publications.

Katz, Steven T. 1978. *Mysticism and Philosophical Analysis.* London: Sheldon Press.

———. 1983. *Buddhist and Western Psychology.* Boulder, Colo.: Prajñā.

Kohlberg, Lawrence. 1984. *The Psychology of Moral Development.* Vol. 2 of *Essays on Moral Development.* San Francisco: Harper & Row.

Kramer, Joel, and Diana Altstad. 1993. *The Guru Papers: Masks of Authoritarian Power.* Berkeley, Calif.: North Atlantic Books/Frog Ltd.

Krishna, Gopi. 1971. *The Biological Basis of Religion and Genius.* New York: Harper & Row.

———. 1972. *Kundalini: The Secret of Yoga.* New York: Harper & Row.

———. 1973. *The Biological Basis of Religion and Genius.* London: Turnstone.

———. 1978. *The Dawn of a New Science.* New Delhi: Kundalini Research and Publication Trust.

———. 1979. *The Real Nature of Mystical Experience.* New Delhi: Kundalini Research and Publication Trust.

Krishna, Gopi, and James Hillman. 1971. *Kundalini: The Evolutionary Energy in Man.* Berkeley, Calif.: Shambhala Publications.

Kuhn, Thomas S. 1962. *The Structure of Scientific Revolutions.* Chicago: University of Chicago.

LaBerge, Stephen. 1986. *Lucid Dreaming: The Power of Being Awake and Aware in Your Dreams.* New York: Ballantine Books.

Lakatos, Imre, and Alan Musgrave. 1970. *Criticism and the Growth of Knowledge.* Cambridge: Cambridge University Press.

Lamotte, Étienne. 1944 and 1949. *Le traité de la grande vertu de sagesse de Nāgārjuna.* 2 vols. Louvain, Belgium: Institut Orientalist.

Larson, Gerald. 1969. *Classical Sāmkhya*. New Delhi: Motilal Banarsidass.

Larson, Gerald, and Ram Shankar Bhattacharya. 1987. *Samkhya: A Dualist Tradition in Indian Philosophy*. Princton, N.J.: Princeton University Press.

Laski, Marghanita. 1961. *Ecstasy: A Study of Some Secular and Religious Experiences*. London: Cresset Press.

Laszlo, Ervin. 2007. *Science and the Akashic Field: An Integral Theory of Everything*. 2nd revised ed. Rochester, Vt.: Inner Traditions.

Laszlo, Ervin, ed. 2009. *The Akashic Experience: Science and the Cosmic Memory Field*. Rochester, Vt.: Inner Traditions International.

Laubry, Charles, and Therese Brosse. 1936. "Data Gathered in India on a Yogi with Simultaneous Registration of the Pulse, Respiration and Electrocardiogram," *Presse Medicale* 44:1601–4.

Leadbeater, C. W. 1927. *The Chakras: A Monograph*. Adyar, India: Theosophical Publishing House.

Leary, Timothy. 1968. *The Politics of Ecstasy*. New York: Putnam.

Lepp, Ignace. 1969. *Death and Its Mysteries*. London: Burns & Oates.

Levine, Marvin. 2000. *The Positive Psychology of Buddhism and Yoga: Paths to Mature Happiness*. London: Routledge.

Lewis, Penny. 1984. *Theoretical Approaches in Dance Movement Therapy*. 2 vols. Dubuque, Iowa: Kendall Hunt.

Lilly, John C. 1972. *The Center of the Cyclone*. New York: Julian Press.

Lindquist, Sigurd. 1935. *Siddhi und Abhiññā* [Skt.: *abhijnā*]: *Eine Studie über die klassischen Wunder des Yoga* [Siddhi and Abhiññā: A Study of the Classical Miracles of Yoga]. Uppsala, Sweden: Uppsala Universitets Arsskrift.

Lockhart, Maureen. 2010. *The Subtle Energy Body: The Complete Guide*. Rochester, Vt.: Inner Traditions International.

Love, Robert. 2010. *The Great Oom: The Improbable Birth of Yoga in America*. New York: Viking.

Maharishi Mahesh Yogi. 1969. *On the Bhagavad Gītā*. Baltimore, Md.: Penguin Books.

Mandell, Arnold J. 1980. "Toward a Psychobiology of Transcendence: God in the Brain." In *The Psychobiology of Consciousness,* edited by Richard J. Davidson and Julian M. Davidson. New York: Plenum Publishing Corp.

Marchand, Peter, ed. 2006. *The Yoga of the Nine Emotions: The Tantric Practice of Rasa Sadhana*. Rochester, Vt.: Destiny Books.

Maslow, Abraham H. 1971. *The Farther Reaches of Human Nature*. New York: Viking.

May, Rollo. 1953. *Man's Search for Himself*. New York: Dell.

Meekums, B. 2002. *Dance Movement Therapy: A Creative Psychotherapeutic Approach.* London: Sage.

Mehta, Rohit. 1975. *Yoga, the Art of Integration: Commentaries on the Yogasutras of Patanjali.* Adyar, India: Theosophical Publishing House.

Miller, Jeanine. 1974. *The Vedas: Harmony, Meditation, and Fulfilment.* London: Rider.

———. 1980. "Agni." *Bulletin of the Yoga Research Centre* 4:17–30.

———. 1985. *The Vision of Cosmic Order in the Vedas.* Foreword by Raimundo Panikkar. London: Routledge & Kegan Paul.

Mishlove, Jeffrey. 1975. *The Roots of Consciousness.* New York: Random House.

Mitchell, Edgar D., and John Warren White. 1974. *Psychic Exploration: A Challenge for Science.* New York: Putnam.

Motoyama, Hiroshi. 1978a. "An Electrophysiological Study of Prana (Ki)." *IARP Journal* 4(1):1–27.

———. 1978b. *Science and the Evolution of Consciousness: Chakras, Ki, and Psi.* With Rande Brown. Brookline, Mass.: Autumn Press.

———. 1988. *Theories of the Chakras: Bridge to Higher Consciousness.* Foreword by Swami Satyananda. Wheaton, Ill.: Quest Books.

———. 1990. *Toward a Superconsciousness: Meditational Theory and Practice.* Translated by Shigenori Nagatomo and Clifford R. Ames. Berkeley, Calif.: Asian Humanities Press.

Mukerji, Swami A. P. 1922. *The Doctrine and Practice of Yoga: Including the Practices and Exercises of Concentration, Both Objective and Subjective, and Active and Passive Mentation, an Elucidation of Maya, Guru Worship, and the Worship of the Terrible, Also the Mystery of Will-Force.* Chicago: Yogi Publication Society.

Mullin, Glenn H., trans. and ed. 2005. *The Six Yoga of Naropa.* Ithaca, N.Y.: Snow Lion Publications.

Murphy, Gardner. 1958. *Human Potentialities.* New York: Basic Books.

Nagapriya. 2004. *Exploring Karma and Rebirth.* Birmingham, England: Windhorse Publications.

Nakamura, Hajime. (1983) 1990. *A History of Early Vedānta Philosophy,* part 1. New Delhi: Motilal Banarsidass.

Ñāṇamoli and Bodhi. 1995. *The Middle Length Discourses of the Buddha: A New Translation of the Majjhima Nikaya.* Boston: Wisdom Publications in association with the Barre Center for Buddhist Studies.

Naranjo, Claudio, and Robert E. Ornstein. 1972. *On the Psychology of Meditation.* London: George Allen & Unwin.

Norbu, Namkhai Chogyal. 1992. *Dream Yoga and the Practice of Natural Light.* Introduced and edited by Michael Katz. Ithaca, N.Y.: Snow Lion Publications.

Nordau, Max. 1883. *Die Conventionellen Lügen der Kulturmenscheit* [The Conventional Lies of Civilized Humanity]. Leipzig, Germany: B. Elischer.

Nyanaponika. 1962. *The Heart of Buddhist Meditation: Satipaṭṭhāna: A Handbook of Mental Training Based on the Buddha's Way of Mindfulness: With an Anthology of Relevant Texts Translated from the Pali and Sanskrit.* London: Rider.

Odajnyk, V. Walter. 1993. *Gathering the Light: A Psychology of Meditation.* Boston: Shambhala Publications.

O'Flaherty, Wendy Doniger. 1981. *Śiva: The Erotic Ascetic.* Oxford: Oxford Paperbacks/Oxford University Press.

Pabongka Rinpoche. 1991. *Liberation in the Palm of Your Hand.* Boston: Wisdom Publications.

Pathak, P. V. 1932. *The Heyapaksha of Yoga.* New Delhi: Asian Publishing Services.

Payne, Helen, ed. 2006. *Dance Movement Therapy: Theory, Research and Practice.* 2nd ed. East Sussex, England, and New York: Routledge.

Peers, E. Allison, ed. and trans. 1974. *The Interior Castle ("The Mansions"),* by Saint Teresa of Avila. London: Sheed & Ward.

Pilarzyk, Tom. 2008. *Yoga Beyond Fitness.* Wheaton, Ill.: Quest Books.

Poortman, J. J. 1978. *Vehicles of Consciousness: The Concept of Hylic Pluralism (Ochêma).* 4 vols. Utrecht: Theosophical Society in the Netherlands.

Popper, Karl, and John C. Eccles. 1977. *The Self and Its Brain.* New York: Springer Verlag.

Poussin, Charles de la Vallée. 1931. "Le Bouddha et les Abhijñās." *Le Muséon.*

Preece, Rob. 2006. *The Psychology of Buddhist Tantra.* Foreword by Stephen Bachelor. Ithaca, N.Y.: Snow Lion Publications.

Price, G. R. 1955. "Science and the Supernatural." *Science* 122 (3165): 359–67.

Pruett, Gordon E. 1987. *The Meaning and End of Suffering for Freud and the Buddhist Tradition.* Lanham, Md.: American University Press.

Quarnström, Olle. 2002. *The Yogaśāstra of Hemacandra: A Twelfth Century Handbook on Śvetāmbara Jainism.* Cambridge, Mass.: Harvard University Press.

Radhakrishnan, Sarvepalli. 1960. *The Brahma Sūtra.* London: George Allen & Unwin.

———. 2007. *Eastern Religions and Western Thought.* New York: Oxford University Press.

Ramana, Maharshi, and Saraswati Ramananda. 1955. *Talks with Sri Ramana Maharshi (in Three Volumes).* Tiruvannamalai, India: T. N. Venkataraman.

Rampuri. 2010. *Autobiography of a Sadhu: A Journey into Mystic India.* 2nd ed. Rochester, Vt.: Destiny Books.

Rao, K. R. 2010. *Yoga and Parapsychology: Empirical Research and Theoretical Studies.* New Delhi: Motilal Banarsidass.

Ray, Reginald. 2001. *Secret of the Vajra World.* Boston: Shambhala Publications.

Reat, N. Ross. 1990. *Origins of Indian Psychology.* Berkeley, Calif.: Asian Humanities Press.

Rele, V. G. 1927. *The Mysterious Kundalini: The Physical Basis of the "Kundalini (hatha) Yoga" According to Our Present Knowledge of Western Anatomy and Physiology.* Bombay: D. B. Taraporevala.

Rensch, Bernhard. 1968. *Biophilosophie auf erkenntnistheoretischer Grundlage* [Biophilosophy on Epistemological Basis]. Stuttgart, Germany: G. Fischer Verlag.

Rhine, J. B. 1934. *Extra-Sensory Perception.* Boston: Boston Society for Psychic Research.

Rhine, J. B., and J. G. Pratt. (1957) 1967. *Parapsychology: Frontier Science of the Mind: A Survey of the Field, the Methods, and the Facts of ESP and PK Research.* Springfield, Ill.: Charles C. Thomas Publishers.

Rhys Davids, Caroline. (1914) 1936. *The Birth of Indian Psychology and Its Development in Buddhism.* London: Luzac & Co.

Ring, Kenneth. 1980. *Life at Death.* New York: William Morrow and Company.

Ring, Kenneth, and Sharon Cooper. 1999. *Mindsight: Near-Death and Out-of-Body Experiences in the Blind.* Palo Alto, Calif.: William James Center for Consciousness Studies.

Rösel, Richard. 1928. *Die psychologischen Grundlagen des Yoga* [The Psychological Foundations of Yoga]. Stuttgart, Germany: Kohlhammer Verlag.

Rowlands, Mark, ed. 1982. *Abhidhamma Papers.* Samatha Trust. http://samatha .org/images/stories/abhidhamma-papers-final.pdf.

Rubik, Beverly, ed. 1989. *The Interrelationship between Mind and Matter: Proceedings of a Conference.* Philadelphia, Pa.: Temple University.

Ryle, Gilbert. 1949. *The Concept of Mind.* London: Hutchinson's University Library.

Sacks, Oliver. 1990. *The Man Who Mistook His Wife for a Hat.* New York: Harper-Collins.

Saddhatissa, H. 1970. *Buddhist Ethics: Essence of Buddhism.* London: George Allen & Unwin.

Salmon, Don, and Jan Maslow. 2007. *Yoga Psychology and the Transformation of Consciousness: Seeing through the Eyes of Infinity.* New York: Paragon House.

Sangharakshita. 1967. *The Three Jewels: An Introduction to Buddhism*. London: Rider.

———. 1980. *A Survey of Buddhism*. Boulder, Colo.: Shambhala Publications.

———. 2000. *Wisdom beyond Words: The Buddhist Vision of Ultimate Reality*. Birmingham, England: Windhorse Publications.

Sannella, Lee. 1987. *The Kundalini Experience: Psychosis or Transcendence?* Lower Lake, Calif.: Integral Publishing.

Sarachchandra, Ediriweera R. 1958. *Buddhist Psychology of Perception*. Colombo, India: Ceylon University Press.

Satprakashananda. 1965. *Methods of Knowledge: Perceptual, Non-Perceptual, and Transcendental According to Advaita Vedānta*. London: George Allen & Unwin.

Schmitz, Oscar A. H. 1923. *Psychoanalyse und Yoga* [Psychoanalysis and Yoga]. Darmstadt, Germany: Otto Reichl Verlag.

Schumann, Hans Wolfgang. 1973. *Buddhism: An Outline of Its Teachings and Schools*. Wheaton, Ill.: Quest Books.

Schwartz, Gary E., and William L. Simon. 2002. *The Afterlife Experiments: Breakthrough Scientific Evidence of Life after Death*. New York: Pocket.

Schweitzer, Albert. (1923) 1961. *Civilization and Ethics*. London: George Allen & Unwin.

Shamdasani, Sonu, ed. 1996. *The Psychology of Kundalini Yoga: Notes of the Seminar Given in 1932 by C. G. Jung*. Princeton, N.J.: Princeton University Press.

Shear, J. 2006. *The Experience of Meditation: Experts Introduce the Major Traditions*. St. Paul, Minn.: Paragon House.

Siegel, Elaine V. 1984. *Dance Movement Therapy: Mirror of Ourselves: The Psychoanalytic Approach*. New York: Human Science Press.

Singleton, Mark. 2010. *Yoga Body: The Origins of Modern Posture Practice*. Oxford: Oxford University Press.

Skolimowski, Henryk. 1994. *The Participatory Mind: A New Theory of Knowledge and of the Universe*. London and New York: Arkana/Penguin.

Snelling, John. 1991. *The Buddhist Handbook: A Complete Guide to Buddhist Schools, Teaching, Practice, and History*. Rochester, Vt.: Inner Traditions International.

Sovatsky, Stuart. 1998. *Words from the Soul: East/West Spirituality and Psychotherapeutic Narrative*. Revised edition. Albany, N.Y.: SUNY Press.

Staal, Frits. 1975. "Drugs and Powers." In *Exploring Mysticism*, edited by F. Staal. Harmondsworth, England: Penguin Books.

Stanton-Jones, K. 1992. *An Introduction to Dance Movement Therapy in Psychiatry*. London: Routledge.

Sternberg, Robert J., ed. 1990. *Wisdom: Its Nature, Origins, and Development.* Cambridge and New York: Cambridge University Press.

Stevenson, Ian. 1966. *Twenty Cases Suggestive of Reincarnation.* Charlottesville: University of Virginia Press.

Storr, Anthony. 1996. *Feet of Clay: Saints, Sinners, and Madmen—A Study of Gurus.* New York: FreePress Paperbacks.

Sukhthankar, Vishnu S., ed. 1933. *The Mahabharata.* Poona, India: Bhandarkar Oriental Research Institute.

Taimni, I. K. 1961. *The Science of Yoga.* Wheaton, Ill.: Quest Books.

Tart, Charles T. 1974. "Out-of-the-Body Experiences." In *Psychic Exploration: A Challenge for Science,* ed. Edgar Mitchell and John White, pp. 349ff. New York: Putnam.

——. 1975a. *States of Consciousness.* New York: E. P. Dutton.

——. 1975b.*Transpersonal Psychologies.* New York: Harper & Row.

——. 1987. *Waking Up: Overcoming the Obstacle to Human Potential.* Boston: New Science Library.

——. 1997. *Body, Mind, Spirit: Exploring the Parapsychology of Spirituality.* Charlottesville, Va.: Hampton Roads Publishers.

——. 2009. *The End of Materialism: How Evidence of the Paranormal Is Bringing Science and Spirit Together.* Foreword by Huston and Kendra Smith. Oakland, Calif.: New Harbinger/Noetic Books.

Taylor, Kathleen. 2001. *Sir John Woodroffe, Tantra and Bengal: "An Indian Soul in a European Body."* London: Curzon Press.

Thurman, Robert A. F. 1993. *The Tibetan Book of the Dead: Liberation through Understanding in the Between.* New York: Bantam Books.

Tomkins, Silvan S. 1962.*Affect, Imagery, Consciousness.* New York: Springer Verlag.

Traleg Kyabgon. 2007. *The Practice of Lojong: Cultivating Compassion through Training the Mind.* Boston: Shambhala Publications.

Tsongkhapa. 1995. *Preparing for Tantra: The Mountain of Blessings.* Translated by Khen Rinpoche. Howell, N.J.: Mahayana Sutra and Tantra Press.

Underhill, Evelyn. 1961. *Mysticism: A Study in the Nature and Development of Man's Spiritual Consciousness.* New York: E. P. Dutton.

Unno, Mark, ed. 2006. *Buddhism and Psychotherapy across Cultures: Essays on Theories and Practices.* Boston: Wisdom Publications.

Valiaveetil, Chacko. 1980. *Liberated Life: Ideal of Jīvanmukti in Indian Religions Specially in Saiva Siddhānta.* Karumathur, India: Arul Anandar College.

van Gorkom, Nina. 1997. *Abhidhamma in Daily Life.* London: Triple Gem Press.

van Lommel, Pim. 2010. *Consciousness beyond Life: The Science of the Near-Death Experience.* New York: HarperOne.

van Lommel, P., R. van Wees, V. Meyers, and I. Elfferich. 2001. "Near-Death Experience in Survivors of Cardiac Arrest: A Prospective Study in the Netherlands." *The Lancet* 358 (9298):2039–45.

Venkatesananda, Swami. 1993. *Vasiṣṭha's Yoga.* Albany, N.Y.: SUNY Press.

Vivekananda, Swami. 1896. "On Professor Max Müller." *Brahmâvadin* (June 6).

———. 1972. *Collected Works: Mayavati Memorial Edition.* Vol. 6. Calcutta: Advaita Ashrama.

von Glasenapp, Helmuth. (1942) 1991. *Doctrine of Karman in Jain Philosophy.* Varanasi, India: P. V. Research Institute.

Wald, George. 1980. *The Origin of Life: Molecules to Living Cells.* San Francisco: W. H. Freeman & Co.

Walsh, Maurice, trans. 1987. *The Long Discourses of the Buddha.* Boston: Wisdom Publications.

Walsh, Roger. 2007. *The World of Shamanism: New Views of an Ancient Tradition.* Woodbury, Minn.: Llewellyn Publications.

Walsh, Roger, and Frances E. Vaughan. 1996. "Comparative Models of the Person and Psychotherapy." In *Transpersonal Psychotherapy,* edited by Seymore Boorstein. Albany, N.Y.: SUNY Press.

———, eds. 1980. *Beyond Ego: Transpersonal Dimensions in Psychology.* Los Angeles: J. P. Tarcher.

Wangyal, Tenzin, Rinpoche. 1998. *The Tibetan Yogas of Dream and Sleep.* Ithaca, N.Y.: Snow Lion Publications.

Washburn, Michael. 2003. *Embodied Spirituality in a Sacred World.* Albany, N.Y.: SUNY Press.

Wasson, R. Gordon. 1972. *Soma: Divine Mushroom of Immortality.* New York: Harcourt, Brace Jovanovich.

Weintraub, Amy. 2004. *Yoga for Depression.* New York: Broadway Books.

Weizsäcker, Carl Friedrich von. 1972. Introduction to *The Biological Basis of Religion and Genius,* by Gopi Krishna. New York: Harper & Row.

Whicher, Ian. 1998. *The Integrity of the Yoga Darśana.* Albany, N.Y.: SUNY Press.

Whicher, Ian, and David Carpenter, eds. 2003. *Yoga: The Indian Tradition.* London and New York: Routledge/Curzon.

White, David Gordon. 1996. *The Alchemical Body: Siddha Traditions in Medieval India.* Chicago: University of Chicago Press.

White, John Warren. 1974. *What Is Meditation?* Garden City, N.Y.: Anchor.

Whitehead, Alfred North. 1919. *An Enquiry Concerning the Principles of Natural Knowledge*. Cambridge: Cambridge University Press.

Wilber, Ken. 1977. *The Spectrum of Consciousness*. Wheaton, Ill.: Theosophical Publishing House.

———. 1980. *The Atman Project*. Wheaton, Ill.: Quest Books.

———. 1996. *Up from Eden*. Wheaton, Ill.: Quest Books.

———. 1998. *The Eye of Spirit*. Boston: Shambhala Publications.

———. 2000a. *Integral Psychology: Consciousness, Spirit, Psychology, Therapy*. Boston: Shambhala Publications.

———. (1995) 2000b. *Sex, Ecology, Spirituality: The Spirit of Evolution*. Boston: Shambhala Publications.

Wood, Ernest. 1948. *Practical Yoga, Ancient and Modern*. New York: E. P. Dutton.

———. 1954. *Great Systems of Yoga*. New York: Philosophical Library.

Woodroffe, Sir John. *See* Arthur Avalon.

Wosien, Maria-Gabriele. 1974. *Sacred Dance: Encounter with the Gods*. London: Avon Books.

Young, Serinity. 1999. *Dreaming in the Lotus*. Boston: Wisdom Publications.

Zaehner, R. C. 1957. *Mysticism: Sacred and Profane*. Oxford and London: Clarendon Press and Oxford University.

Index

Abhedananda, Swami, 8
Abhinavagupta, 178
abnormal psychology, 21
Adler, Alfred, 4
affects. *See* emotions/affects
Agamya Paramahansa, Sri Mahatma,
  9–10
ākāsha (ether-space), 88–89
Alexander the Great, 251, 252, 254, 255
alpha standpoint, 117
Alstad, Diana, 184
Alter, Joseph S., 15
Ambrose, Saint, 253
Ammonius Sakkas, 253
Analysis, 163–64
Ananda Acharya, 11, 186
ananugami ("nonaccompanying"
  avadhi), 70
anavasthita ("unstable" *avadhi*), 70
Anaximander, 251
Anaximenes, 251
Antequil-Duperron, Abraham-
  Hyacinthe, 188
anugami ("accompanying" *avadhi*), 70
Apollonius of Tyana, 253
Aquinas, Thomas, 1–2
Arbman, Ernst, 195–96
archaic structure of consciousness,
  81–84
Aristotle, 1, 61, 86, 90, 251, 252
Aristoxenus, 252
Arnold, Edwin, 24
Aronson, Harvey, 105
Ārtabhāga, Jāratkārava, 40
Asanga, 57
Asrani, U. A., 196
Assagioli, Roberto, 67, 68, 140–41,
  143–44, 163–64
Atkinson, William Walker (Yogi
  Ramacharaka), 10, 120
Augustine, Saint, 1, 197
authoritarianism, 182–85

authority (*adhikāra*), 182, 223. See also
  gurus
avadhi, 70, 94
avadhi-jnāna, 69. *See also* suprasensory
  capacity
Avalon, Arthur. *See* Woodroffe, John
avasthita ("stable" *avadhi*), 70
awareness, 142–45
  self-consciousness, self-observation,
    and, 159–60
  See also conscious intensity, layers of;
    consciousness

Bādarāyana, 156
Baier, Karl, x, 187–88, 207
Bardesanes of Edessa, 253
Bardo Thödol (Tibetan Book of the
  Dead), 24, 217
Beauregard, Marlo, 22
behaviorism, 4, 135, 138
being, categories of, 42–43
Bentov, Itzhak, 129–30
Bergson, Henri, 124
Bernard, Pierre ("Oom the
  Omnipotent"), 10, 12, 120
beta standpoint, 117
Bhagavad-Gītā, 106, 119, 223, 225
  Bhakti-Yoga and, 113
  on brahma-*nirvāna*, 222
  on death and dying, 178, 213–14
  ecstatic realization in, 30–31
  on emotions, 93, 106–7
  God consciousness and, 177
  on liberation, 220
  Panentheism and, 156
  principles, 106–7
  on suffering, 37
  on Yoga, 39–40
  yuga doctrine and, 78–79
Bhakti-Yoga, 166
  nine sentiments of, 113
Bharati, Baba, 9

introspection, 12, 27, 135–36
Irenaeus, Bishop, 197
Īshvara Krishna, 52, 67, 100, 147, 154, 227

Jaeschke, Heinrich August, 256
Jaina and Hindu yogic ecstasies, the
　ladder of, 198–99
Jaina ladder to perfection, 173–74
Jaina Yoga, 134, 238–40
　emotional aspects, 114–16
　knowledge, wisdom, and gnosis in, 134
　subtle body in, 122–23
Jainism
　art of dying in, 218
　Buddhism and, 57
　Hinduism and, 57, 239
　jīvanmukta in, 228–29
　karma in, 42–43
　meditation in, 179–80, 194
　omniscience and, 44, 70, 134, 173–74,
　　212, 228
　perception in, 94–95
　serpent power in, 131
　on suffering, 38
James, William, 3–4, 46, 60–61, 136, 140
Janaka, King, 220
Janet, Pierre, 97, 195
jīvanmukta, 174, 223–28
　in Jainism, 228–29
jīvanmukti, 219, 229
　in Vedānta and Classical Yoga, 226–28
Jīvanmukti in Transformation (Fort), 227
Jīvanmukti-Viveka, 224, 227
Jnāna-Yoga (practice) of Vedānta and
　other Hindu traditions, 167–69
Jones, William, 257
Judge, William Quine, 208
Julian, Emperor, 253
Jung, Carl Gustav, 4–5, 235
　active imagination technique, 236
　on Christianity, 163, 235, 236
　on consciousness and the
　　unconscious, 96, 97, 137, 138
　on ego and self, 137–38, 153
　vs. Freud, 97, 137
　on individuation, 137–38
　kundalinī and, 6, 125, 126
　on psychoanalysis, 6
　on religion, 183–84
　Roberto Assagioli and, 5

Tantra and, 106
　on West and East, 6, 16–18
　on Yoga, 16, 18, 21, 235

Kabat-Zinn, Jon, 36
Kalanos, 6–7, 252
kali-yuga, 78
Kant, Immanuel, 2, 59, 150
karma, 50
　defined, 40
　"law" of, 40–46
　types of, 42, 44, 46
Katz, Steven T., 144
Kellner, Carl, 9–10
Kepler, Johann, 90
kevala-jnāna, 70
Kilner, Walter J., 121
Kittel, Ferdinand, 256
knowledge, defined, 132
knowledge, wisdom, and gnosis, 132
　in Buddhist Yoga, 133–34
　in Hindu Yoga, 132–33
　in Jaina Yoga, 134
Kohlberg, Lawrence, 82
Koren, Stanley, 211
Kramer, Joel, 184
Krishna, Gopi, 125–30
Krishnamurti, J., 24
Krishnānanda Vidyāvāgīshvara, 206–7
Kuhn, Thomas S., 60, 61
Külpe, Oswald, 136
kundalinī, 29–30, 124–25
　Gopi Krishna and modern research
　　on, 125–29
　in Hindu Yoga, 130–31
　in Jainism, 131
　Jung and, 6, 125, 126
　physio-kundalinī, 129–30
　prāna and, 128–29

Lacan, Jacques, 98
Lancelin, Charles, 209
Larson, Gerald James, 38, 54, 228
Laski, Marghanita, 139
Laszlo, Ervin, 5, 86, 88–89
Laubry, Charles, 189
Leadbeater, Charles W., 208
Leary, Timothy, 210
Leibniz, Gottfried Wilhelm, 96
Lepp, Ignace, 213

spiritual practice, unhealthy motivations in, 105–6
Sri Aurobindo, 25–26, 51, 84, 186
Staal, Frits, 204
standpoints (metaphysical perspectives), 117–18
Stenberg, Esther, 236
Sthiramati, 115
Storr, Anthony, 182–83
Streitfeld, Harold, 129
Structures of Consciousness (Feuerstein), xi
subtle body, 117–23
   19th- and 20th-century research on, 119–20
suffering (*duhkha*), 34–40, 170
   Patanjali on, 34, 36, 38, 40, 108–10
   types of, 38, 39
superconscious, 68, 141. See also *buddhi*
supernatural abilities. *See* paranormal abilities
suprasensory capacity, 69, 70
Sureshvara, 225
Suzuki, D. T., 14, 24–25
Swedenborg, Immanuel, 120

Tantra, 106, 123, 124, 206
   paranormal abilities and, 206–7
Tart, Charles T., 142–43, 215, 231
   on consciousness/awareness, 67, 143
   on consensus trance, 72, 76, 142, 143
   on death, 213
   on ego, 153
   on out-of-body experiences (OBEs), 209
   on science, scientism, and spirituality, 203
   States of Consciousness, 143, 210
temperament, 108–9
Temple, Paul N., 202
Tenhaeff, Wilhelm H. C., 117
Tenzin Wangyal, 71–72
Teresa of Avila, 197
Teresi, Dick, 85
Thales of Miletus, 251
Theosophical Society, 7, 13, 24, 120, 189, 207, 208
Tibetan Buddhism, 14, 133–34
   dying in, 217
   tulkus in, 49, 230–31

Tibetan Dream Yoga, 74
Tilak, Gangadhar, 186
Tomkins, Silvan S., 152
Traleg Kyabgon Rinpoche, 216
Transcendental Meditation (TM), 27, 176–77
transcendental Reality, 27, 45, 71, 149, 151, 152, 154–55, 159
transcendental Witness, 112, 149–51, 159–60
transconceptual ecstasy, 147, 148, 160, 167
transpersonal psychology, 22, 140–42.
   See also self-transcendence
Trumpp, Ernst, 256
Trungpa Rinpoche, Chögyam, 149, 193
truth, 31, 61–63
   characteristics, 62
   See also reality
Tsongkhapa, Je, 39, 45
tulkus, 49, 230–31
Tull, Hermann W., 41
Tūrān Shāh, 254

Uddālaka Āruni, 261n2
Umāsvāti, 194
unconscious
   collective, 67, 97, 137, 242
   conscious, subconscious, and, 102–3
   in modern depth psychology, 96–98
   in Yoga and other Indian traditions, 98–102
Underhill, Evelyn, 195, 197

Vācaspati Mishra, 107, 199, 205
values, 31–32
van Gogh, Vincent, 24
van Lommel, Pim, 86, 209
vardhamana ("growing"/increasing *avadhi*), 70
Vasubandhu, 58
Vaughan, Frances E., 140, 141
Vedānta, 167–69
   values and qualities aspired to in, 31–32
Venkatesananda, Swami, 223
Victoria, Queen, 7–8
Vidyāranya, 71, 101, 223–24, 227
Vijnāna Bhikshu, 56, 199
vision-logic, 77, 82, 83
Vivekananda, Swami, x, 8, 13, 15, 24

Voltaire, François Marie Arouet de, 256
von Hartmann, Karl Robert Eduard, 96
Vyāsa, 38, 42, 58, 107

Wagner, Richard, 24
waking state, 71–72
Wald, George, 86
Walsh, Roger, 132, 140, 141
Washburn, Michael, 237
Wasson, R. Gordon, 210–11
Weizsäcker, Carl Friedrich von, 126–28
West and East
    in antiquity, 251–57
    meeting of, 5–18
Western Yoga, toward a, 235–37
White, John, 187
Whitehead, Alfred North, 86
Wholeness or Transcendence?
    (Feuerstein), 82
Wiedenmann, Baptist, 256–57
Wilber, Ken, 144
    on Aurobindo, 26
    Gebserian structures of consciousness
        and, 77, 83
    Great Nest of Being, 27
    integral psychology, 22, 25, 67, 83
    on Integral Yoga, 25–26
    on meditation and contemplation, 187
    Roberto Assagioli and, 141
    spectrum model, 77, 82, 83, 140, 144
    speculative psychology, 83
    on transpersonal bands of
        consciousness, 140, 141
    vision-logic, 77, 82
    yuga doctrine and, 78
Wilkins, Charles, 257
Windischmann, Carl Joseph
    Hieronymus, 188–89
Windish, Ernst, 23
wisdom, 132
    types of, 133–34
Witness, 158–59

witnessing Self, 76, 115, 150
    veiling the, 151–52
Wittgenstein, Ludwig, 59
Woodhouse, Mark B., 135
Woodroffe, John (aka Arthur Avalon), 11,
    120, 125–26, 130
Worrall, Olga, 121
Wundt, Wilhelm, 3, 136

Yādavaprakāsha, 222
Yājnavalkya, 40–41, 47, 220, 261n2
Yesudian, Selvarajan, 11–12
Yoga
    defined, 39–40, 111, 131
    early writings on, 9, 256–57
    historical perspective on, 6–15
    as "living fossil," 26
    nature of, 56
    and other spiritual traditions, 145–48
    types/branches of, 23, 179–80
    See also specific topics
*Yoga Morality: Ancient Teachings at a
    Time of Global Crisis* (Feuerstein), 165
Yoga psychology
    concept of, 6
    initiatory structure and training,
        28–30
    literature on, 241–50
    methodology, 27
    vs. modern psychology, 23–33
*Yoga Tradition: Its History, Literature,
    Philosophy, and Practice, The*
    (Feuerstein), 239
Yogananda, Paramahamsa, 11
Yogeshananda, Swami, 9
Young, Serinity, 73
Young, Thomas, 90
yuga, defined, 78
yuga doctrine, 78–79

zeta standpoint, 117
Ziegenbalg, Bartholomaeus, 256

292 · INDEX